Atlas of Cardiovascular Magnetic Resonance

Editor-in-Chief

Warren J. Manning, MD

Section Chief
Non-Invasive Cardiac Imaging
Beth Israel Deaconess Medical Center
Professor of Medicine and Radiology
Harvard Medical School
Boston, Massachusetts

Series Editor

Eugene Braunwald, MD, MD (Hon), ScD (Hon)

Distinguished Hersey Professor of Medicine
Harvard Medical School
Chairman, TIMI Study Group
Brigham and Women's Hospital
Boston, Massachusetts

With 49 Contributors
Developed by Current Medicine Group, LLC
Philadelphia

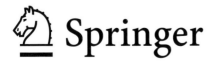 Springer

CURRENT MEDICINE GROUP LLC, PART OF SPRINGER SCIENCE+BUSINESS MEDIA LLC

400 Market Street, Suite 700 • Philadelphia, PA 19106

Developmental Editors . . . . Lenora Thrower, Anthony Mirra
Editorial Assistants . . . . Juleen Deaner, Bridget Jordan
Design and Layout . . . . William Whitman, Jr., Dan Britt
Illustrators . . . . Dan Britt, Kim Broadbent, Marie Dean, Heather Hoch, Wieslawa Langenfeld, Jacqueline Leonard, Maureen Looney, Deborah Lynam
Production Coordinator . . . . Carolyn Naylor
Indexer . . . . Holly Lukens

Library of Congress Cataloging-in-Publication Data

Atlas of cardiovascular magnetic resonance / editor-in-chief, Warren J. Manning ; with 49 contributors. -- 1st ed.
    p. ; cm.
  Includes bibliographical references and index.
  ISBN-13: 978-1-57340-299-6 (alk. paper)
  ISBN-10: 1-57340-299-0 (alk. paper)
  1. Cardiovascular system--Magnetic resonance imaging--Atlases. I. Manning, Warren J. II. Title: Cardiovascular magnetic resonance.
  [DNLM: 1. Cardiovascular Diseases--diagnosis--Atlases. 2. Magnetic Resonance Imaging--methods--Atlases. WG 17 A88153 2008]

  RC670.5.M33A83 2008
  616.1'07548--dc22

            2007051345

  ISBN-13: 978-1-57340-299-6
  ISBN-10: 1-57340-299-0

www.springer.com

For more information, please call 1 (800) 777-4643
or email us at orders-ny@springer.com

www.currentmedicinegroup.com

10 9 8 7 6 5 4 3 2 1

Printed in China by L. Rex Printing Company LTD

This book was printed on acid-free paper

PREFACE

Spring 1997 was a decisive period for me. At the former Beth Israel Hospital in Boston, we had a weekly cardiology catheterization conference during which we typically focused on hemodynamics, invasive angiography, and novel coronary interventions. At the conclusion of one session in the Spring of 1997, Dr. Sven Paulin, a pioneer in cardiovascular radiology and our Chief of Radiology, offered to show us an interesting video he had recently received from his colleagues at the University of Pennsylvania MR Center. With Sven's usual flair, he prefaced the VHS video presentation with, "I don't know what will become of this new imaging modality, but the images are certainly impressive!" Had there been a camera to capture the event, it would have documented a stunned first year cardiology fellow gazing at his first cine cardiovascular magnetic resonance (CMR). The patient had severe aortic regurgitation. The anatomic detail was far superior to anything I had seen before. With Sven, and subsequently Bob Edelman as my CMR mentors, I embarked on a two decade long foray into CMR that continues to this day.

During the past two decades, we have seen a near revolution in noninvasive cardiac imaging. The pendulum in cardiology has swung from the era of intervention to the era of noninvasive imaging. In the process, CMR has developed from a promising research tool available at a few specialized academic sites, to a multifaceted clinical imaging tool now widely available across the globe. CMR and cardiac CT now join the more established imaging modalities of echocardiography and nuclear cardiology to form the four pillars of noninvasive cardiac imaging. In this atlas, an internationally recognized group of authors presents the current state of CMR in pictorial form. No dynamic imaging field can be completely summarized in such a text, but we have tried to be comprehensive in scope, incorporating CMR physics and basics of image construction and extending to clinical applications of stress, viability, valvular function, congenital disease, coronary imaging, and interventional CMR. Our goal is to provide value for both the novice and the experienced CMR user, the adult and the pediatric imager, the cardiologist and the radiologist, the imager of today, and those who want a glimpse of what CMR will offer tomorrow. To put CMR in perspective, we conclude with a chapter comparing and contrasting CMR with the other noninvasive imaging methods. Though a multiauthored text, we have tried to present the text and figures with a uniform style and abbreviation set.

This atlas would not have been possible without the vision of the series editor, Dr. Eugene Braunwald, my mentor since a third year medicine clerkship at the Brigham and Women's Hospital, and Abe Krieger, former president of Current Medicine Group. I also thank Lenora Thrower, Developmental Editor at Current Medicine, Megan Charlton, Managing Editor at Current Medicine, and Iris Wasserman, my administrative assistant for nearly two decades, for their efforts in seeing this atlas to fruition. Most importantly, I thank my wife, Susan Gail, and children, Anya, Sara, and Isaac for their love and unwavering support for undertaking this project despite an already full day.

Warren J. Manning, MD

DEDICATION

To Sven and Bob
– for their teaching, guidance, friendship, and warm welcome to the world of CMR.

Rajiv Agarwal, MD
Cardiovascular Association, PLLC
Houston, Texas

Evan Appelbaum, MD, MMSci, FACC
Division of Cardiology, Non-Invasive Section
Co-Director, PERFUSE CMR Core Laboratory
Beth Israel Deaconess Medical Center
Harvard Medical Center
Boston, Massachusetts

Ravi Assomull, MRCP
CMR Fellow
Cardiovascular Magnetic Resonance Unit
Royal Brompton Hospital
London, United Kingdom

Robert W. W. Biederman, MD,
  FACC, FASA
Associate Professor of Medicine
Department of Medicine
Drexel University College of Medicine
Philadelphia, Pennsylvania
Director
Cardiovascular Magnetic Resonance Imaging
Division of Cardiovascular Disease
Center for Cardiac Magnetic
  Resonance Imaging
Allegheny General Hospital
Pittsburgh, Pennsylvania

David A. Bluemke, MD, PhD, FAHA
Radiologist-in-Chief
Warren G. Magnuson Clinical Center
National Institutes of Health
Bethesda, Maryland
Professor of Radiology and Medicine
Johns Hopkins University School of Medicine
Baltimore, Maryland

René M. Botnar, PhD
Professor of Cardiovascular Imaging
King's College London
Division of Imaging Sciences
The Rayne Institute
St. Thomas' Hospital
London, United Kingdom

Daniel N. Costa, MD
Radiologist
Department of Radiology
Hospital Sírio-Libanês
São Paulo, Brazil

Kevin J. Duffy Jr, MD
Clinical Assistant Professor
Department of Cardiovascular Medicine
University of Pennsylvania
Staff Cardiologist
Department of Medicine
Philadelphia VA Medical Center
Philadelphia, Pennsylvania

Hale Ersoy, MD
Assistant Professor of Radiology
Brigham and Women's Hospital
Harvard Medical School
Boston, Massachusetts

Victor A. Ferrari, MD
Professor of Medicine and Radiology
Department of Cardiovascular Medicine
University of Pennsylvania School of Medicine
Associate Director
Non-Invasive Imaging Laboratory
Hospital of the University of Pennsylvania
Philadelphia, Pennsylvania

Otavio Rizzi Coelho Filho, MD
Research Fellow
Cardiac Magnetic Resonance Imaging
Cardiovascular Division
Department of Medicine
Brigham and Women's Hospital
Harvard Medical School
Boston, Massachusetts

Scott D. Flamm, MD
Head
Cardiovascular Imaging
Imaging Institute
Cleveland Clinic
Cleveland, Ohio

Matthias G. Friedrich, MD, FESC
Director, Stephenson CMR Centre at the
  Libin Cardiovascular Institute of Alberta
Associate Professor of Medicine
Departments of Cardiac Sciences
  and Radiology
University of Calgary
Calgary, Alberta, Canada

Tal Geva, MD
Professor
Department of Pediatrics
Harvard Medical School
Chief
Division of Noninvasive Cardiac Imaging
Department of Cardiology
Children's Hospital Boston
Boston, Massachusetts

Thomas H. Hauser, MD, MMSc, MPH
Assistant Professor
Department of Medicine
Harvard Medical School
Director of Nuclear Cardiology
Department of Medicine
Cardiovascular Division
Beth Israel Deaconess Medical Center
Boston, Massachusetts

Daniel A. Herzka, PhD
Senior Member Research Staff
Clinical Sites Research Program
Philips Research North America
Briarcliff Manor, New York

Kraig V. Kissinger, BS, RT (R) (MR)
Senior MR Technologist
Cardiac MR Center
Beth Israel Deaconess Medical Center
Boston, Massachusetts

Christopher M. Kramer, MD
Professor
Departments of Medicine and Radiology
Director, Cardiovascular Imaging Center
University of Virginia Health System
Charlottesville, Virginia

Raymond Y. Kwong, MD, MPH, JACC
Assistant Professor of Medicine
Director of Cardiac Magnetic
  Resonance Imaging
Cardiovascular Division
Department of Medicine
Harvard Medical School
Boston, Massachusetts

Robert J. Lederman, MD
Cardiovascular Branch
Clinical Research Program
Division of Intramural Research
National Heart, Lung, and Blood Institute
National Institutes of Health
Bethesda, Maryland

Warren J. Manning, MD
Chief, Non-Invasive Cardiac Imaging
Co-Director, Cardiac MR Center
Beth Israel Deaconess Medical Center
Professor of Medicine
Professor of Radiology
Harvard Medical School
Boston, Massachusetts

Robert Manka, MD
German Heart Institute Berlin
Department of Internal
  Medicine/Cardiology
Berlin, Germany

Martin S. Maron, MD
Assistant Professor of Medicine
Division of Cardiology
Department of Medicine
Tufts School of Medicine
Boston, Massachusetts

Elliot R. McVeigh, PhD
Professor and Director
Department of Biomedical Engineering
Johns Hopkins University School of Medicine
Baltimore, Maryland

Eike Nagel, MD, PhD
Professor of Clinical Cardiovascular Imaging
King's College London
Division of Imaging Sciences
The Rayne Institute
St. Thomas' Hospital
London, United Kingdom

Krishna S. Nayak, PhD
Assistant Professor
Ming Hsieh Department of
  Electrical Engineering
Viterbi School of Engineering
University of Southern California
Assistant Professor
Keck School of Medicine
University of Southern California
Los Angeles, California

Stefan Neubauer, MD, FRCP,
  FACC, FMedSci
Professor
Department of Cardiovascular Medicine
University of Oxford
Oxford, United Kingdom

Reza Nezafat, PhD
Instructor in Medicine
Department of Medicine
Harvard Medical School
Assistant Scientific Director,
  Cardiac MR Center
Division of Cardiology
Department of Medicine
Beth Israel Deaconess Medical Center
Boston, Massachusetts

Jon-Fredrik Nielsen, PhD
Postdoctoral Research Associate
Ming Hsieh Department of
  Electrical Engineering
University of Southern California
Los Angeles, California

Rory O'Hanlon, MRCP
CMR Fellow
Cardiovascular Magnetic Resonance Unit
Royal Brompton Hospital
London, United Kingdom

Nael Osman, PhD
Department of Radiology
Division of Magnetic Resonance Research
Department of Electric and
  Computer Engineering
Johns Hopkins University
Baltimore, Maryland

Rajan A. G. Patel, MD
Fellow
Cardiovascular Division
Department of Medicine
University of Virginia Health System
Charlottesville, Virginia

Ivan Pedrosa, MD
Assistant Professor of Radiology
Harvard Medical School
Director of Body MR Imaging
Beth Israel Deaconess Medical Center
Boston, Massachusetts

Sanjay K. Prasad, MD, MRCP
Consultant Cardiologist
National Heart and Lung Institute
Imperial College
Cardiovascular Magnetic Resonance Unit
London, United Kingdom

Martin R. Prince, MD
Professor of Radiology
Weill Medical College of Cornell University
Columbia College of Physicians
  and Surgeons
Chief of MRI
New York Hospital
New York, New York

Vikas K. Rathi, MD
Assistant Professor of Medicine
Department of Internal Medicine
Drexel University College of Medicine
Division of Cardiology
Allegheny General Hospital
Pittsburgh, Pennsylvania

Neil M. Rofsky, MD
Associate Professor of Radiology
Harvard Medical School
Director of MRI
Beth Israel Deaconess Medical Center
Boston, Massachusetts

Carolina Sant'Anna Henry, MD
Weill Medical College of Cornell University
New York, New York

Michael Schar, PhD
Department of Radiology
Division of Magnetic Resonance Research
Johns Hopkins University
Baltimore, Maryland
Philips Medical Systems
Cleveland, Ohio

Brian J. Schietinger, MD
Fellow
Cardiovascular Division
Department of Medicine
University of Virginia Health System
Charlottesville, Virginia

Richard Eldridge Slaughter,
  MB, BS, FRANZCR
Adjunct Professor
School of Physical and Chemical Science
Queensland University of Technology
Chair
Division of Medical Imaging
The Prince Charles Hospital
Brisbane, Queensland, Australia

Kevin E. Steel, DO
Advanced Cardiac Imaging Director
Department of Cardiology
Wilford Hall Medical Center
San Antonio, Texas

Oliver Strohm, MD, FESC
Cardiologist
Deputy Director, Stephenson CMR Centre
Associate Professor
Departments of Cardiac Sciences
 and Radiology
University of Calgary
Calgary, Alberta, Canada

Matthias Stuber, PhD
Associate Professor
Department of Radiology
Division of Magnetic Resonance Research
Department of Electric and
 Computer Engineering
Johns Hopkins University
Baltimore, Maryland

Harikrishna Tandri, MD
Department of Medicine and Radiology
Johns Hopkins School of Medicine
Baltimore, Maryland

Robert G. Weiss, MD
Professor
Department of Medicine
Division of Magnetic Resonance Research
Johns Hopkins University
Baltimore, Maryland
Philips Medical Systems
Cleveland, Ohio

Andrea J. Wiethoff, PhD
Philips Medical Systems
Best, Netherlands

Honglei Zhang, MD
Weill Medical College of Cornell University
New York, New York

Xiaoming Zhang, MD, PhD
Research Fellow
Department of Radiology
Weill Medical College of Cornell University
New York, New York
Attending Radiologist
Department of Radiology
QiLu Hospital of Shandong University
Jinan, Shandong, China

CONTENTS

COMMON ABBREVIATIONS

3D	Three-dimensional		LVOT	Left ventricular outflow tract
ARVC	Arrhythmogenic right ventricular cardiomyopathy		MI	Myocardial infarction
ASD	Atrial septal defect		MIP	Maximal image projection
CAD	Coronary artery disease		MO	Microvascular obstruction
CS	Coronary sinus		MPA	Main pulmonary artery
CCT	Cardiovascular computed tomography		MRA	Magnetic resonance angiography
CE	Contrast enhanced		MRI	Magnetic resonance imaging
CMR	Cardiovascular magnetic resonance		NAV	Navigator
CMRS	Cardiovascular magnetic resonance spectroscopy		PA	Pulmonary artery
CNR	Contrast-to-noise ratio		PC	Phase contrast
CO	Cardiac output		PR	Pulmonic regurgitation
CT	Computed tomography		PS	Pulmonic stenosis
DCM	Dilated cardiomyopathy		PV	Pulmonary vein
EF	Ejection fraction		RA	Right atrium
EKG	Electrocardiogram		RAA	Right atrial appendage
Gd	Gadolinium		RCA	Right coronary artery
GRE	Gradient recalled echo		RF	Radiofrequency
HCM	Hypertrophic cardiomyopathy		RV	Right ventricle
HR	Heart rate		RIPV	Right inferior pulmonary vein
IVC	Inferior vena cava		RSPV	Right superior pulmonary vein
LA	Left atrium		RVOT	Right ventricular outflow tract
LAA	Left atrial appendage		SE	Spin echo
LAD	Left anterior descending coronary artery		SNR	Signal-to-noise ratio
LCX	Left circumflex coronary artery		SSFP	Steady state free precession
LGE	Late gadolinium enhancement		SV	Stroke volume
LIPV	Left inferior pulmonary vein		SVC	Superior vena cava
LM	Left main coronary artery		T	Tesla
LSPV	Left superior pulmonary vein		TE	Echo time
LV	Left ventricle		VSD	Ventricular septal defect
LVEF	Left ventricular ejection fraction			

1

CHAPTER

Physics

Reza Nezafat and Daniel A. Herzka

Magnetic resonance imaging (MRI) is a noninvasive imaging modality that can be used to measure anatomic, functional, metabolic, and chemical characteristics of cardiovascular systems. MRI is based on the nuclear MR phenomenon initially observed by two Nobel Prize winners: Felix Block and Edward Purcell. When nuclei with a net magnetic dipole moment were placed in a magnetic field, they absorbed energy in the radiofrequency range of the electromagnetic spectrum and emitted this energy when the nuclei transferred to their original state. The strength of the magnetic field and the frequency of the absorption and emission of energy matched each other. The ability of nuclear MR

to generate images using the signal radiated by nuclei was pioneered by two other Nobel Prize winners—Paul Lauterbur and Sir Peter Mansfield—who created two-dimensional images by introducing spatial gradients in the magnetic fields.

At the center of an MRI system is a very strong magnet. What happens to protons (hydrogen atoms) within the magnetic field permits the noninvasive interrogation of the organic tissue. Because the human body is composed of a large fraction (approximately 70%) of water that contains two protons, MRI presents an excellent and flexible imaging modality. In this chapter, we review the fundamentals of MRI physics.

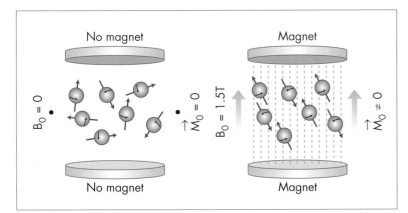

Figure 1-1. Normally the protons in a sample are in a random array without any net magnetization. However, when tissue or other organic matter is placed in a magnetic field (B_0), the protons (hydrogen atoms) align along or against the static magnetic field. A slightly higher number of protons are aligned parallel to the field, yielding a net magnetization of the sample (M_0), which is also aligned with B_0. At equilibrium, the magnitude of this magnetization vector is proportional to the magnitude of B_0.

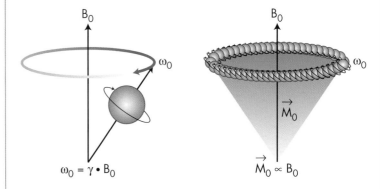

Figure 1-2. The spinning protons or "spins" do not exactly align with the magnetic field. Instead, they align to a fixed angle to B_0, and rotate or precess around that magnetic field at a rate or frequency ξ_0. The central relationship in MRI is shown by the equation that states that spins will precess at a frequency ξ_0 when placed in a magnetic field with strength B_0. Gyromagnetic ratio, γ, is a constant that for protons is 42.56 MHz/T. ξ_0 is referred to as the Larmor or resonance frequency. Furthermore, because there are so many spins in the imaging volume and they are randomly distributed around B_0, they can be added into a single large equilibrium magnetization vector M_0.

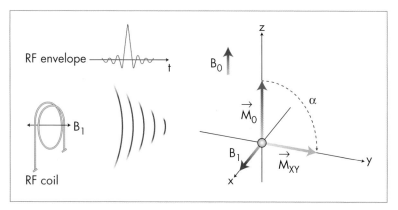

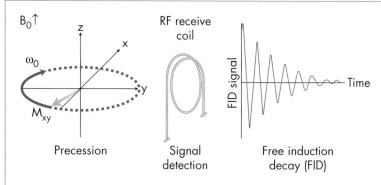

Figure 1-3. The equilibrium magnetization M_0 can be disturbed by the use of a radiofrequency (RF) energy burst or pulse applied at the Larmor frequency ξ_0. The RF pulse, created by an RF coil, produces a new magnetic field B_1, which changes the direction of the effective magnetic field. The RF pulse rotates the existing magnetization from the longitudinal direction (z) to the transverse direction (x-y plane), converting M_0 into M_{XY}. Such magnetization is then termed the *transverse component M_{XY}*. The angle of rotation of the magnetization is called the flip angle, α.

Figure 1-4. After the transmission of the radiofrequency (RF) pulse has ceased the effective magnetic field is again B_0. The magnetization in the transverse plane M_{XY} precesses about B_0 until it has reached the equilibrium again. The precession of the magnetization induces a current in a receiver coil and that is the signal an MR scanner detects. If we examine the signal over time, we see a feature referred to as the free induction decay, which displays the return of M_{XY} to M_Z. Note that when M_{XY} is perpendicular to the coil, no signal is detected, whereas when M_{XY} points directly toward or away from the coil, the signal is maximal. Over time M_{XY} returns to equilibrium and the free induction decay decays away.

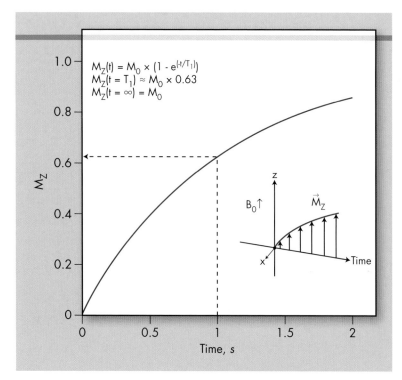

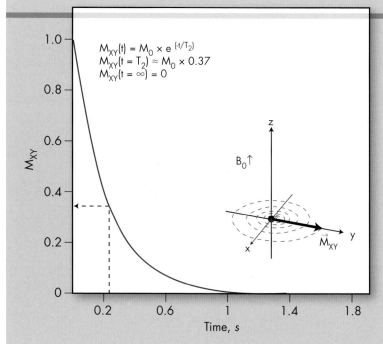

Figure 1-5. There are two different and independent processes that drive the magnetization toward equilibrium. The first one is longitudinal or T_1 relaxation, which causes the regrowth of longitudinal magnetization M_Z toward M_0. T_1, the relaxation time constant, is measured in microseconds, is a property of the tissue, and reflects the underlying interaction between the spins and the surrounding "lattice" or molecular environment. After a radiofrequency excitation in which all M_Z is tipped into transverse magnetization M_{XY}, it takes approximately T_1 microseconds to recover 63% of the original equilibrium M_0. After approximately $5T_1$, 99.9% of the magnetization is recovered.

Figure 1-6. The second process, which returns magnetization toward equilibrium, is T_2 or transverse relaxation. T_2, measured in microseconds, decays the magnitude of the transverse magnetization M_{XY} to zero. Note that after radiofrequency excitation, it takes T_2 microseconds for only 37% of magnetization to remain. T_2 is a reflection of the underlying interaction between spins. When combined with a T_1 relaxation, we see that the magnetization vector effectively spirals around B_0, decays with time constant T_2, and regrows with time constant T_1. Note that the two relaxation processes are independent of each other and are tissue dependent.

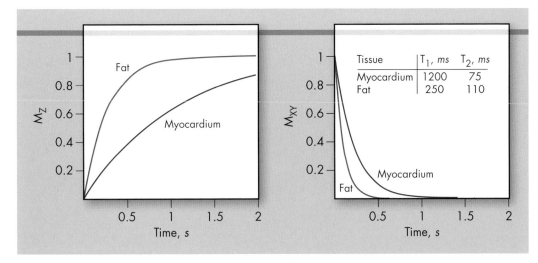

Tissue	T_1, ms	T_2, ms
Myocardium	1200	75
Fat	250	110

Figure 1-7. T_1 and T_2 represent a major mechanism for contrast generation in MRI. In this example, we see the T_1 and T_2 relaxation curves for protons in fat and myocardial muscle. Because T_1 and T_2 are properties of tissue, fat, which has a shorter T_1 than myocardium, relaxes faster. Fat also has a shorter T_2 than myocardium and therefore decays faster. Capturing an image at particular times in these relaxation curves can yield high or low contrast.

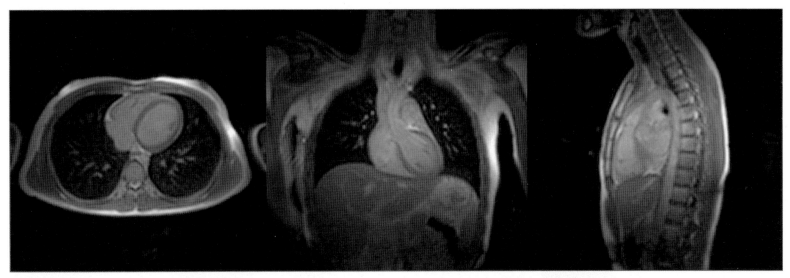

Figure 1-8. One of the strengths of MRI is its ability to image any slice or volume at any orientation within the magnet. Unlike CT, MRI is not limited to axial planes but can instead acquire flexible image orientations. There are three main processes involved in image formation: *slice encoding (left), frequency encoding (middle),* and *phase encoding (right).* All of these processes rely on an extra time-dependent magnetic field gradient (G) superimposed on the static magnetic field B_0.

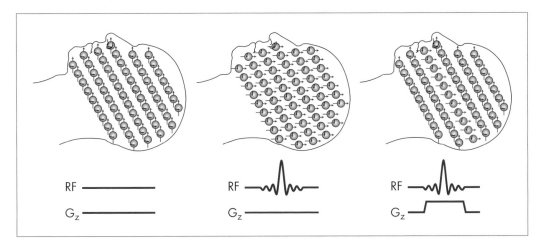

Figure 1-9. Slice selection is the first process used in image formation. In the presence of a static magnetic field B_0, all the spins within the tissue align with the field, as shown by the diagram on the *left*. If radiofrequency (RF) excitation is used without an accompanying gradient, all the spins will be tipped into transverse plane, a process called *nonselective excitation*. Finally, if a gradient is applied during the RF pulse, a small subset of spins—a slice—is selected for imaging. RF excitation in the presence of a gradient G_z is called *selective excitation*.

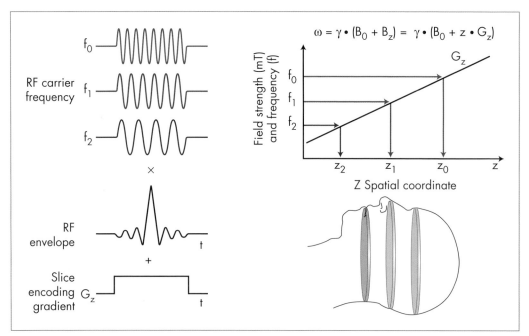

Figure 1-10. The carrier frequency of the radiofrequency (RF) pulse determines the location of the excited spins in the slice selection process. Because the RF pulse only excites a spin whose resonance frequency matches the carrier frequency, a small subset of spins is excited. The amplitude of the gradient waveform determines the position and thickness of the excited slice. In this example, three different frequencies are used in the RF excitation process that results in excitation of three parallel slices along z direction.

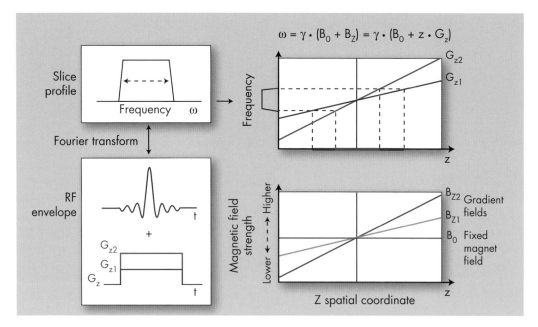

Figure 1-11. The radiofrequency (RF) pulse also has bandwidth, a frequency width that it can affect (*upper left*). The bandwidth of the RF pulse in combination with the amplitude of the concurrent gradient G_z together determine the thickness and profile of the slice of spins being excited and therefore imaged. For a constant bandwidth RF pulse, the larger the gradient ($G_{Z2} > G_{Z1}$), the larger the superimposed magnetic field $B_{Z'}$, and the smaller the slice thickness selected for imaging.

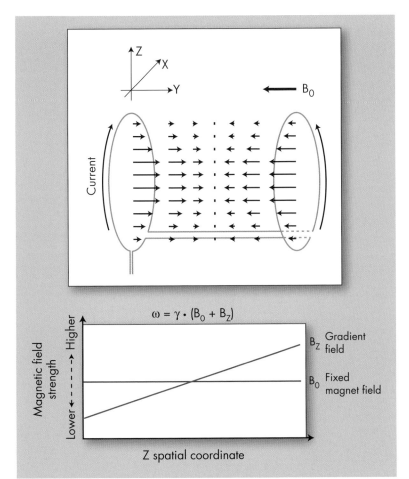

$$\omega = \gamma \cdot (B_0 + B_Z)$$

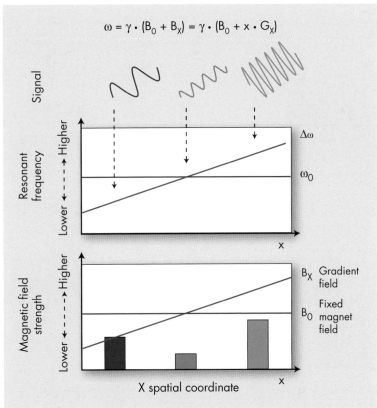

$$\omega = \gamma \cdot (B_0 + B_X) = \gamma \cdot (B_0 + x \cdot G_X)$$

Figure 1-12. The process of slice encoding needs a gradient in the magnetic field in the direction of the main field B_0. This is typically achieved with a gradient insert—a pair of coils—as shown here. The coils generate a magnetic field when a strong current is pushed through them. By pairing the coils and running the same current through both, it is possible to generate a symmetric magnetic field. In this example, the B_z magnetic field is generated. Note that the field is strongest near the center of the coils, and that it drops off linearly for the paired fields.

Figure 1-13. Frequency encoding is the second process for localization of the imaging process within a selected plane and it also takes advantage of the central equation in MRI: $\xi = \gamma B$. When frequency encoding, a linear spatial gradient B_X is superimposed on the fixed magnetic field B_0. In this example, three different objects rest at three different locations along x within the magnet. While B_X is applied, the spin located at the three different positions has three different resonance frequencies. During the signal detection process, only one mixed signal is detected. Note that the gradient field strength is given by the product of the position x and the strength of the applied gradient G_X, measured in mT/m.

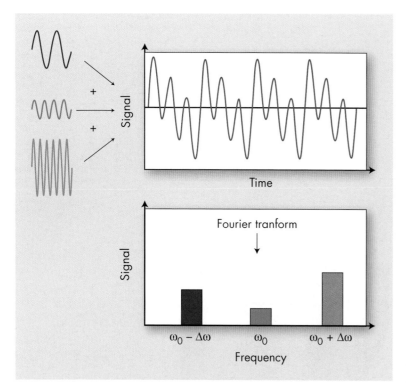

Figure 1-14. The signal detected from the three objects is actually the sum of their three different frequencies. Using a process called the *fast Fourier transform (FFT)*, it is possible to separate and distinguish the three signals and their relative amplitudes. FFT translates a signal, time in this case, into a map of the relative strengths of the individual frequency components in the signal. Frequency encoding is used to localize the origin of the signal in X direction commonly referred to as read-out direction.

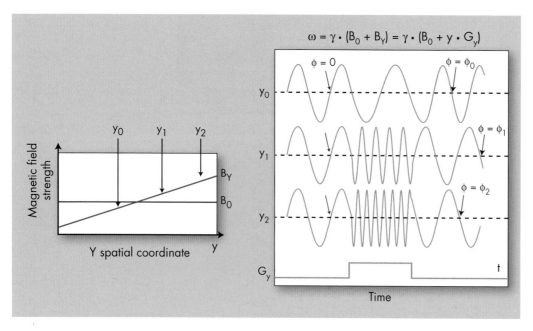

Figure 1-15. The second step used in signal localization within a selected plane is phase encoding. During phase encoding, a temporary gradient G_Y is applied. During this gradient, spins at different y-coordinates resonate at different frequencies. By controlling the duration and amplitude of G_Y, the amount of relative phase ϕ, defined by the zero crossings, can be controlled. At the end of phase encoding, different positions in Y will have different accumulated phase ϕ.

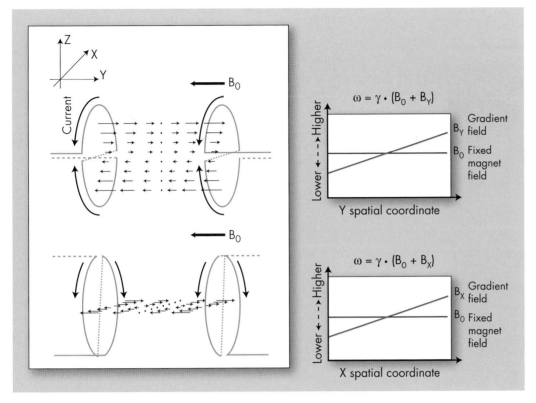

Figure 1-16. The process of in-plane signal localization using phase encoding and frequency encoding requires extra gradients G_Y and G_X in the magnetic field. This is typically achieved with a gradient insert—a pair of coils—as shown here. The coils generate a magnetic field when a strong current is pushed through them. These gradients are turned on and off during formation of an image to localize the source of an MR image within a plane.

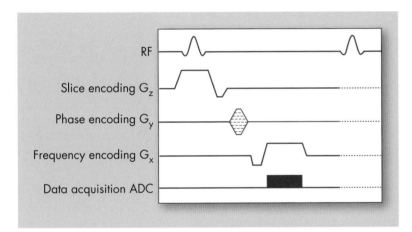

Figure 1-17. When we combine all the gradients necessary for an imaging experiment, we get a pulse sequence. In this example, radiofrequency (RF) excitation is accompanied by a slice selection gradient for slice-selective excitation. Afterward, one of a multiplicity of phase encoding steps is applied. Finally the readout gradient, along with its prewinder, is applied. The image data are acquired during the readout gradient via analog-to-digital converters (ADCs). The whole process is repeated until all necessary image data are acquired.

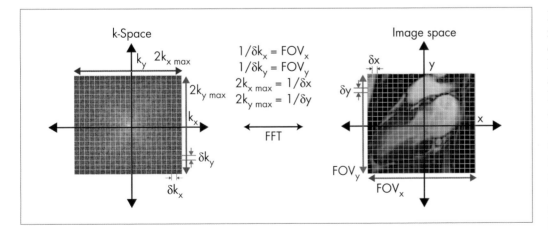

Figure 1-18. k-space is a spatial-frequency map of the image of interest. The k-space of an image can be obtained by using a fast Fourier transform (FFT), and equivalently an image can be obtained by applying an FFT to k-space. In MRI, clinicians do not acquire images directly. Instead, we acquire the k-space of an image and later reconstruct the image. Several interesting relationships between k-space and image space are highlighted here. Primarily, the field of view (FOV) of the image defines the samples spacing or resolution in k-space: δk_x and δk_y. Similarly, the desired image resolution specifies the maximum values needed in k-space: ky_{max} and kx_{max} in this two-dimensional example. Therefore, the size of an image the clinician wants specifies how densely k-space must be sampled, and the higher the resolution desired, the further out k-space must be sampled.

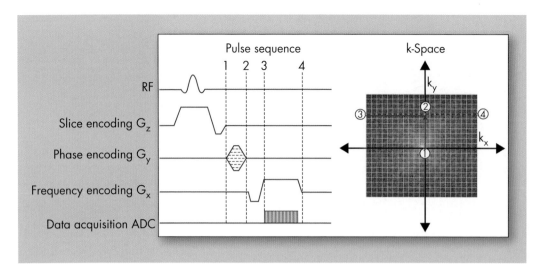

Figure 1-19. There is also a direct relationship between *k*-space sampling and the pulse sequence diagrams we have seen before. The position in *k*-space is determined by the area under the gradient waveforms. Therefore, as the pulse sequence is applied, *k*-space is traversed and sample points are collected to fill it in. After traversing all of *k*-space, the image is reconstructed. If one line of *k*-space each of radiofrequency (RF) excitation is acquired, then the whole process needs to be repeated multiple times, each with a different phase encoding gradient amplitude. At the end of the process, when *k*-space is fully sampled, an image can be reconstructed. ADC—analog-to-digital converter.

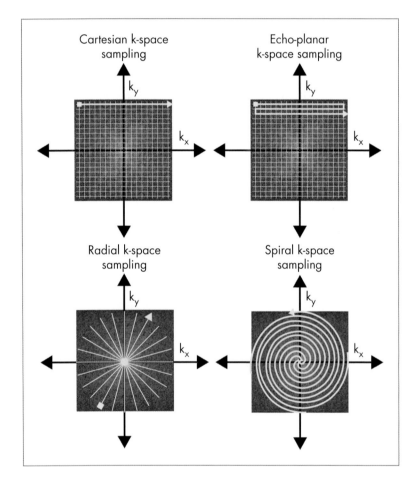

Figure 1-20. There are various sampling strategies for *k*-space. The most common technique is to acquire one Cartesian "line" of *k*-space after each excitation, as previously shown. Other strategies acquire multiple Cartesian lines of *k*-space per radiofrequency excitation. On the *top right* side, an example known as echo-planar imaging is shown. Further examples acquire lines based on a different grid, such as radial imaging (*bottom left*) and spiral imaging (*bottom right*). There are advantages and disadvantages of using each of sampling strategies in terms of speed, imaging artifacts, and so forth. However, all attempt to cover *k*-space as uniformly as possible.

2

CMR Imaging Methods

Krishna S. Nayak and Jon-Fredrik Nielsen

Cardiovascular magnetic resonance (CMR) imaging methods utilize the following features: 1) Fourier-based image acquisition, 2) synchronization with underlying physiology, and 3) additional contrast preparation. This chapter introduces the three elements of CMR imaging, discusses their advantages and disadvantages, and provides illustrative examples.

The first section of this chapter, titled "Imaging Sequences," introduces balanced steady-state free precession, gradient-recalled echo, phase contrast, and rapid acquisition with relaxation enhancement pulse sequences, as well as alternative k-space sampling schemes and parallel imaging. The second section, titled "Synchronization with Physiology," discusses cardiac and respiratory synchronization. The third section, titled, "Contrast Preparation Sequences," introduces methods for fat and blood suppression, enhancement of T1 and T2 contrast, and application of spatial tags. The final section, titled, "Representative Examples," covers the assembly of these components into routinely used CMR protocols for assessing myocardial scarring, intracardiac flow, myocardial perfusion, and the lumen of coronary arteries.

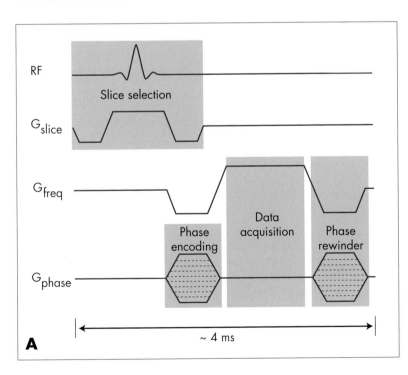

A

Figure 2-1. Balanced steady-state free precession (SSFP, also known as True-FISP, FIESTA, and balanced-FFE) is a pulse sequence routinely used for rapid imaging of cardiac function. SSFP has exceptionally high signal-to-noise ratio efficiency and strong T2/T1 weighting, producing images with high blood-myocardium contrast. In SSFP pulse sequence (**A**), the net gradient area is zero on all axes and spins are refocused every repetition time (TR) interval. This results in maximally efficient use of the magnetization (*ie*, no magnetization is spoiled or "wasted"). However, the SSFP signal is sensitive to local resonance offset Δf, and reaches zero for $\Delta f = \pm 1/2TR$ and periodically thereafter, producing well-known "banding" artifacts [1]. These can be avoided by minimizing the TR, which maximizes the SSFP band spacing $1/TR$, and by performing careful shimming over the region of interest (ROI), such that the ROI is placed near the center of the SSFP band.

Continued on the next page

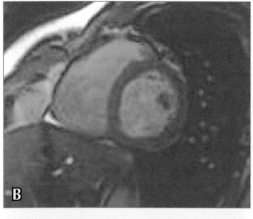

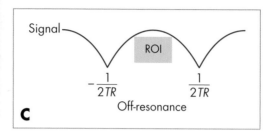

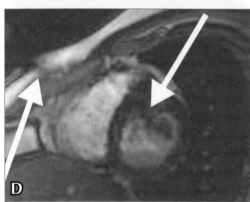

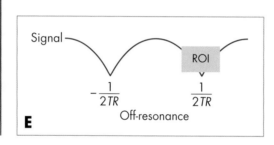

Figure 2-1. *(Continued)* In an example of a successful SSFP image acquisition (**B**), shown with corresponding spectral profile (**C**), the scan has been properly calibrated such that the local resonance offset in the ROI is in the center of the SSFP band. In the case of an unsuccessful example (**D**), also shown with corresponding spectral profile (**E**), improper shimming has placed the ROI directly over a null, resulting in visible artifacts (*arrows*). SSFP imaging becomes increasingly difficult at higher static field strengths because the dominant sources of off-resonance scale linearly with B0. Although cardiac SSFP imaging at 1.5T can be performed reasonably robustly using a TR of 6 ms or less (bandwidth $1/TR \geq 167$ Hz), the corresponding protocol at 3T would need to use a TR of 3 ms or less ($1/TR \geq 333$ Hz) to avoid banding artifact [2]. G_{freq}—frequency-encode gradient; G_{phase}—phase-encode gradient; G_{slice}—slice gradient; RF—radiofrequency.

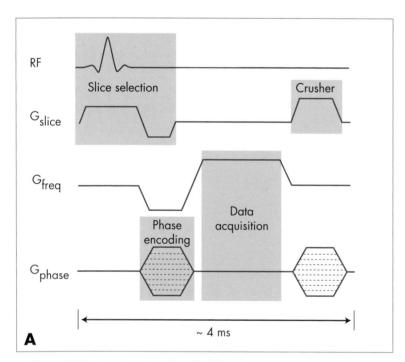

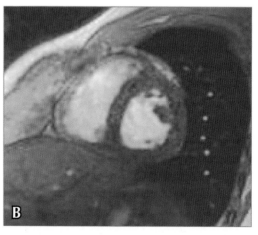

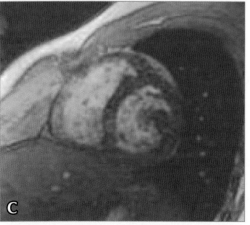

Figure 2-2. Gradient-recalled echo (GRE) is a rapid imaging sequence that spoils (removes) the transverse magnetization at the end of each repetition time (TR) interval. In the pulse sequence timing diagram (**A**), a "crusher" gradient pulse is played at the end of the TR to remove residual transverse magnetization. GRE sequences are not as signal-to-noise ratio efficient as other imaging methods, but have an advantage in that they do not suffer from banding artifacts. The steady-state signal strength for a flip angle α is proportional to $[1-e^{-TR/T1}]\sin\alpha/[1-e^{-TR/T1}\cos\alpha]$, which produces T1-weighted images. Tissue and fluids (*eg*, blood) that move into and out of the imaging volume appear relatively bright because such spins are not in a steady state. This results in "inflow enhancement," which causes blood-myocardium contrast to vary with cardiac phase. As seen in cardiac short-axis images from early diastole (**B**) and late diastole (**C**), inflow of unsaturated ("fresh") spins gives rise to the relatively bright blood signal in early (**B**) but not in late (**C**) diastole. G_{freq}—frequency-encode gradient; G_{phase}—phase-encode gradient; G_{slice}—slice gradient; RF—radiofrequency.

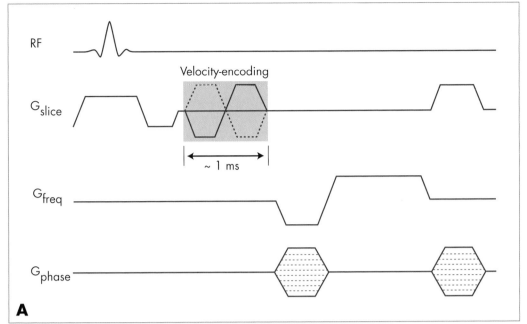

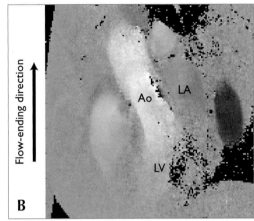

A

B

Figure 2-3. Phase contrast (PC) is an approach used to obtain velocity information on a pixel-by-pixel basis. Velocity is encoded into the phase of the image by inserting a bipolar gradient pulse between excitation and data acquisition [3]. In the PC pulse sequence timing example (**A**), a bipolar pulse is placed on the through-slice ("z") axis, which causes spins with velocity component v_z along the z-axis to acquire a phase $\phi = \gamma m_1 v_z$, where m_1 is the first moment of the bipolar waveform. Scanner hardware–related factors, such as complex receive coil sensitivities and off-resonance, also contribute to image phase. For this reason, two images with different velocity-encoding (VENC) gradients must be obtained (*eg*, by using bipolars with opposite signs or turning off the bipolar for one of the images; both are indicated by *dotted lines* in **A**). The phase difference $\Delta\phi$ between these two images is used to calculate the velocity component $v_z = \Delta\phi/(\gamma\Delta m_1)$. The key parameter when prescribing a PC sequence is the VENC value, which corresponds to the largest unaliased velocity (*ie*, the velocity v that makes $\Delta\phi = \pi$, or VENC = $\pi/\gamma\Delta m_1$). To avoid 2π phase wraps in the phase image,

it is therefore necessary to set the VENC at least as large as the maximum velocity. However, the VENC should not be set unnecessarily large because the signal-to-noise ratio in the PC images scales inversely with the VENC. Note that a reduced VENC corresponds to a larger bipolar pulse. To obtain the velocity component v_x along the x-axis (frequency-encoding direction), a separate image with the bipolar placed on the x-axis must be obtained. Similarly, measuring v_y requires another acquisition with the bipolar gradient on the y-axis (phase-encoding direction). Therefore, measuring the full three-dimensional velocity-vector $\mathbf{v} = v_x\hat{x} + v_y\hat{y} + v_z\hat{z}$ requires a minimum of four separate acquisitions: one reference scan (*eg*, with the bipolar turned off) and three acquisitions with the bipolar gradient successively placed on the x, y, and z gradient axes [4]. **B,** Velocity and magnitude images from a three-chamber view in a healthy volunteer were obtained at peak systole, with VENC along the readout direction. Ao—aorta; G_{freq}—frequency-encode gradient; G_{phase}—phase-encode gradient; G_{slice}—slice gradient; LA—left atrium; LV—left ventricle; RF—radiofrequency.

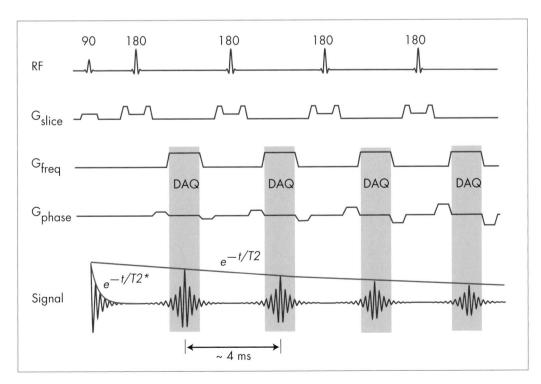

Figure 2-4. Rapid acquisition with relaxation enhancement (RARE, also known as fast-spin echo or turbo-spin echo) is a pulse sequence consisting of a selective tip-down, followed by a train of large-tip spin-echo refocusing pulses (usually 180°) [5]. Each spin-echo pulse is followed by the acquisition of a single phase-encode line. The purpose of the spin-echo pulses is to refocus the transverse magnetization at the center of each data acquisition (DAQ) window regardless of resonance frequency offset. Therefore, the echo amplitude decays as $e^{-t/T2}$ (*green curve*), with the time origin ($t = 0$) at the center of the selective 90° tip-down pulse. This means that the initial magnetization at $t = 0$ "survives" for a duration of approximately T2, during which it can be imaged. In other words, the resulting image is effectively a snapshot of the magnetization at $t = 0$.

Continued on the next page

Figure 2-4. *(Continued)* The figure shows an echo-train length (ETL) of 4, although longer ETLs are possible. The echo spacing (time between adjacent echoes) is determined by the time required to play the imaging and crusher gradients, and is typically 4 to 10 ms. RARE sequences involve relatively high radiofrequency (RF) power deposition, a problem that increases with increasing static magnetic field strength. Refocusing pulses of 150° or lower are often used in practice to mitigate RF heating constraints. G_{freq}—frequency-encode gradient; G_{phase}—phase-encode gradient; G_{slice}—slice gradient.

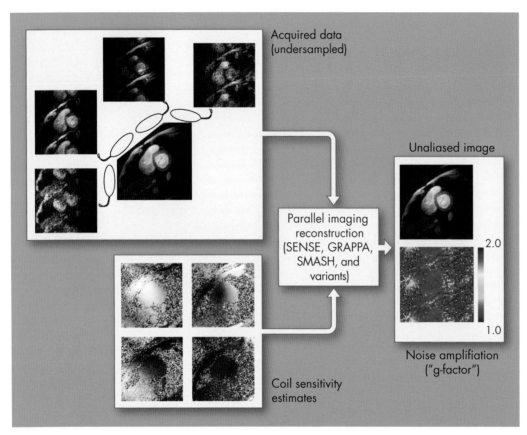

Figure 2-5. Parallel imaging is a robust and widely used approach for accelerating image acquisition. There are several variants, all of which share a common theme [6–8]. Individual elements in a receiver coil array capture the object of interest with a unique spatial weighting, which is considered an "encoding" additional to Fourier encoding. When k-space is undersampled (*eg*, by acquiring only every other phase encode), aliasing is a direct consequence. Parallel imaging techniques utilize knowledge of the coil sensitivity pattern to reconstruct alias-free (full field-of-view) images from aliased undersampled data. With knowledge of the coil sensitivities and undersampled k-space data from all coils, it is possible to either estimate the missing k-space data prior to performing the inverse Fourier transform (generalized autocalibrating partially parallel acquisitions [GRAPPA], simultaneous acquisition of spatial harmonics [SMASH]), or remove the aliasing directly in image space (sensitivity encoding [SENSE]). The so-called reduction factor (or acceleration factor) is always less than the number of independent coils. Parallel imaging also produces spatially varying signal-to-noise ratio loss, called "g-factor," which depends on the coil sensitivity pattern, sampling pattern, and scan plane orientation.

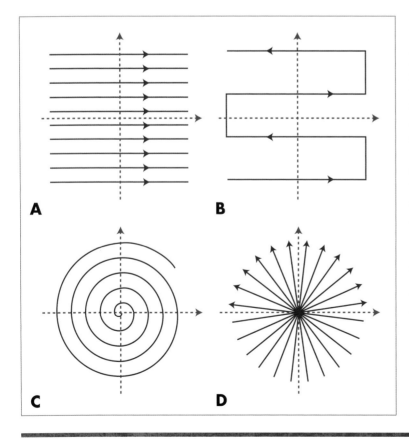

Figure 2-6. The vast majority of cardiovascular magnetic resonance (CMR) imaging sequences cover k-space using a Cartesian two-dimensional Fourier transform sampling pattern (**A**), consisting of parallel phase-encode lines. Other k-space trajectories are used in niche applications and may have a more substantial role in the future. Following each excitation, echo-planar imaging (EPI) (**B**) samples several phase encodes in a faster fashion. This sampling pattern reduces the total imaging time, but is sensitive to ghosting caused by misalignment between odd (left-right) and even (right-left) echoes and warping caused by off-resonance. Artifacts can be minimized by keeping the echo train length (ETL) short. Cardiac EPI using ETLs of 3 and 4 has been successfully demonstrated [9]. Spiral trajectories (**C**) sample k-space in a spiraling pattern, which is time efficient and robust to flow artifacts [10]. Spirals can produce blurring in the presence of off-resonance, but accurate shimming and short-segmented readouts can be used in many CMR applications, including function [11] and flow [12]. Radial trajectories (also known as projection reconstruction) (**D**) can achieve the shortest readout duration for a given resolution requirement, and are used frequently in angiography [13] and imaging of ultra-short T2 species [14]. Spiral and radial data require a modified reconstruction involving resampling to a Cartesian grid [15] or direct inverse Fourier transformation.

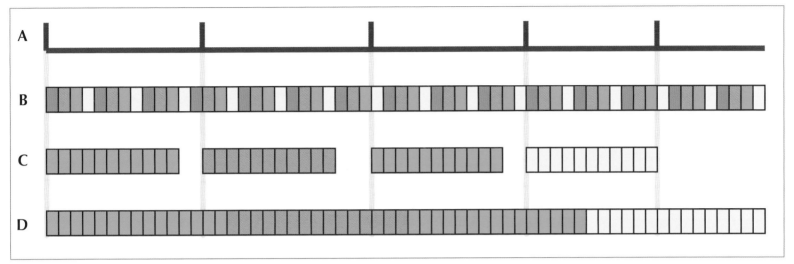

Figure 2-7. Cardiac phase is typically determined using an external "trigger" signal (**A**), which can be derived from a photoplethysmograph or electrocardiograph (ECG) R-wave, or a processed version of these signals (*eg*, vector ECG). Three basic methods for cardiac synchronization are real-time imaging, prospective gating, and retrospective gating. The k-space data needed to form a single image can be divided into segments that are represented by colored blocks. In real-time imaging (**B**), k-space data are collected continuously and at the highest rate possible, without considering the trigger signal. In prospectively gated imaging (**C**), one segment of data is acquired repeatedly in each heartbeat.

The pulse sequence responds to each trigger by moving to the next k-space segment. In retrospectively gated imaging (**D**), data are acquired continuously and are marked with the cardiac phase from which they were acquired. Data from the same cardiac phase are retrospectively assembled to produce a single "CINE" movie. Real-time imaging is the most robust because it does not assume periodicity of motion, but has limited spatial resolution and signal-to-noise ratio due to the limited acquisition time per frame [16]. Gated imaging is capable of achieving high spatial and temporal resolution and unique types of image contrast, but is susceptible to beat-to-beat variations.

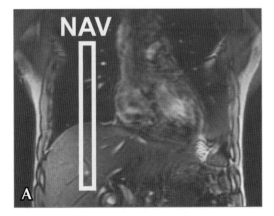

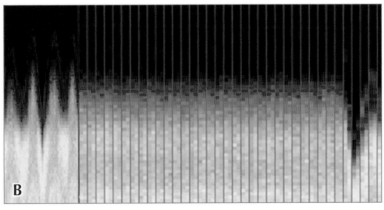

Figure 2-8. Respiratory phase is typically determined using bellows (which detect abdominal circumference) or navigator echoes [17]. The most common navigator-echo acquisition involves a one-dimensional cylinder passing through the right hemidiaphragm (**A**). A single excitation and one-dimensional data readout (~ 10 ms total duration) is used to produce a profile from which diaphragm position is derived. This can be used to retrospectively assemble acquired data from the same respiratory phase, prospec-

tively acquire data from a desired respiratory phase, or monitor the performance of a breath-hold (**B**). There are many variants, including using extra navigators over the heart, using navigators before and after imaging, and adapting the scan plane/volume based on the navigator acquisition. A typical assumption when performing motion compensation is that the shift in cardiac position is 60% of the shift in diaphragm position. NAV—navigator echo. (**B** *courtesy of* C. Jahnke.)

A major strength of cardiovascular magnetic resonance is its ability to generate many different types of image contrast. Image contrast is influenced by intrinsic properties of the imaging sequence (described above), and by optional contrast preparation sequences (described below) that may be used prior to image acquisition.

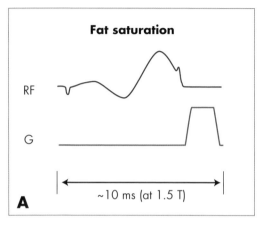

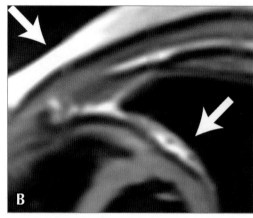

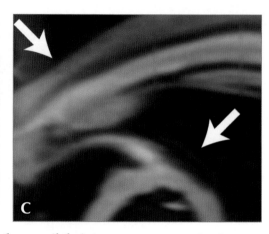

Figure 2-9. Fat signal can be suppressed using a pre-pulse (called "fat saturation" [FATSAT]). It is often necessary to suppress fat because it produces high signal due to its short T1 and may obscure neighboring structures of interest. ¹H in lipid molecules experience a resonance frequency chemical shift of approximately -3.5 parts-per-million relative to ¹H in water and lean tissue. This translates to -220 Hz at 1.5T, and -440 Hz at 3T. A common method for suppressing fat is to excite all fat spins with a frequency-selective excitation pulse, and then spoil their transverse magnetization with a large gradient, called a "crusher" (**A**). Note that the saturation is frequency selective and not spatially selective. Performance is illustrated in black-blood short-axis imaging without (**B**) and with (**C**) FATSAT (*arrows*). Because lipid protons typically have short T1, the benefits of saturated fat signal are available for only a limited time. Therefore, FATSAT is used in non–time-resolved imaging. G—gradient; RF—radiofrequency.

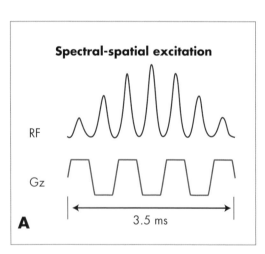

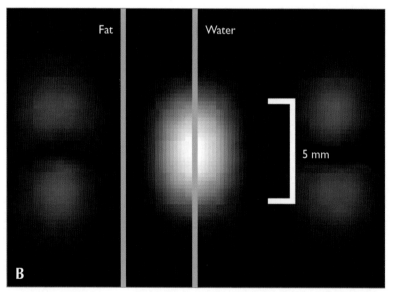

Figure 2-10. Spectral-spatial pulses utilize the chemical shift between water and fat to excite only water spins (or only lipid spins) within a slice or volume of interest [18]. The radiofrequency (RF) waveform is divided into several subpulses that are synchronized with an oscillating gradient (**A**). The resulting excitation profile (**B**) is selective in both space (*vertical axis*) and resonant frequency (*horizontal axis*). This approach is used in continuous CINE and real-time imaging. Gz—slice selection gradient.

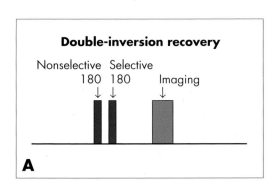

Double-inversion recovery

Nonselective Selective
180 180
↓ ↓
Imaging
↓

A

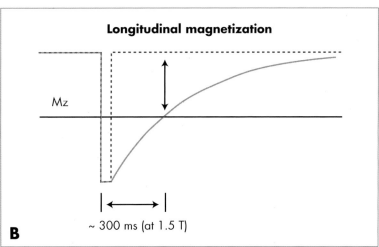

Longitudinal magnetization

M_z

~ 300 ms (at 1.5 T)

B

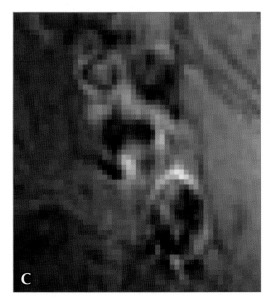

C

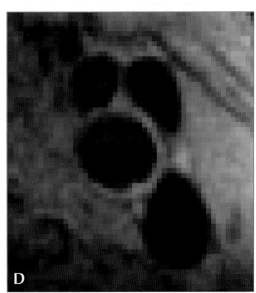

D

Figure 2-11. Double-inversion recovery (DIR) is a method for suppressing blood signal based on its flow and T1 properties [19]. Nonselective and slice-selective inversion pulses are played consecutively in order to invert all spins outside of the imaging slice (**A**). Imaging is performed at the null-time (**B**) of the spins being suppressed (*eg*, blood). At the imaging time, there is excellent contrast between in-slice static tissue (*dashed purple*) and blood that has flown into the imaging slice (*black*). This approach is often used to image cardiac and vascular morphology. For illustration, rapid-acquisition with relaxation enhancement carotid wall images are shown without (**C**) and with (**D**) DIR preparation. M_z—longitudinal magnetization.

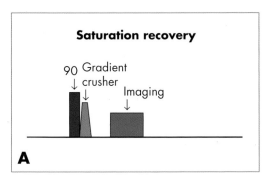

Saturation recovery

90 Gradient
↓ crusher
↓
Imaging
↓

A

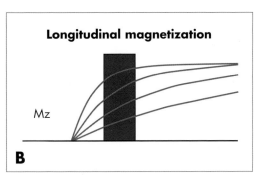

Longitudinal magnetization

M_z

B

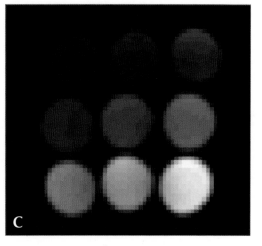

C

Figure 2-12. Saturation recovery (SR) is a method for increasing T1 contrast in images (spins with long T1 are suppressed). A nonselective 90° excitation is followed by a gradient crusher and a delay (T_{SR}) before imaging (**A**). The longitudinal magnetization prior to imaging (**B**) is highly dependent on T1. This is illustrated in a T1 phantom with test tubes containing doped water with T1s of 1300, 850, 600, 500, 325, 250, 150, 100, and 65 ms with $T_{SR} = 100$ ms (**C**). In this range, signal intensity is roughly proportional to 1/T1. SR is often used in first-pass myocardial perfusion imaging. M_z—longitudinal magnetization.

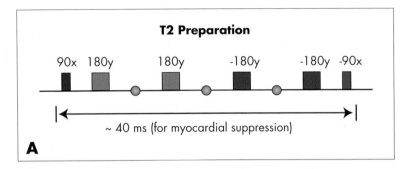

T2 Preparation

90x 180y   180y   -180y   -180y -90x

~ 40 ms (for myocardial suppression)

A

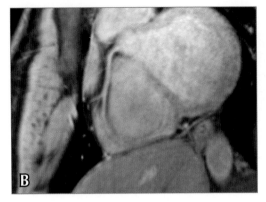

B

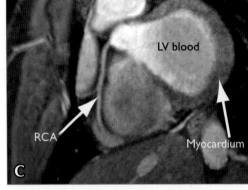

LV blood

RCA

Myocardium

C

Figure 2-13. T2 preparation is a method for increasing the T2 contrast in images (spins with short T2 are suppressed) [20]. A 90° excitation that tips spins to the transverse plane is followed by a train of 180° refocusing pulses and a 90° tip-up pulse (**A**). Spin magnetization decays with T2 while in the transverse plane. The refocusing pulses create spin echoes (*green circles*) and ensure that magnetization is coherently tipped up by the final pulse. Larger numbers of refocusing pulses (the minimum number is one) make the method more resistant to motion and spin diffusion and provide a purer T2 weighting. This approach is frequently used for myocardial suppression. For illustration, coronary artery images are shown without (**B**) and with (**C**) T2 preparation. LV—left ventricle; RCA—right coronary artery. (Images B and C *courtesy of* Nezafat R.)

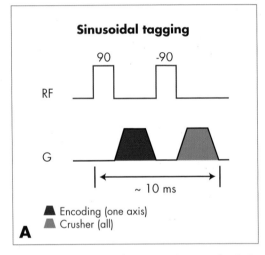

Sinusoidal tagging

90   -90

RF

G

~ 10 ms

▲ Encoding (one axis)
▲ Crusher (all)

A

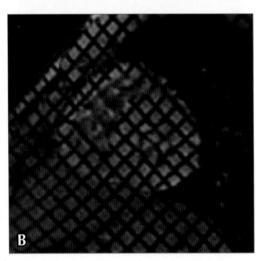

B

cycle. Sinusoidal spatial tags (**A**) are the simplest variety. Excitations with a 90° and -90° gradient in between provides sinusoidal longitudinal magnetization as a function of position along the axis of the encoding gradient (*purple*). A gradient crusher (*green*) eliminates residual transverse magnetization. This can be repeated along two encoding axes to provide a two-dimensional grid of tags (**B**). Motion of these tags during the cardiac cycle can provide valuable information, such as regional myocardial strain. G—gradient; RF—radiofrequency.

Figure 2-14. Spatial tagging is a method that provides additional information about the motion of spins. Spins in a particular location or locations are saturated, making them appear dark. The motion of these dark regions can be tracked throughout the cardiac

REPRESENTATIVE EXAMPLES

The following four examples are intended to illustrate how physiologic synchronization, contrast preparation, and imaging sequences are assembled to form clinically useful imaging methods.

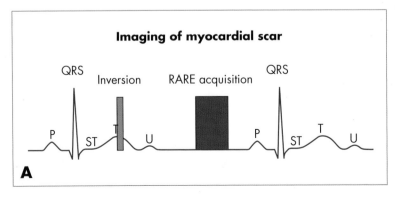

Imaging of myocardial scar

QRS   Inversion   RARE acquisition   QRS

P   ST   T   U   P   ST   T   U

A

Figure 2-15. Imaging of myocardial scarring using inversion recovery rapid acquisition with relaxation enhancement (RARE) 10 to 15 minutes after administration of gadolinium-DTPA. Acquisitions are typically performed during a breath-hold to freeze respiratory motion and are cardiac gated to freeze cardiac motion. After each trigger, a nonselective inversion pulse inverts the longitudinal magnetization (Mz) of all spins, and RARE imaging is performed at the null-time of normal myocardium (**A**).

Continued on the next page

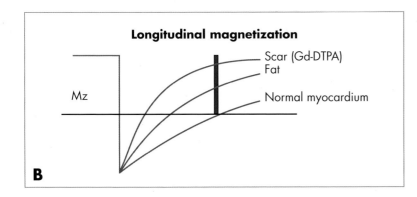

B

Longitudinal magnetization

Mz

Scar (Gd-DTPA)
Fat
Normal myocardium

Figure 2-15. *(Continued)* Myocardial scar, which collects gadolinium (Gd)-DTPA several minutes after administration, exhibits bright signal due to its short T1 (**B**). Fat is also somewhat bright because its T1 is shorter than that of normal myocardium. The repetition time is typically 2 R-R intervals to allow for near complete relaxation.

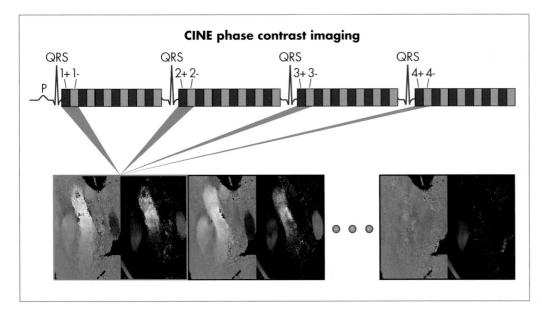

CINE phase contrast imaging

Figure 2-16. Intracardiac flow using CINE gradient-recalled echo (GRE) phase contrast. Acquisitions are typically performed during a breath-hold and are cardiac gated. After each trigger, one k-space segment (*eg*, 1 through 4) is repeatedly acquired with two different flow encodings (*eg*, + and -, representing bipolar and inverted bipolar, or bipolar on and off). Images are formed by assembling data from the same cardiac phase (*red*). Velocity images or color-flow overlay images can be generated.

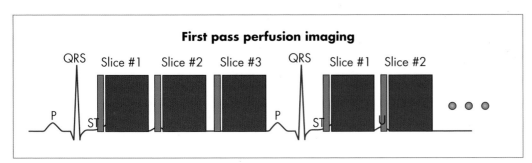

First pass perfusion imaging

Figure 2-17. Myocardial perfusion imaging using multislice saturation recovery gradient-recalled echo (GRE) with a bolus of gadolinium-DTPA. Acquisitions are typically cardiac gated and are performed during free-breathing. Contrast passage takes 30 to 45 seconds, precluding the use of a breath-hold. After each trigger, three slices are imaged using a saturation pulse and series of imaging excitations. GRE, steady-state free precession, and GRE–echo-planar imaging are the most common acquisitions. The slices may be arbitrarily oriented (*eg*, three short-axis slices, or two short-axis slices and one long-axis slice). Note that although the images come from different cardiac phases, there is consistency. Images of slice 1 are always from systole, whereas images of slice 3 are always in diastole. This illustration shows three slices per R-R interval. However, these settings may be changed (*eg*, four slices every two R-R) in response to the patient's heart rate, or by changing the desired spatial resolution.

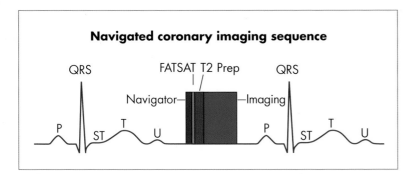

Navigated coronary imaging sequence

Figure 2-18. Imaging of the coronary artery lumen using respiratory navigated fat saturated (FATSAT) T2-prepared gradient-recalled echo (GRE). Acquisitions are typically cardiac gated and performed during free-breathing (using navigator echo–based motion compensation). Each R-R interval contains a navigator echo acquisition, fat saturation, T2 preparation, and GRE imaging. Imaging is performed during a stable diastolic window typically identified using a calibration scan. If a steady-state free precession acquisition is used, the imaging is preceded by an initial preparation that reduces transient signal oscillations during the approach to steady state.

REFERENCES

1. Carr HY: Steady-state free precession in nuclear magnetic resonance. *Phys Rev* 1958, 112:1693–1701.

2. Schär M, Kozerke S, Fischer SE, Boesiger P: Cardiac SSFP imaging at 3 Tesla. *Magn Reson Med* 2004, 51:799–806.

3. Hahn EL: Detection of sea-water motion by nuclear precession. *J Geophys Res* 1960, 65:776–777.

4. Pelc NJ, Bernstein MJ, Shimakawa A, Glover GH: Encoding strategies for three-direction phase-contrast MR imaging of flow. *J Magn Reson Imaging* 1991, 1:405–413.

5. Hennig J, Nauerth A, Freidburg H: RARE imaging: a fast imaging method for clinical MR. *Magn Reson Med* 1986, 3:823–833.

6. Pruessmann KP, Weiger M, Scheidegger MB, Boesiger P: SENSE: sensitivity encoding for fast MRI. *Magn Reson Med* 1999, 42:952–962.

7. Griswold MA, Jakob PM, Heidemann RM, *et al.*: Generalized auto-calibrating partially parallel acquisitions (GRAPPA). *Magn Reson Med* 2002, 47:1202–1210.

8. Sodickson DK, Manning WJ: Simultaneous acquisition of spatial harmonics (SMASH): fast imaging with radiofrequency coil arrays. *Magn Reson Med* 1997, 38:591–603.

9. Epstein FH, Wolff SD, Arai AE: Segmented k-space fast cardiac imaging using an echo-train readout. *Magn Reson Med* 1999, 41:609–613.

10. Nishimura DG, Irarrazabal P, Meyer CH: A velocity k-space analysis of flow effects in echo-planar and spiral imaging. *Magn Reson Med* 1995, 33:549–556.

11. Yang PC, Kerr AB, Liu AC, *et al.*: New real-time interactive magnetic resonance imaging complements echocardiography. *J Am Coll Cardiol* 1998, 32:2049–2056.

12. Nayak KS, Pauly JM, Kerr AB, *et al.*: Real-time color flow MRI. *Magn Reson Med* 2000, 43:251–258.

13. Peters DC, Korosec FR, Grist TM, *et al.*: Undersampled projection reconstruction applied to MR angiography. *Magn Reson Med* 2000, 43:91–101.

14. Gatehouse PD, Bydder GM: Magnetic resonance imaging of short T2 components in tissue. *Clin Radiol* 2003, 58:1–19.

15. Jackson JI, Meyer CH, Nishimura DG, Macovski A: Selection of a convolution function for Fourier inversion using gridding. *IEEE Trans Med Imaging* 1991, 10:473–478.

16. Nayak KS, Hu BS: The future of real-time cardiac magnetic resonance imaging. *Curr Cardiol Rep* 2005, 7:45–51.

17. Ehman RL, Felmlee JP: Adaptive technique for high-definition MR imaging of moving structures. *Radiology* 1989, 173:255–263.

18. Meyer CH, Pauly JM, Macovski A, Nishimura DG: Simultaneous spatial and spectral selective excitation. *Magn Reson Med* 1990, 15:287–304.

19. Edelman RR, Chien D, Kim D: Fast selective black blood MR imaging. *Radiology* 1991, 181:655–660.

20. Brittain JH, Hu BS, Wright GA, *et al.*: Coronary angiography with magnetization-prepared T2 contrast. *Magn Reson Med* 1995, 33:689–696.

3

CHAPTER

Contrast Agents

Andrea J. Wiethoff and René M. Botnar

Signal intensity in MRI primarily depends on the local values of the longitudinal (1/T1) and transverse (1/T2) relaxation rate of water protons. Depending on the pulse sequence, the signal usually tends to increase with shorter T1 (higher 1/T1), and decrease with shorter T2 (higher 1/T2) relaxation times. The environment in which the nucleus is located determines the MR signals created. Therefore, by manipulating the chemical environment around the protons, the signal can be altered. MR contrast agents were developed as a way to modulate the chemical environment inside an organism. The relaxivities R1 and R2, which are commonly expressed in $(mM \times s)^{-1}$ indicate the increase in 1/T1 and 1/T2 per concentration of contrast agent with $T1_0$ and $T2_0$ the relaxation times of native tissue (*ie*, tissue devoid of exogenous contrast agent).

$$1/T1 = 1/T1_0 + R1 \text{ [contrast agent]}$$
$$1/T2 = 1/T2_0 + R2 \text{ [contrast agent]}$$

Gadolinium-based contrast agents usually increase 1/T1 and 1/T2 in similar amounts ($R2/R1 \cong 1–2$), whereas iron particle-based contrast agents have a much stronger effect on increasing 1/T2 ($R2/R1 > 10$). Gadolinium-based contrast agents lead to a positive contrast effect (detected as an increase in signal intensity or brightness), whereas iron particle-based contrast agents usually cause a negative contrast effect (detected as a decrease in signal intensity or darkness). MR pulse sequences that emphasize differences in T1 and T2 are commonly referred to as T1- and T2-weighted sequences. Apart from their effect in increasing 1/T2, iron particles also increase 1/T2* because of their effect on the local magnetic field B_0, thus causing local field inhomogeneities ΔB_0. This additional effect leads to even more rapid signal decay.

$$1/T2^* = 1/T2 + \gamma \Delta B_0$$

Iron-based contrast agents are therefore typically imaged using T2*-weighted imaging sequences. More recent approaches for iron-oxide–based nanoparticle particle visualization directly image the dipole field by means of water suppression [1] or the background gradients caused by those particles [2–4]. For signal quantification, T2-multi echo spin echo or T2* multigradient echo sequences can be used to generate T2 or T2* maps. Typical R1 and R2 values of currently approved gadolinium-based contrast agents are in the range of $R1 = 3$ to 5 $(mM \times s)^{-1}$, and $R2 = 5$ to 6 $(mM \times s)^{-1}$. The relaxivities of iron-based contrast agents are significantly higher $R1 = 20$ to 25 $(mM \times s)^{-1}$ and $R2 = 100$ to 200 $(mM \times s)^{-1}$. Because of the low concentrations at which molecular imaging targets are generally found, relaxivity is important in the design of molecular contrast agents.

Extracellular Gadolinium Contrast Agents (Rapid Blood Clearance)

Agent	Characteristics	Cardiovascular Indication Approved/Under Trial
Magnevist (Bayer Healthcare, Wayne, NJ) [5]	Gd-DTPA, ionic, linear chelate; $R1 = 5.3$ mM^{-1}s^{-1} (2T); $R2 = 6.8$ mM^{-1}s^{-1}	MRA; delayed enhancement; and perfusion
Gadovist (Bayer Healthcare, Wayne, NJ) [6]	Gd-DO3A-butriol, nonionic, macrocyclic chelate; $R1 = 6.1$ mM^{-1}s^{-1} (2T)	MRA; delayed enhancement; and perfusion
MultiHance (Bracco, Milan, Italy) [7]	Gd-BOPTA, ionic, linear, some albumin binding; $R1 = 9.7$ mM^{-1}s^{-1} (1T); $R2 = 12.5$ mM^{-1}s^{-1}	MRA; delayed enhancement; and perfusion
ProHance (Bracco, Milan, Italy) [8]	Gd-HP-DO3A, nonionic, macrocyclic chelate; $R1 = 3.7$ mM^{-1}s^{-1} (1T); $R2 = 4.8$ mM^{-1}s^{-1}	MRA; delayed enhancement; and perfusion
Omniscan (GE Healthcare, Princeton, NJ) [9]	Gd-DTPA-BMA, nonionic, linear chelate; $R1 = 3.9$ mM^{-1}s^{-1} (1T); $R2 = 4.3$ mM^{-1}s^{-1}	MRA; delayed enhancement; and perfusion
OptiMARK (Mallinckrodt, St. Louis, MO) [10]	Gd-DTPA-BMEA, nonionic, linear chelate; $R1 = 5.2$ mM^{-1}s^{-1} (1.5T)	MRA; delayed enhancement; and perfusion

Figure 3-1. Extracellular gadolinium contrast agents (rapid blood clearance). Gd-BOPTA—gadobenate dimeglumine; Gd-DO3A—gadobutrol; Gd-DTPA— gadopentetate dimeglumine; Gd-DTPA-BMA—gadodiamide; Gd-DTPA-BMEA—gadoversetamide; Gd-HP-DO3A—gadoteridol; MRA—magnetic resonance angiography.

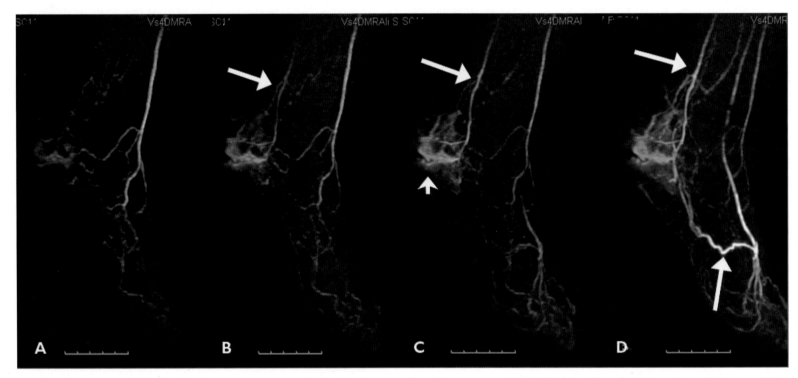

Figure 3-2. A–D, Patient with type II diabetes and lower limb occlusive disease, Fontaine stage IV. Preoperative evaluation of pedal vessel before bypass surgery using time-resolved contrast-enhanced steady-state gradient echo angiography (4 s/frame, four-dimensional TREAT) after the administration of 0.1 mmol/kg Magnevist (Bayer Healthcare, Wayne, NJ). (*Courtesy of* Elmar Speuntrup, MD, RWTH, Aachen, Germany.)

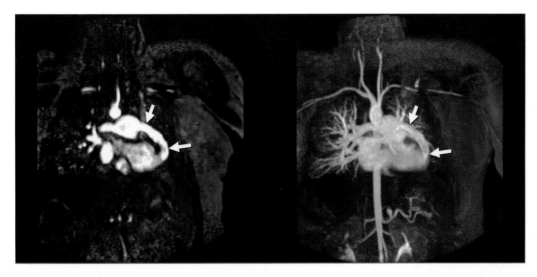

Figure 3-3. Left ventricle (LV) to pulmonary artery (PA) conduit. First pass angiography using a steady state T1-weighted gradient echo technique in a patient with a LV/PA conduit after administration of 0.1 mmol/kg Magnevist (Bayer Healthcare, Wayne, NJ). *Left panel*: Raw data. *Right panel*: Maximum intensity projection of large vessels and LV/PA conduit. (*Courtesy of* Heiko Stern, MD, Deutsches Herzzentrum München, Munich, Germany.)

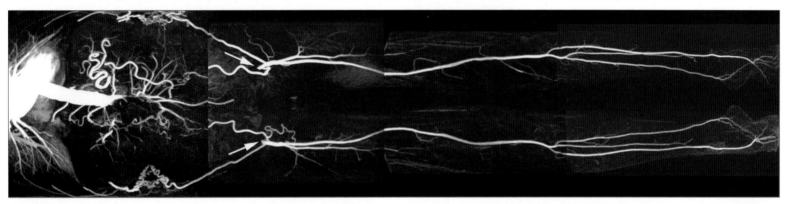

Figure 3-4. Peripheral MR angiography with Magnevist (Bayer Healthcare, Wayne, NJ) of a 63-year-old man with complaints of bilateral intermittent claudication, absent pulsations in the groin, and impotence. The full-volume maximum intensity projection of this four-station contrast-enhanced MR angiography acquisition reveals occlusion of the infrarenal aorta, common iliac, and external iliac arteries on both sides, confirming the diagnosis of Leriche syndrome. Both superficial femoral arteries are reconstituted by collaterals arising from the intercostal arteries and retrogradely filling the circumflex iliac arteries (*arrows*). Note exquisite image quality of the arteries all the way down to the toes. There is a low-grade nonsignificant stenosis in the right anterior tibial artery (TR/TE/SENSE factor: 3.8 / 1.3 / 2x [aortoiliac] and 3x [upper and lower legs]). (*Courtesy of* Tim Leiner, MD, Maastricht University Hospital, The Netherlands.)

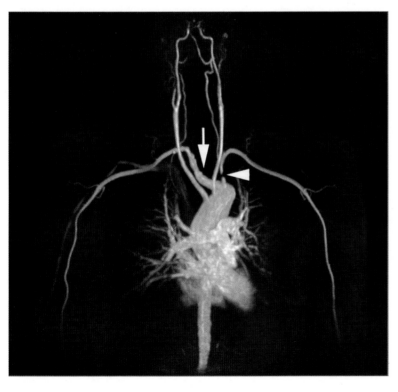

Figure 3-5. Aorta and subclavian MR angiography with Magnevist (Bayer Healthcare, Wayne, NJ) of a 45-year-old man with complaints of numbness in the left hand. The full volume maximum intensity projection reveals a high-grade stenosis in the left subclavian artery (*arrowhead*) and an aberrant right subclavian artery (*arrow*) (TR/TE/SENSE factor: 4.0 / 1.5 / 2x). (*Courtesy of* Tim Leiner, MD, Maastricht University Hospital, The Netherlands.)

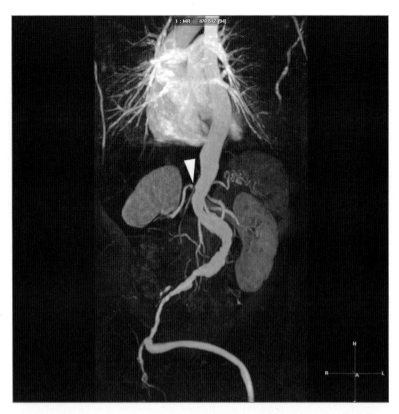

Figure 3-6. Renal artery MR angiography with Magnevist (Bayer Healthcare, Wayne, NJ) of a 67-year-old woman with hypertension refractory to medical treatment with multiple antihypertensive drugs. The patient previously underwent femorofemoral crossover bypass surgery because of peripheral arterial occlusive disease of the left iliac arteries. The maximum intensity projection shows a high-grade stenosis of the right renal artery (*arrowhead*). (TR/TE/SENSE factor 3.9 /1.3 / 2x). (*Courtesy of* Tim Leiner, MD, Maastricht University Hospital, The Netherlands.)

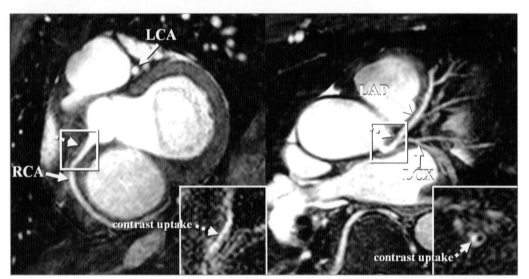

Figure 3-7. Coronary magnetic resonance plaque imaging with Magnevist (Bayer Healthcare, Wayne, NJ). T1-weighted electrocardiogram-triggered and navigator-gated inversion recovery fast gradient echo coronary artery images in a patient without a history of heart disease. Delayed enhancement images of the proximal right coronary artery (RCA) and left anterior descending (LAD) artery (*large white boxes*) demonstrate focal contrast uptake in the coronary vessel wall, which is most likely caused by the presence of a fibrous-rich plaque. LCA—left coronary artery; LCX—left circumflex artery.

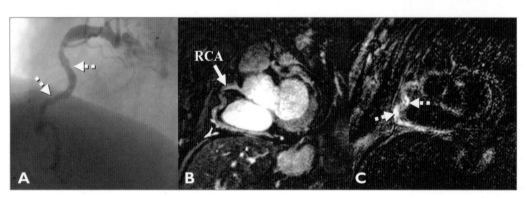

Figure 3-8. Coronary magnetic resonance plaque imaging with Magnevist (Bayer Healthcare, Wayne, NJ). A, Radiograph coronary angiography in a patient with an acute coronary syndrome with two lesions (*arrows*) in the right coronary artery (RCA). B, MR coronary angiography reveals low blood signal in the RCA suggestive of slow flow or occlusion of the RCA. Delayed enhancement coronary MRI after administration of 0.2 mmol/kg. C, Magnevist demonstrates two focal hotspots (*dotted arrows*) suggestive of two coronary lesions.

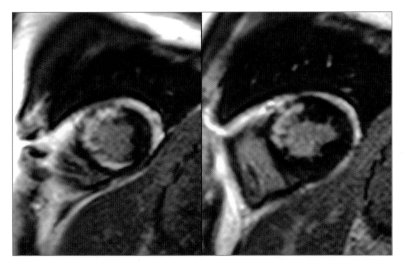

Figure 3-9. Subendocardial infarct. Late gadolinium enhancement imaging of a subendocardial antero- to inferoseptal infarct using a two-dimensional T1-weighted inversion recovery segmented gradient echo technique approximately 10 minutes after administration of 0.1 mmol/kg Gadovist (Bayer Healthcare, Wayne, NJ).

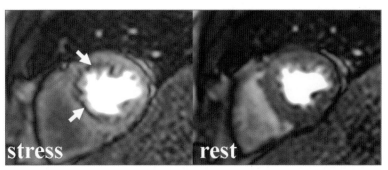

Figure 3-10. Inducible perfusion deficit. First pass myocardial perfusion imaging using a two-dimensional T1-weighted saturation recovery segmented gradient echo technique during rest and adenosine stress (140 μg/min/kg) after administration of 0.025 mmol/kg Gadovist (Bayer Healthcare, Wayne, NJ). Note that the perfusion deficit (*arrows*) does not persist during the rest study.

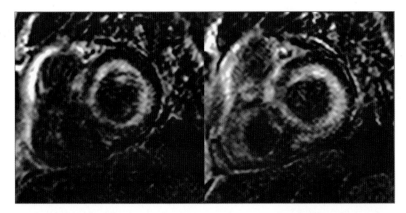

Figure 3-11. Amyloidosis. Late gadolinium enhancement imaging of a patient with advanced amyloidosis using a two-dimensional T1-weighted inversion recovery segmented gradient echo technique approximately 10 minutes after administration of 0.2 mmol/kg Magnevist (Bayer Healthcare, Wayne, NJ).

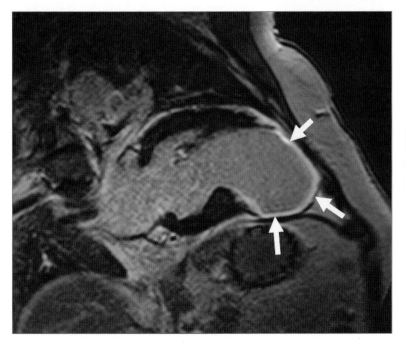

Figure 3-12. Left ventricular (LV) aneurysm. Late gadolinium enhancement imaging of an LV aneurysm (*arrows*) using a two-dimensional T1-weighted inversion recovery segmented gradient echo technique approximately 10 minutes after administration 0.2 mmol/kg Magnevist (Bayer Healthcare, Wayne, NJ).

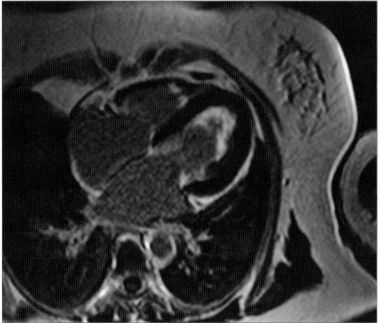

Figure 3-13. Loeffler's endocarditis. Late gadolinium enhancement imaging of a patient with Loeffler's endocarditis using a two-dimensional T1-weighted inversion recovery segmented gradient echo technique and 0.2 mmol/kg Magnevist (Bayer Healthcare, Wayne, NJ).

Blood Pool Gadolinium Contrast Agents (Slow Blood Clearance)

Agent	Characteristics	Cardiovascular Indication Approved/Under Trial
Vasovist (EPIX Pharmaceuticals, Lexington, MA) [11,12]	Gd, binds to albumin; $R1 = 19$ mM^{-1}s^{-1}	Peripheral MRA
B 22956 (Bracco, Milan, Italy) [13–15]	Gd, binds to albumin; $R1 = 27$ mM^{-1}s^{-1} (0.5T)	Coronary angiography studies (discontinued)
Gadomer-17 (Bayer Healthcare, Wayne, NJ) [16]	Gd dendrimer; $R1 = 14.7$ mM^{-1}s^{-1} (2T); $R2 = 21.4$ mM^{-1}s^{-1}	MRA (discontinued?)

Figure 3-14. Blood pool gadolinium (Gd) contrast agents (slow blood clearance). MRA—magnetic resonance angiography.

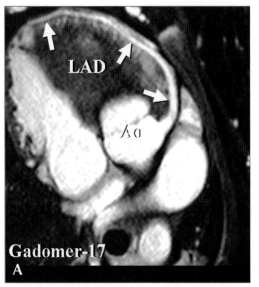

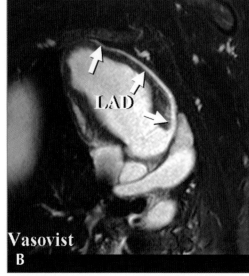

Figure 3-15. Coronary artery imaging using blood pool agents. MR coronary angiography of the left anterior descending artery (LAD) in a domestic swine using a T1-weighted inversion recovery fast gradient echo sequence and Gadomer-17 (Bayer Healthcare, Wayne, NJ) (**A**) and Vasovist (Bayer Healthcare, Wayne, NJ) (**B**). Gadomer-17 is a 24-gadolinium cascade polymer, whereas Vasovist is an albumin-binding gadolinium-based contrast agent. Good delineation of the LAD can be observed with these intravascular contrast agents.

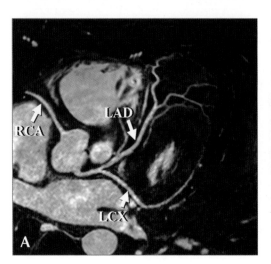

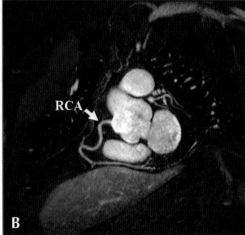

Figure 3-16. Coronary artery imaging using B-22956 (Bracco, Milan, Italy). MR coronary angiogram using the whole heart technique of the left main artery, left anterior descending artery (LAD), and left circumflex artery (LCX) (**A**) and the right coronary artery (RCA) (**B**) in a patient after injection of B-22956, an albumin-binding intravascular contrast agent. Good delineation of the major coronary arteries can be observed with good suppression of the myocardium. Image acquisition was performed using an electrocardiogram-triggered and navigator-gated three-dimensional inversion recovery fast gradient echo technique. (*Courtesy of Volker Rasche, PhD, University Hospital Ulm, Germany.*)

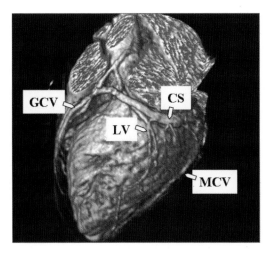

Figure 3-17. Coronary vein imaging using B-22956 (Bracco, Milan, Italy). Three-dimensional rendered MR coronary veinogram using the whole heart technique after injection of B-22956, an albumin-binding intravascular contrast agent. Good delineation of the coronary sinus (CS) and the great cardiac vein (GCV) can be observed. Image acquisition was performed using an electrocardiogram-triggered and navigator-gated three-dimensional inversion recovery fast gradient echo technique. LV—left ventricle; MCV—middle cardiac vein. (*Courtesy of* Volker Rasche, PhD, University Hospital Ulm, Germany.)

Liver Iron Oxide Contrast Agents (Rapid Blood Clearance)

Agent	Characteristics	Cardiovascular Indication Approved/Under Trial
Feridex/Endorem (Bayer Healthcare, Wayne, NJ) [17]	Fe, SPIO (IV), dextran coating; R1 = 40 mM^{-1}s^{-1} (0.47T); R2 = 160 mM^{-1}s^{-1}; size = ~80–150 nm	Approved liver agent; stem cell labeling
Resovist (Bayer Healthcare, Wayne, NJ) [18]	Fe, SPIO, carboxydextran coating; R1 = 19.4 mM^{-1}s^{-1} (0.47T); R2 = 185.8 mM^{-1}s^{-1}; size = 60 nm	Approved liver agent; stem cell labeling

Figure 3-18. Liver iron oxide contrast agents (rapid blood clearance). Fe—iron; IV—intravenous; SPIO—superparamagnetic iron oxide.

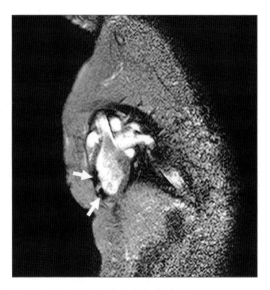

Figure 3-19. Feridex-labeled (Bayer Healthcare, Wayne, NJ) endothelial progenitor cells. Cine gradient echo image of Feridex-labeled endothelial progenitor cells (*arrows*) in the anterior wall of a rat heart. Note the excellent differentiation between myocardium, blood, and labeled cells.

Blood Pool Iron Oxide Contrast Agents (Slow Blood Clearance)

Agent	Characteristics	Cardiovascular Indication Approved/Under Trial
Supravist (Bayer Healthcare, Wayne, NJ) [19]	Fe, USPIO, carboxydextran coating; R1 = 7.8 mM^{-1}s^{-1} (2T); R2 = 86.8 mM^{-1}s^{-1}; size = ~30 nm	MRA; perfusion
VSOP-C184 (Ferropharm, Teltow, Germany) [20]	Fe, VSOP, citrate coating; R1 = 14 mM^{-1}s^{-1} (1.4T); R2 = 33.5 mM^{-1}s^{-1}; size = ~7 nm	Early clinical and pre-clinical studies for MRA; plaque imaging
Combidex/Sinerem (Advanced Magnetics, Cambridge, MA) [21,22]	Fe, USPIO, dextran coating; R1 = 23 mM^{-1}s^{-1} (0.5T); R2 = 53 mM^{-1}s^{-1}; size = ~30 nm	MRA; plaque imaging
Monocrystalline iron oxide (MION-47) [23]	Fe, USPIO, polymer coating; R1 = 16.5 mM^{-1}s^{-1} (0.5T); R2 = 34.8 mM^{-1}s^{-1}; size = ~20 nm	Experimental nanoparticle

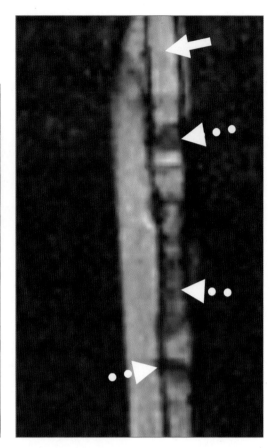

Figure 3-20. Blood pool iron oxide contrast agents (slow blood clearance). Fe—iron; MRA—magnetic resonance angiogram; USPIO—ultrasmall superparamagnetic iron oxide.

Figure 3-21. Macrophage imaging using ferumoxtran-10. Gradient echo aortic angiogram (*arrow*) in an atherosclerotic Watanabe rabbit 5 days after administration of 1000 μmol Fe/kg ferumoxtran-10. The black dots (*dotted arrows*) in the arterial vessel wall correspond to ferumoxtran-10 internalized in macrophages present in the atherosclerotic plaque. (*Courtesy of* Claire Corrot, PhD, Guerbet, Paris, France.)

Targeted Contrast Agents

Agent	Characteristics	Cardiovascular Indication Approved/Under Trial
GadofluorineM (Bayer Healthcare, Wayne, NJ) [24,25]	Gd-GlyMe-DOTA-perfluorooctyl-mannose interacts with hydrophobic plaque materials and predominantly accumulates in extracellular matrix; R1 = 17.4 $mM^{-1}s^{-1}$ (1.5T)	Preclinical development; atherosclerosis
Fluorinated nanoparticles (Kereos, St. Louis, MO) [26–28]	Gd-DTPA-BOA nanoparticles (10,000–50,000 Gd3+/particle) decorated with F(ab)' fragment against fibrin or with peptidomimetic vitronectin antagonist against $\alpha v \beta 3$; R1 = 0.18–0.54 mL s-1 pmol-1/nanoparticle (fibrin-binding nanoparticle); R1 = 19.1 $mM^{-1}s^{-1}$ (0.47T); R2 = 22.9 $mM^{-1}s^{-1}$ ($\alpha v \beta 3$-binding nanoparticle)	Preclinical for cardiovascular indications/angiogenesis; plaque detection
EP-2104R (EPIX Pharmaceuticals, Lexington, MA) [29,30]	Gd-DOTA bound to small peptide; binds to fibrin	Phase II feasibility study of fibrin imaging completed
EP-3600 (EPIX Pharmaceuticals, Lexington, MA)	Gd-based bound to small peptide; binds to fibrin	Preclinical studies for perfusion
Gd-DTPA-B(sLe^x)A [31]	Gd-DTPA-B(sLe^x)A binds to E- and P-selectin	Preclinical studies for imaging endothelial activation
Crosslinked iron oxide (CLIO) [32]	Fe, USPIO, crosslinked derivative of MION; R1 = ~30 $mM^{-1}s^{-1}$ (0.5T); R2 = ~150 $mM^{-1}s^{-1}$	Preclinical studies for targeted imaging (eg, VCAM-1, E-selectin)
Recombinant HDL-like nanoparticles [33]	Gd-DTPA-DMPE, rHDL nanoparticle; R1 = 10.4 $mM^{-1}s^{-1}$ (1.5T); size = ~7–12 nm	Preclinical studies for plaque imaging
Immunomicelles [34]	~6200 Gd per immunomicelle; antibody against macrophage scavenger receptor; R1 = ~10–12 $mM^{-1}s^{-1}$; size ~100–110 nm	Preclinical studies for plaque imaging
Liposomes [35]	Gd-DTPA-BSA or Gd-DTPA-BOA; cyclic RGD peptide against $\alpha v \beta 3$; R1 = 5.5 $mM^{-1}s^{-1}$ (1.5T); size = ~150 nm	Preclinical studies for angiogenesis

Figure 3-22. Targeted contrast agents. Gd-DOTA—gadoterate; Gd-DTPA—gadopentetate dimeglumine; Gd-DTPA-BOA—gadolinium diethylene-triamine-pentaacetic acid-bis(oleate); Gd-DTPA-BSA—Gd-DTPA-bis(stearyl amide); Gd-DTPA-DMPE—Gd-DTPA-1, 2-dimyristoyl-sn-glycero-3-phosphoethenolamine; HDL—high-density lipoprotein; MION—monocrystalline iron oxide nanocompound; rHDL—reconstituted high-density lipoprotein; RGD—arginine-glycine-aspartic acid; USPIO—ultrasmall superparamagnetic iron oxide; VSOP—very small superparamagnetic iron oxide particles.

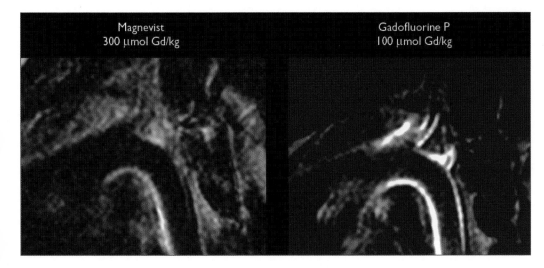

Figure 3-23. Plaque imaging with Gadofluorine P (Bayer Schering Pharma Aktiengesellschaft, Berlin, Germany). MRI of atherosclerotic aortic arch of a WHHL rabbit, acquired with a two-dimensional T1-weighted inversion recovery TurboFLASH sequence before and at 9 hours after intravenous injection of 0.3 mmol Gd/kg Magnevist (Bayer Healthcare, Wayne, NJ) or 0.1 mmol Gd/kg Gadofluorine P. (Siemens Magnetom Allegra, head scanner, 1.5 T; two-dimensional T1-weighted inversion recovery TurboFLASH sequence IR tbfl; TR/TE/TI 300/4/120 ms, α = 20°.) (*Courtesy of* B. Misselwitz, PhD, Bayer-Schering Pharma AG, Berlin, Germany.)

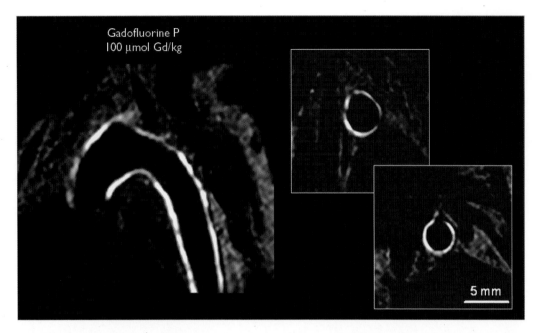

Figure 3-24. Plaque imaging with Gadofluorine P (Bayer Schering Pharma Aktiengesellschaft, Berlin, Germany). MRI of atherosclerotic aortic arch of a WHHL rabbit, acquired with a two-dimensional T1-weighted inversion recovery fast gradient echo sequence before and at 6 hours after intravenous injection of 0.1 mmol Gd/kg Gadofluorine P. (Siemens Magnetom Allegra, head scanner, 1.5 T; two-dimensional T1-weighted inversion recovery fast gradient echo sequence IR tbfl; TR/TE/TI 300/4/120 ms, $\alpha = 20°$.) (*Courtesy of* B. Misselwitz, PhD, Bayer-Schering Pharma AG, Berlin, Germany.)

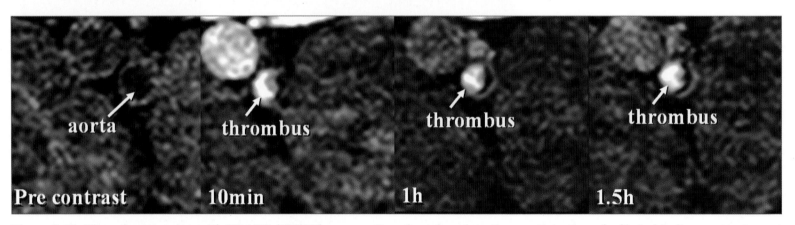

Figure 3-25. Thrombus imaging with EP-1873 (EPIX Pharmaceuticals, Lexington, MA). T1-weighted fast gradient echo images with inferior and superior saturation bands demonstrating noninvasive thrombus detection postinjection of a fibrin-binding contrast agent (2 µmol/kg) in a rabbit model of plaque rupture. Note the rapid blood clearance of the agent at 1 hour postinjection.

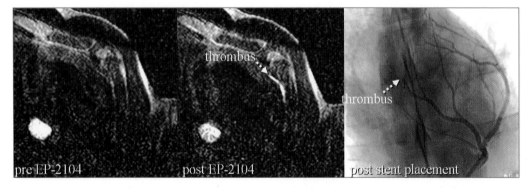

Figure 3-26. Thrombus imaging with EP-2104 (EPIX Pharmaceuticals, Lexington, MA). T1-weighted electrocardiogram-triggered and navigator-gated inversion recovery fast gradient echo images in a pig model of coronary in-stent thrombosis. Previous to injection of the fibrin-binding contrast agent, the in-stent thrombus is hardly visible; however, after administration of 4 µmol/kg EP-2104, thrombus delineation is excellent. Radiograph coronary angiography confirms the presence of a thrombus in the left anterior descending artery.

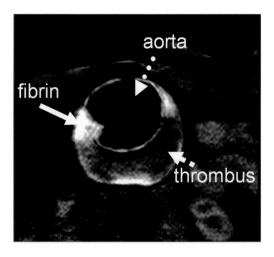

Figure 3-27. Thrombus imaging with EP-2104 (EPIX Pharmaceuticals, Lexington, MA). T1-weighted fast gradient echo images in a patient with an aortic aneurysm after administration of 4 μmol/kg EP-2104. Contrast agent accumulation can be observed in the shoulders of the thrombus and at the 6 o'clock position. The presence of fibrin in the shoulder regions of the thrombus suggests loss of vessel wall integrity and the presence of a potentially rupture-prone aneurysm.

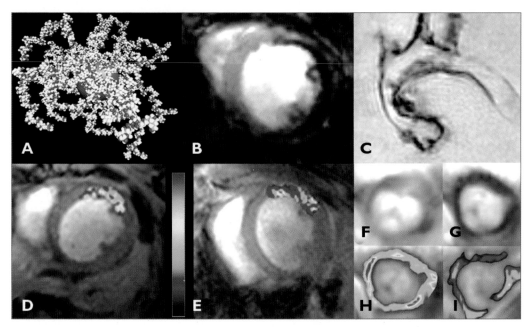

Figure 3-28. Molecular MRI with magneto-fluorescent iron oxide nanoparticle (MNFP). **A,** An iron-oxide nanoparticle containing a central core of iron oxide measuring 3 nm to 5 nm in diameter, surrounded by a dextran coat. **B,** Molecular MRI of myocardial macrophage infiltration in a healing myocardial infarction. The image shown was acquired in a mouse infarct model at 9.4 T and shows significant negative contrast enhancement in the injured anterolateral wall. Fluorescence microscopy of the MNFP cross-linked iron oxide (CLIO)-Cy5.5 and immunohistochemistry confirmed the uptake of the agent by macrophages penetrating the healing infarct. **C,** Accumulation of CLIO-Cy5.5 in macrophage-rich atheromatous plaque in an apoE-/- mouse. The image shown is a T2*-weighted gradient echo acquired ex vivo at 14 T. **D** and **E,** Molecular MRI of cardiomyocyte apoptosis in a mouse model of transient coronary ligation with the annexin-based probe Anx-CLIO-Cy5.5. T2* maps have been created in vivo at 9.4 T in areas of myocardial hypokinesis. A mouse injected with the unlabeled control probe (CLIO-Cy5.5) is shown (**D**) and a mouse injected with the active AnxCLIO-Cy5.5 probe is shown (**E**). T2* (scale = 0–20 ms) is significantly lower in the mouse given the active probe. **F–I,** Molecular MRI of VCAM-1 expression in the aortic root of apoE-/- mice. MRI of the aortic root acquired before (**F**) and 48 hours after (**G**) the injection of a VCAM-1 targeted MNFP. Significant negative contrast, consistent with probe accumulation, has occurred in the aortic root (**H**). A large amount of probe uptake, reflecting robust VCAM-1 expression, is seen in an apoE-/- mouse fed a high cholesterol diet (**I**). However, significantly less probe uptake is seen in a mouse fed a high-cholesterol diet, but treated concurrently with atorvastatin.

(Panel **A** *adapted from* Harisinghani *et al.* [36]; panel **B** *adapted from* Sosnovik *et al.* [37]; panel **C** *adapted from* Aikawa *et al.* [38]; panels **D** and **E** *adapted from* Sosnovik *et al.* [39]; panels **F** and **G** *adapted from* Nahrendorf *et al.* [40]; panels **H** and **I** *courtesy of* David Sosnovik, MD, Harvard Medical School, Boston, MA.)

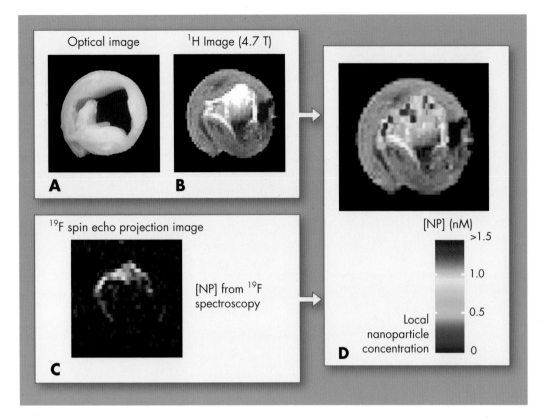

Figure 3-29. **A–D**, Fluorine imaging of unstable plaque. A 1H image (**B**) of carotid endarterectomy specimen (**A**) of an unstable plaque acquired with the following imaging parameters: 256 × 256 matrix; 0.5 s TR; 7.6 ms TE; 1-mm slice thickness; and two signal averages. The corresponding fluorine image (**C**) acquired after administration of a fibrin-binding perfluorocarbon nanoparticle demonstrates quantitatively the fibrin-binding sites (**D**). Imaging parameters of the 19 F image included 64 × 32 matrix; 1.0 s TR; 4.5 ms TE; 26-mm slice thickness; and two signal averages. (*Courtesy of* Sam Wickline, MD, Washington University, St. Louis, MO.)

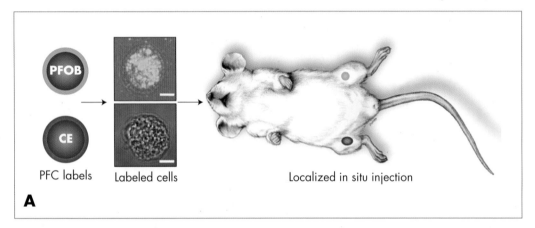

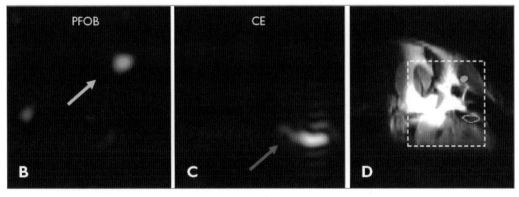

Figure 3-30. Dual-label 19-fluorine MRI of endothelial precursor cells. **A**, Stem/progenitor cells labeled with perfluorooctyl bromide (PFOB) (*green*) or perfluoro-15-crown-5 ether (CE) (*red*) nanoparticles and injected into mouse thigh skeletal muscle. **B–D**, Frequency selective excitation of the perfluoronanoparticles (4 × 106) allows background-free cell visualization at 11.7 T (**B** and **C**). Overlay of the fluorine signal onto a conventional 1H image (**D**) reveals PFOB- and CE-labeled cells localized to the left and right leg, respectively (*dashed line* indicates 3 × 3 cm² field of view for 19 F images). (*Courtesy of* Sam Wickline, MD, Washington University, St. Louis, MO.)

1. Stuber M, Gilson WD, Schaer M, *et al.*: Shedding light on the dark spot with IRON: a method that generates positive contrast in the presence of superparamagnetic nanoparticles. In *Proceedings of the International Society of Magnetic Resonance in Medicine*; 2005; Miami Beach, FL. Abstract 2608.

2. Seppenwoolde JH, Viergever MA, Bakker CJ: Passive tracking exploiting local signal conservation: the white marker phenomenon. *Magn Reson Med* 2003, 50:784–790.

3. Mani V, Briley-Saebo KC, Itskovich VV, *et al.*: Gradient echo acquisition for superparamagnetic particles with positive contrast (GRASP): sequence characterization in membrane and glass super-paramagnetic iron oxide phantoms at 1.5T and 3T. *Magn Reson Med* 2006, 55:126–135.

4. Dahnke H, Liu W, Frank JA, Schaeffter T: Optimal positive contrast of labeled cells via conventional 3D imaging. In *Proceedings of the International Society of Magnetic Resonance in Medicine*; 2006; Seattle, WA. Abstract 361.

5. Weinmann HJ, Laniado M, Mutzel W: Pharmacokinetics of Gd DTPA/dimeglumine after intravenous injection into healthy volunteers. *Physiol Chem Phys Med NMR* 1984, 16:167–172.

6. Volger H, Platzek J, Schuhmann-Giampieri G, *et al.*: Pre-clinical evaluation of Gadobutrol: a new, neutral, extracellular contrast agent for magnetic resonance imaging. *Eur J Radiol* 1995, 21:1–10.

7. MultiHance drug information. Magnetic Resonance TIP: MRI database. http://www.mr-tip.com/serv1.php?type=db1&dbs=multihance.

8. ProHance drug information. Magnetic Resonance TIP: MRI database. http://www.mr-tip.com/serv1.php?type=db1&dbs=prohance.

9. Omniscan GE drug information. Magnetic Resonance TIP: MRI database. http://www.mr-tip.com/serv1.php?type=db1&dbs=Relaxivity&set=8.

10. Lin S-P, Brown JJ: MR contrast agents: physical and pharmacological basics. *J Magn Reson Imaging* 2007, 25:884–899.

11. Hartmann M, Wiethoff AJ, Hentrich HR, Rohrer M: Initial imaging recommendations for Vasovist angiography. *Eur Radiol* 2006, 16(Suppl 2):B15–B23.

12. Caravan P, Cloutier NJ, Greenfield MT, *et al.*: The interaction of MS-325 with human serum albumin and its effect on proton relaxation rates. *J Am Chem Soc* 2002, 124:3152–3162.

13. Preda A, Novikov V, Moglich M, *et al.*: MRI monitoring of Avastin anti-angiogenesis therapy using B22956/1, a new blood pool contrast agent, in an experimental model of human cancer. *J Magn Reson Imaging* 2004, 20:865–873.

14. La Noce A, Stoelben S, Scheffler K, *et al.*: B22956/1, a new intravascular contrast agent for MRI: first administration to humans: preliminary results. *Acad Radiol* 2002, 9(Suppl 2):S404–S406.

15. Cavagna FM, Lorusso V, Anelli PL, *et al.*: Preclinical profile and clinical potential of gadocoletic acid trisodium salt (B22956/1), a new intravascular contrast medium for MRI. *Acad Radiol* 2002, 9(Suppl 2): S491–S494.

16. Clarke SE, Weinmann HJ, Dai E, *et al.*: Comparison of two blood pool contrast agents for 0.5 T MR angiography: experimental studies in rabbits. *Radiology* 2000, 214:787–794.

17. Feridex/EndoremT drug information. Magnetic Resonance TIP: MRI database. http://www.mr-tip.com/serv1.php?type=db1&dbs=Relaxivity&set=3.

18. Lawaczeck R, Bauer H, Frenzel T, *et al.*: Magnetic iron oxide particles coated with carboxydextran for parenteral administration and liver contrasting: preclinical profile of SH U555A. *Acta Radiol* 1997, 38:584–597.

19. Simon GH, von Vopelius-Feldt J, Wendland MF, *et al.*: MRI of arthritis: comparison of ultrasmall superparamagnetic iron oxide vs Gd-DTPA. *J Magn Reson Imaging* 2006, 23:720–727.

20. Taupitz M, Wagner S, Schnorr J, *et al.*: Phase I clinical evaluation of citrate-coated monocrystalline very small superparamagnetic iron oxide particles as a new contrast medium for magnetic resonance imaging. *Invest Radiol* 2004, 39:394–405.

21. Herborn C, Vogt FM, Lauenstein TC, *et al.*: Magnetic resonance imaging of experimental atherosclerotic plaque: comparison of two ultrasmall superparamagnetic particles of iron oxide. *J Magn Reson Imaging* 2006, 24:388–393.

22. Ruehm SG, Corot C, Vogt P, *et al.*: Magnetic resonance imaging of atherosclerotic plaque with ultrasmall superparamagnetic particles of iron oxide in hyperlipidemic rabbits. *Circulation* 2001, 103:415–422.

23. Shen T, Weissleder R, Papisov M, *et al.*: Monocrystalline iron oxide nanocompounds (MION): physicochemical properties. *Magn Reson Med* 1993, 29:599–604.

24. Meding J, Urich M, Licha K, *et al.*: Magnetic resonance imaging of atherosclerosis by targeting extracellular matrix deposition with Gadofluorine M. *Contrast Media Mol Imaging* 2007, 2:120–129.

25. Sirol M, Itskovich VV, Mani V, *et al.*: Lipid-rich atherosclerotic plaques detected by gadofluorine-enhanced in vivo magnetic resonance imaging. *Circulation* 2004, 109:2890–2896.

26. Flacke S, Fischer S, Scott MJ, *et al.*: Novel MRI contrast agent for molecular imaging of fibrin: implications for detecting vulnerable plaques. *Circulation* 2001, 104:1280–1285.

27. Winter PM, Caruthers SD, Kassner A, *et al.*: Molecular imaging of angiogenesis in nascent Vx-2 rabbit tumors using a novel alpha(nu)beta3-targeted nanoparticle and 1.5 tesla magnetic resonance imaging. *Cancer Res* 2003, 63:5838–5643.

28. Winter PM, Morawski AM, Caruthers SD, *et al.*: Molecular imaging of angiogenesis in early-stage atherosclerosis with alpha(v)beta3-integrin-targeted nanoparticles. *Circulation* 2003, 108:2270–2274.

29. Botnar RM, Perez AS, Witte S, *et al.*: In vivo molecular imaging of acute and subacute thrombosis using a fibrin-binding magnetic resonance imaging contrast agent. *Circulation* 2004, 109:2023–2029.

30. Botnar RM, Buecker A, Wiethoff AJ, *et al.*: In vivo magnetic resonance imaging of coronary thrombosis using a fibrin-binding molecular magnetic resonance contrast agent. *Circulation* 2004, 110:1463–1466.

31. Barber PA, Foniok T, Kirk D, *et al.*: MR molecular imaging of early endothelial activation in focal ischemia. *Ann Neurol* 2004, 56:116–120.

32. Wunderbaldinger P, Josephson L, Weissleder R: Crosslinked iron oxides (CLIO): a new platform for the development of targeted MR contrast agents. *Acad Radiol* 2002, 9(Suppl 2):S304–S306.

33. Frias JC, Williams KJ, Fisher EA, Fayad ZA: Recombinant HDL-like nanoparticles: a specific contrast agent for MRI of atherosclerotic plaques. *J Am Chem Soc* 2004, 126:16316–16317.

34. Amirbekian V, Lipinski MJ, Briley-Saebo KC, *et al.*: Detecting and assessing macrophages in vivo to evaluate atherosclerosis noninvasively using molecular MRI. *Proc Natl Acad Sci U S A* 2007, 104:961–966.

35. Mulder WJ, Strijkers GJ, Griffioen AW, *et al.*: A liposomal system for contrast-enhanced magnetic resonance imaging of molecular targets. *Bioconjug Chem* 2004, 15:799–806.

36. Harisinghani MG, Barentsz J, Hahn PF, *et al.*: Noninvasive detection of clinically occult lymph-node metastases in prostate cancer. *N Engl J Med* 2003, 348:2491–2499.

37. Sosnovik DE, Nahrendorf M, Deliolanis N, *et al.*: Fluorescence tomography and magnetic resonance imaging of myocardial macrophage infiltration in infarcted myocardium in vivo. *Circulation* 2007, 115:1384–1391.

38. Aikawa E, Nahrendorf M, Sosnovik D, *et al.*: Multimodality molecular imaging identifies proteolytic and osteogenic activities in early aortic valve disease. *Circulation* 2007, 115:377–386.

39. Sosnovik DE, Schellenberger EA, Nahrendorf M, *et al.*: Magnetic resonance imaging of cardiomyocyte apoptosis with a novel magneto-optical nanoparticle. *Magn Reson Med* 2005, 54:718–724.

40. Nahrendorf M, Jaffer FA, Kelly KA, *et al.*: Noninvasive vascular cell adhesion molecule-1 imaging identifies inflammatory activation of cells in atherosclerosis. *Circulation* 2006, 114:1504–1511.

4
CHAPTER

MR Angiography: Principles and Techniques

Daniel N. Costa and Neil M. Rofsky

Technologic developments in the past decade have resulted in impressive advances and increased importance of magnetic resonance (MR) angiography in clinical practice. MR angiography has become a key component of state-of-the-art vascular imaging, with applications ranging from assessment of atherosclerotic disease to plaque characterization. For physicians interpreting medical images, knowledge of the principles and techniques underlying MRI acquisition and processing is important to understand and overcome some of the limitations intrinsic to this modality. MR angiography techniques can be conveniently divided into three broad groups: 1) flow-based techniques (*eg*, time-of-flight and phase contrast); 2) techniques that capitalize on intrinsic signal features (*eg*, black blood and bright blood); and 3) contrast-enhanced techniques.

This chapter provides an illustrated review of general principles and techniques relevant to MR angiography. First, we discuss advantages of MRI over other methods. Examples of pulse sequences and postprocessing techniques relevant to vascular imaging are shown. Strategies to synchronize intravenous contrast passage in the area of interest and scanning are explored. Finally, details about limitations and pitfalls are discussed.

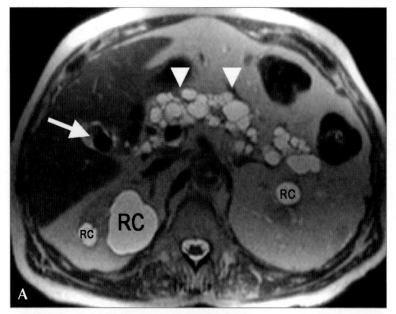

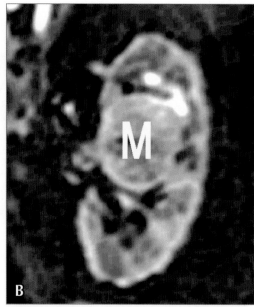

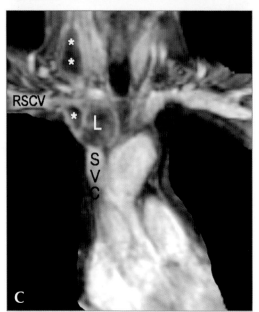

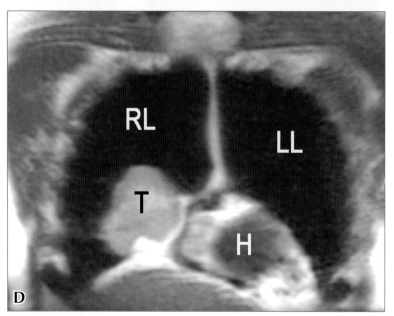

Figure 4-1. Advantages of magnetic resonance (MR) angiography over other modalities. MR angiography has a variety of contrast mechanisms while avoiding iodinated contrast material and ionizing radiation. Furthermore, functional assessments are quite feasible with MRI. With cross-sectional imaging to depict underlying and adjacent soft tissue abnormalities, MR angiography and CT angiography offer supplements to vascular information not available with digital subtraction angiography. Some examples of incidental findings with variable clinical significance are shown.

A, MR angiography was requested to assess for renal artery stenosis in an 81-year-old woman with hypertension. Axial T2-weighted single-shot fast spin-echo (SSFSE) image of the upper abdomen in the MR angiography of the renal arteries shows gallbladder stone (*arrow*), multiple pancreatic cysts (*arrowheads*), and bilateral renal cysts (RCs).

B, MR angiography for suspected abdominal aortic aneurysm in a 76-year-old man. Sagittal oblique thin-slab maximum intensity projection (MIP) image derived from the three-dimensional gradient-echo T1-weighted postcontrast sequence shows a 3-cm enhancing renal mass (M) occupying the middle third of the left kidney. This was subsequently removed and proven to be a renal cell carcinoma.

C, MR angiography for evaluation of the thoracocervical veins in a 65-year-old man with superior vena cava (SVC) syndrome. Coronal oblique restricted volume postcontrast MIP image shows metastatic enlarged paratracheal lymph node (L) obstructing and thrombosing (*asterisk*) the distal segment of the right subclavian vein (RSCV) and right internal jugular vein (*two asterisks*).

D, In this same patient, coronal SSFSE for black-blood imaging revealed the primary lung tumor (T) in right lung (RL) base. H—heart; LL—left lung.

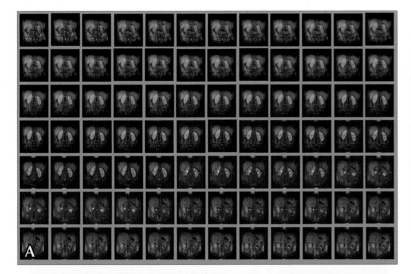

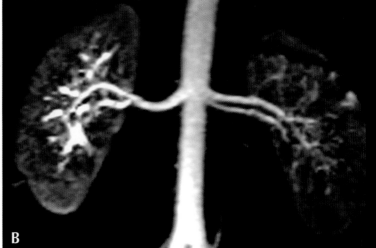

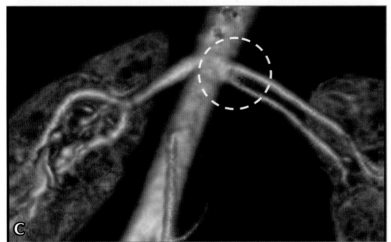

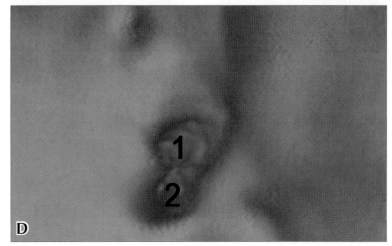

Figure 4-2. Examples of image postprocessing techniques. Regardless of the imaging strategy, image post-processing plays a critical role for interpretation, communication of magnetic resonance (MR) angiographic findings, volumetric quantification, and an understanding of complex anatomic relationships [1].

A, MR angiography of the renal arteries in a 24-year-old man with hypertension. The original stack of thin slices (84 coronal images shown in small scale here) with high spatial resolution can be combined to generate high-quality reconstructions.

B, All the images shown in **A** are here displayed as a single maximum intensity projection image where normal renal arteries can be appreciated. Two main renal arteries are seen on the left as an anatomic variant.

C, Magnified left oblique volume-rendered view gives a better perspective of the origin of the renal arteries on the left, which seem to arise from a common trunk (*dashed circle*). Such techniques that emphasize surface representations display findings in a more intuitive manner to referring physicians.

D, Endoluminal view from the aorta toward the ostia (1 and 2) of the right renal arteries confirms that both arise from a common trunk.

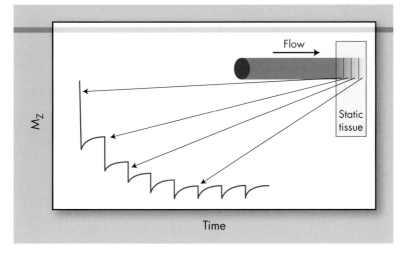

Figure 4-3. Time-of-flight basic principle. Spins subjected to a train of repetitive radiofrequency (RF) pulses (excitations) achieve a steady state in which the longitudinal magnetization (Mz) vector and thus the signal is less than the maximum value. This effect is called signal saturation. Stationary protons within a defined volume are exposed to such a series of pulses during time-of-flight sequences and become saturated. In comparison, protons in flowing blood emanating from outside the excited volume have not experienced prior excitation and enter the imaging volume with full Mz. Time-of-flight exploits the difference in Mz between flowing and stationary tissues to generate images [2]. Selection of the imaging volume must be considered with respect to the velocity of flow. If the transit time for the blood to cross the excited volume is less than the repetition time, the spins will experience more than one RF excitation and will be partially saturated, reducing the contrast between blood and stationary tissue (*see* Fig. 4-15).

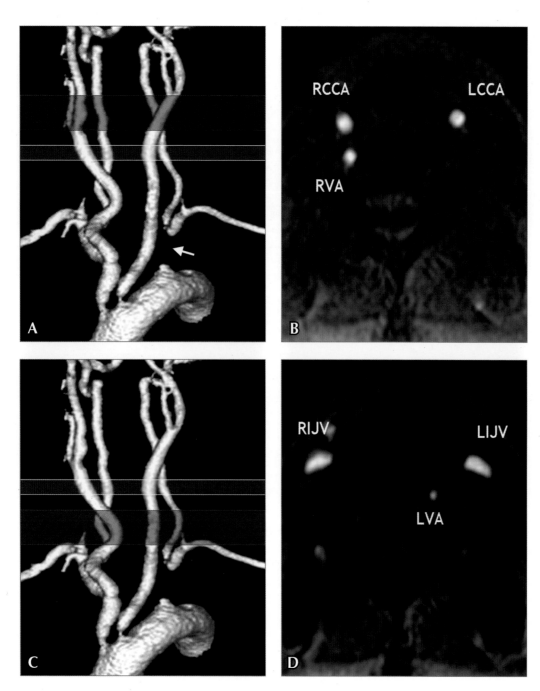

Figure 4-4. Presaturation pulses. Magnetic resonance angiography of the neck in a 72-year-old man with subclavian steal syndrome.

A, Inflow effects creating bright blood: background contrast are bidirectional. Application of a presaturation pulse (*red box*) on one side of the imaging volume suppresses signal of inflowing blood from that direction within the imaging slice (*white box*). For this reason, the saturation pulse is direction specific but not vessel specific [2].

B, Because this saturation pulse is nulling the signal of spins traveling to the slice from the craniocaudal direction, only vessels with blood flowing in the caudocranial direction appear with increased signal. Note a lack of signal in the expected location of the left vertebral artery (*arrow*).

C, When the saturation pulse is applied below the imaging slice the opposite effect occurs and only vessels with flow in the craniocaudal direction are shown (**D**). In this patient, there is occlusion of the proximal left subclavian artery (*arrow* in **A**) that causes reversal of the flow direction in the left vertebral artery. Saturation bands can also be selected for each image slice to optimally saturate blood entering that region, particularly in two-dimensional time-of-flight sequences. These saturation bands are referred to as floating or traveling saturation pulses. LCCA—left common carotid artery; LIJV—left internal jugular vein; LVA—left vertebral artery; RCCA—right common carotid artery; RIJV—right internal jugular vein; RVA—right vertebral artery.

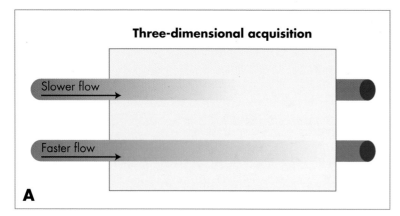

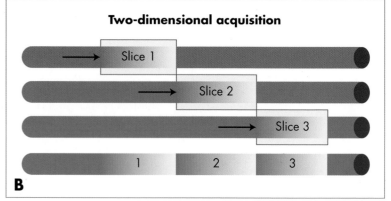

Figure 4-5. Time-of-flight inflow and saturation effects. Inflowing blood with nonsaturated spins produces bright signal. Progressive exposure to radiofrequency pulses in three-dimensional thick slab acquisition (**A**) results in saturation of protons in blood thereby reducing inflow effects and, consequently, contrast. The faster the flow, the further the distance traveled before effective contrast is reduced. The advantages of three-dimensional imaging are improved spatial resolution and signal-to-noise ratio, but at the cost of in-plane and through-plane saturation effects. In the two-dimensional technique (**B**), consecutive thinner slices (usually in the range of 1.5–4.0 mm) are acquired to create a stack of images covering the anatomy of interest. With this strategy, through-plane saturation is minimized.

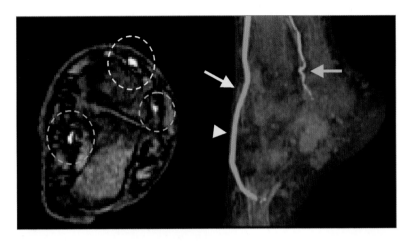

Figure 4-6. Time-of-flight technique. Pedal arteries can be depicted using axial electrocardiogram-triggered two-dimensional images (*left*) that can be combined to generate maximum intensity projection (MIP) reconstructions (*right*). In the source image, distal segments of anterior tibial (*yellow dashed circle*), posterior tibial (*blue dashed circle*), and fibular (*green dashed circle*) arteries are seen. In the MIP reconstruction, both tibial vessels are shown (with respective *colored arrows*) and the major contribution of the anterior tibial artery to the dorsalis pedis (*arrowhead*) artery is noted.

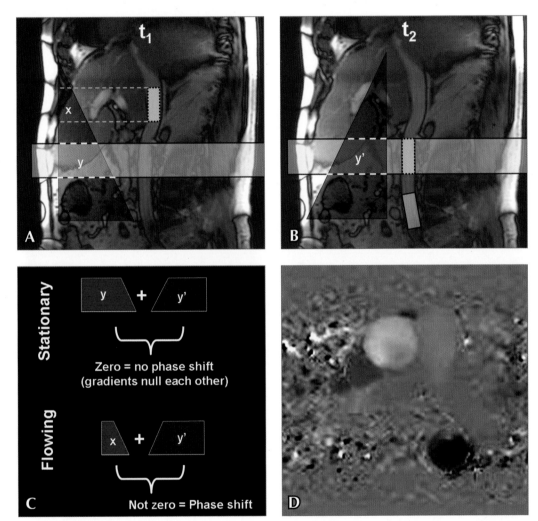

Figure 4-7. Phase-contrast principles. **A,** Spins moving in the presence of a magnetic field gradient (*red triangle*) accumulate additional phase shift, which is proportional to the velocity of the spins. Note that at time t_1 the column of blood in *yellow* is exposed to a lower magnetic field (x) than the stationary tissues in the imaging slice (*green box*, which is under a higher magnetic field labeled y). **B,** After a defined period of time (t_2), the gradient is replaced for another one (*blue triangle*) with the same amplitude but opposite in polarity. At this moment, the column of blood has moved to another position where it is exposed to a higher magnetic field (y', which is equal to y in amplitude but with opposite polarity). **C,** Because the same tissue was exposed to two different forces, a net phase shift will occur. In contradistinction, the stationary tissues in the imaging slice did not move; thus, they will be exposed to a gradient with the same amplitude and opposite polarity, and the phase of those protons will return to the initial status (ie, phase shift is

null). **D,** Images have excellent contrast between flowing blood and static tissue. In this pulse sequence, signal intensity of each pixel is proportional to the velocity of blood flow along the encoding axis. This fact can be used to calculate absolute values of flow after the cross-sectional area of the vessel is known. In this case, flow in the caudocranial direction is positive/bright, such as in the ascending aorta, and negative/dark in the opposite direction, such as in the descending aorta; note that the pulmonary trunk and major pulmonary arteries are not clearly seen because their flow occurs predominantly in the plane of the imaging slice, instead of the plane of the flow-encoding gradient.

Because the gradient change experienced by the flowing tissue is proportional to the distance traveled, its velocity can be derived. Also, because flow depends on velocity and cross-sectional area of the region, knowledge of the latter allows for an absolute flow value to be obtained. One challenging issue with phase-contrast imaging is the selection of gradient strengths appropriate for the velocity of blood in the vascular tree of interest. Each sequence has a tailored velocity encoding factor (V_{enc}, expressed in cm/s) that sets the maximum velocity for which the acquisition is sensitive. Sequences with large V_{enc} are less sensitive to slow flow. Thus, V_{enc} determines the highest and lowest velocities measurable by phase-contrast techniques. Another limitation of this technique is that phase shifts arise exclusively from the component of motion in the direction of the applied flow-encoding gradient pulse. With multidirectional flow, as occurs in the hands and feet, multiple orthogonal flow directions would require the application of additional gradients and thus prolong the total imaging time.

Flow Values

Timeframe	Flow, mL/s
0	-98
34	-61
69	79
103	465
137	662
172	696
206	642
240	603
274	501
309	323
343	80
377	-154
412	-181
446	-164
480	-122
515	-91
549	-90
583	-92
618	-89
652	-89
686	-84
720	-77
755	-82

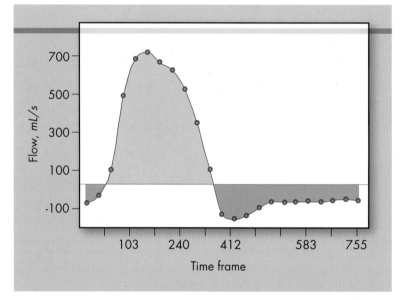

Figure 4-8. Flow measurement using phase-contrast imaging in a 39-year-old man with aortic regurgitation. Using flow values (**A**) calculated with phase-contrast technique at the aortic valve level, it is possible to draw a curve with respect to time (**B**, *purple line*). Anterograde flow has positive value, whereas retrograde flow is negative. The regurgitant fraction can then be calculated as the sum of the *blue areas* over all the areas combined (in this case, moderate-to-severe regurgitation was noted). In stenotic segments, pressure gradients can be estimated using peak velocity values, in a manner analogous to Doppler ultrasonography [3].

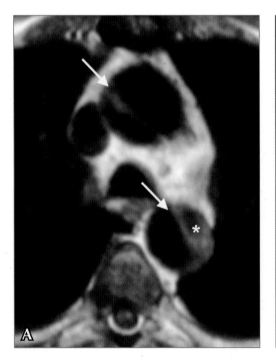

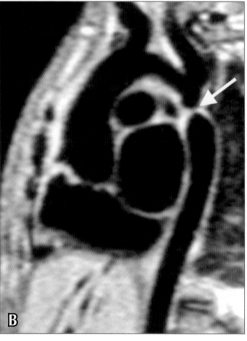

Figure 4-9. Dark-blood imaging. **A**, Note that vessels appear as low signal structures and the intimal flap (*arrows*) of dissection involving both the ascending and descending aorta can be easily seen. Note the signal difference between true and false lumina. Because flow is slow or absent in the false lumen, there is relative increased signal (*asterisk*). **B**, In another patient with aortic coarctation (*arrow*), this technique allows excellent depiction of anatomy. Although contrast-enhanced sequences are well suitable for lumen assessment, dark-blood imaging is superior to detect thrombus and mural abnormalities [4].

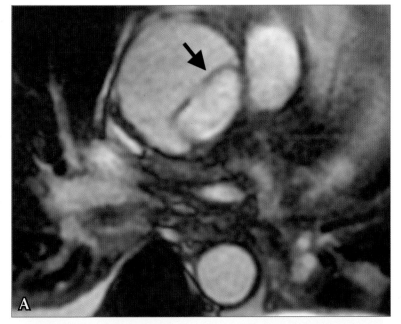

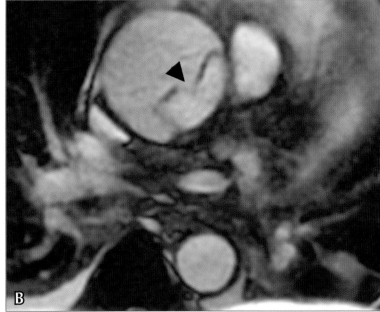

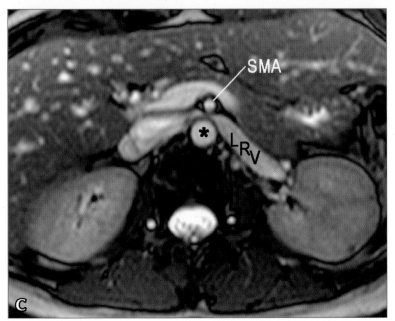

Figure 4-10. Bright-blood electrocardiogram (ECG)-triggered imaging. Time-of-flight technique is not suitable for areas of complex directionality of blood flow (*eg*, in the cardiac chambers). The best options are the balanced steady-state free precession sequences (sometimes referred to as SSFP or using acronyms from different vendors such as TrueFISP, FIESTA, and so forth). Images obtained with these sequences have a high signal-to-noise ratio and little sensitivity to motion but result in bright signal from both arteries and veins. Both stationary and moving fluid are shown with high signal intensity [5]. Multiple images are obtained in different times at the same location so that navigation through images generates a cine view that emulates "real-time" imaging. **A** and **B**, Axial ECG-triggered bright-blood images in a 63-year-old man with recent onset chest pain and acute renal failure. Compare the appearance of the intimal flap (*arrow* in **A**) in the ascending aorta in two different moments of the cardiac cycle: systole (**A**) and diastole (**B**). The intimal discontinuity representing the tear is also seen (*arrowhead* in **B**). **C**, In this other example, axial SSFP image in a 29-year-old woman with abdominal pain shows impingement of the left renal vein (LRV) as it crosses between the abdominal aorta (*asterisk*) and the superior mesenteric artery (SMA), the so-called "nutcracker syndrome." There is engorgement of the vein proximal to the constricted segment.

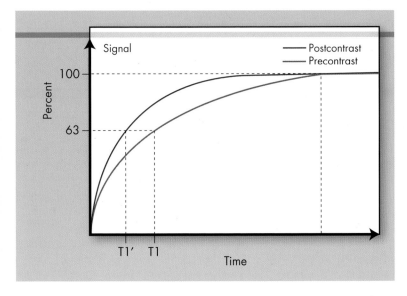

Figure 4-11. Effect of paramagnetic contrast on T1 values and image. Chelates of gadolinium contain unpaired electrons that render them paramagnetic, the latter a term for physical property that yields increased signal. This causes reduction of both T1 (*purple curve*, compared with the *green curve* representing the longitudinal magnetization in respect to time for the same tissue before intravenous contrast administration) and T2 relaxation times [6]. The shorter T1 results in increased signal on T1-weighted images following contrast administration. For magnetic resonance angiography, a short window exists during which the signal brightening selectively affects the arterial structures.

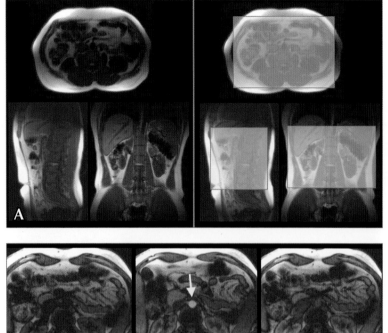

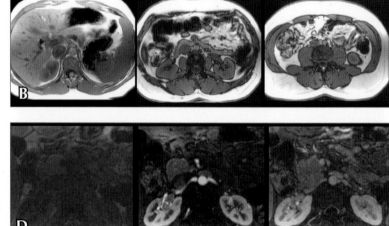

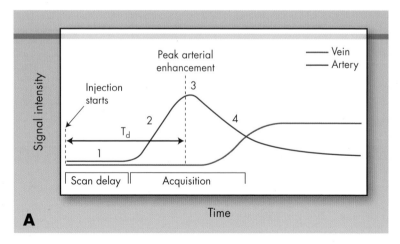

Figure 4-12. Comprehensive protocol. Although a myriad of different strategies can be found in the literature, regardless of the vascular territory of interest, magnetic resonance (MR) angiographic protocols basically consist of the following: **A**, Spatial localizers. These are low-resolution images in all three planes useful for checking proper coil positioning and for initial identification of the area of interest. In this MR angiography of the renal arteries, the area to be covered is roughly represented by the *yellow boxes*.

B, Anatomic precontrast evaluation. Different types of pulse sequences can be used for further detailing the anatomy of the area of interest. Knowledge of anatomy is important to prevent errors in prescription of the coverage area. Non-enhanced sequences, often referred to as dark-blood and bright-blood imaging, can be used in conjunction with these and are discussed later. In body MRI, single-shot fast spin-echo and/or gradient-echo (GRE) imaging is commonly used because of the short acquisition time and good image quality. These images provide soft tissue information that can facilitate a correct diagnosis. In the case shown here, selected T1-weight-ed GRE images show the location of the upper and lower limits of the kidneys, information that will be used for prescription of upcoming sequences.

C, Timing bolus. With contrast-enhanced techniques, a timing bolus sequence is used to determine the arrival time of the intravenous contrast agent in the vessel of interest. This facilitates appropriate timing of the image acquisition to ensure selective visualization of the artery of interest. The timing bolus sequence consists of low spatial and high temporal resolution images repeatedly obtained at the same level in the vessel of interest/reference, in this case, the aorta (*arrow*) at the level of the renal arteries during the injection of a small amount (1–2 cm^3) of contrast media.

D, Precontrast and postcontrast. Contrast-enhanced pulse sequences are the most recently developed techniques [7] but have widespread acceptance due to high reliability and excellent image quality. Because paramagnetic contrast agents preferably shorten T1 values of the tissues, T1-weighted imaging is more suitable to highlight vascular structures. In order to better capture contrast passage in the arterial tree while veins remain with low concentration of gadolinium, fast scanning is essential. For this reason, faster gradients, short repetition time, reduced data sampling, high receiver bandwidth, fractional echo, and zero-filling are useful. Here, precontrast and postcontrast (both the first and second passes) are respectively shown. Following image acquisition, postprocessing is the next step.

Figure 4-13. **A** and **B**, Timing bolus for proper synchronization of contrast injection and image acquisition. This diagram shows the increase in signal intensity in the arterial (*purple curve*) and venous (*green curve*) beds over time after injection of a small volume (1–2 mL) of contrast followed by saline flush. At the same time injection begins, a series of images are quickly and continuously acquired (**B**) showing progressive enhancement of the vessel of interest (abdominal aorta, in this case) and, later, veins (*arrow* points the inferior vena cava in *image 4*), while the aorta fades out. *Numbers* in the curve correspond to images in the bottom, starting from the absence of contrast (*1*), progressive aortic enhancement (*2* and *3*), and venous return with decrease in aortic signal (*4*).

Continued on the next page

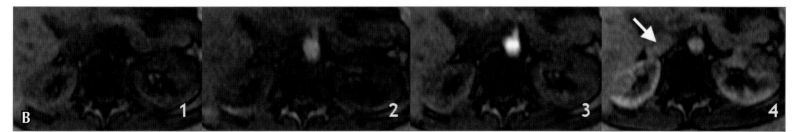

Figure 4-13. *(Continued)* A test bolus is used to establish the time delay between contrast injection and maximum arterial enhancement (T_d) [8], preventing excessively late or early scanning. For each k-space (data matrix) filling approach, there is an optimal scan delay to ensure that the center of k-space is acquired when peak arterial enhancement is present. Other timing strategies are available, including automated bolus detection and operator-dependent real-time bolus detection [9]. More recently, time-resolved sequences in which long-standing continuous image acquisition obviates timing calculations are available [10]. In order to deliver all of the contrast media from the venous circulation into the arterial tree, contrast injection can be followed by saline flush [11]. Another important technical aspect of contrast-enhanced magnetic resonance angiography of the chest and/or neck is to avoid administration of contrast media in the left arm. This is because when the left brachiocephalic vein has high concentration of contrast it may obscure visualization of the arch vessels due to its proximity as the vein crosses mediastinum from left to right [12].

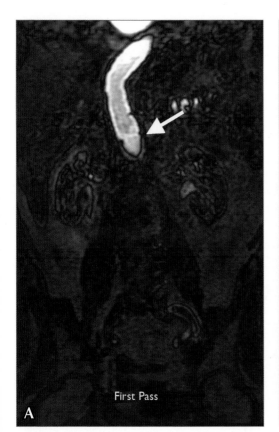

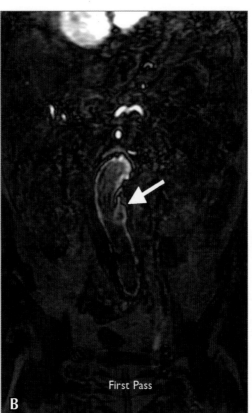

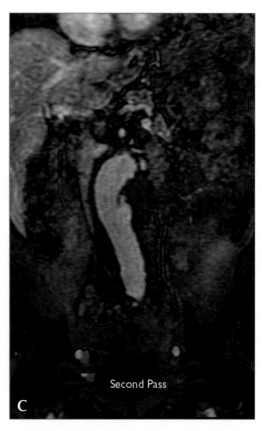

Figure 4-14. Artifacts in early acquired arterial phases in magnetic resonance (MR) angiography for follow-up of abdominal aortic aneurysm in a 90-year-old man.

A, In the first acquisition at the suprarenal abdominal aorta, there is almost uniform contrast with slight edge ringing observed (*arrow*).

B, In the first acquisition at the infrarenal abdominal aorta (slice is more anterior vs **A**), a sufficient concentration of gadolinium has not been achieved; thus the lumen is barely visualized while there is prominent edge enhancement (*arrow*),

findings indicative of the "too early" artifact. This can be seen when acquisition of MR data (central lines of k-space in particular) occurs before contrast bolus arrival [13]. To ensure that diagnostic information is obtained despite this artifact, identical three-dimensional acquisitions in rapid succession are usually performed [12].

C, The second acquisition, obtained very shortly after the first, has good enhancement with a sufficient concentration of gadolinium at the infrarenal aorta when the center of k-space was acquired.

Continued on the next page

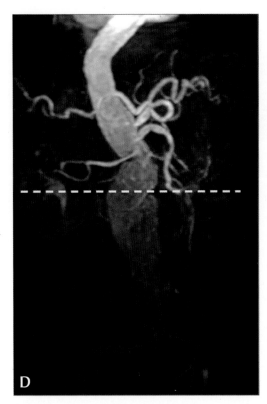
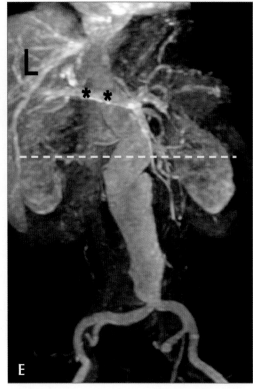
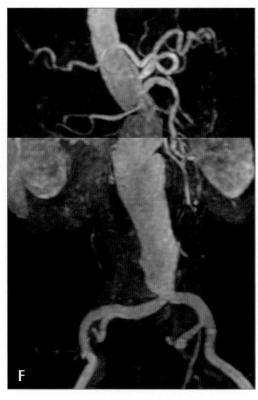

Figure 4-14. *(Continued)* **D**, Maximum intensity projection (MIP) reconstruction of first contrast passage data set demonstrates again poor enhancement in the infrarenal abdominal aorta and iliac arteries (below the *dashed line*), whereas the visualized descending thoracic aorta (above the *dashed line*) shows adequate enhancement diminishing in quality toward the renal arteries.

E, MIP image from the second passage data set shows excellent rendering of the infrarenal abdominal aorta and iliac arteries (below the *dashed line*); however, the suprarenal vascular anatomy is limited by overlying enhancement of visceral structures, *ie*, the liver (L), and veins (*eg*, portal vein [*two asterisks*]).

F, This ideal image is a combination of selected halves of **D** and **E**, with reasonable quality in the entire abdominal aorta.

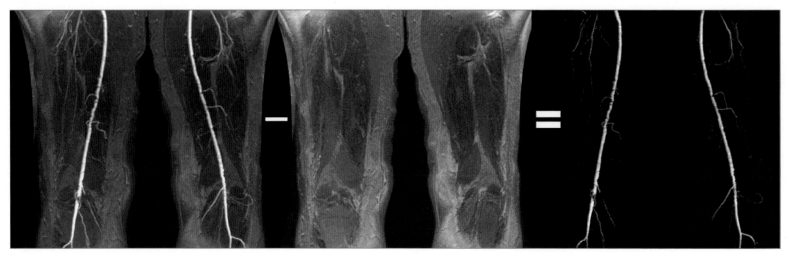

Figure 4-15. Subtraction is a method for suppressing background signal. In order to increase vessel conspicuity with magnetic resonance (MR) angiography, the signal of background tissues needs to be eliminated. The technique most commonly used is subtraction of identical nonenhanced (or mask; *center image*) from contrast-enhanced (CE) [*left*] images to improve vessel-to-background contrast (*right*). Disadvantages are lower signal-to-noise ratio in the subtracted images and reliance of coregistration of the mask and CE data sets. Whenever nonvascular landmarks are needed, such as for therapeutic planning, these structures can be reintroduced [14,15].

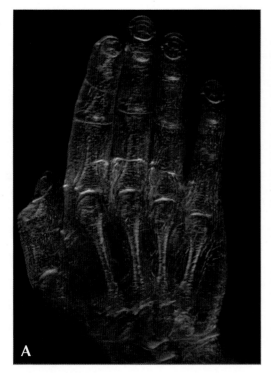 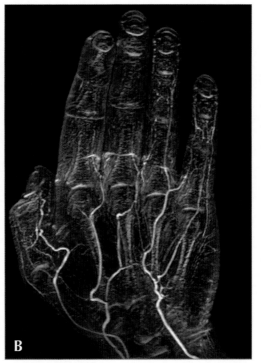 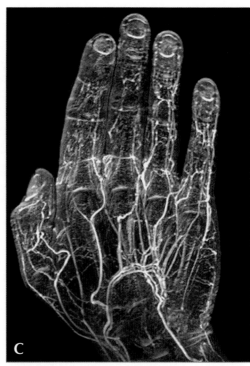

Figure 4-16. Time-resolved magnetic resonance angiography of the left hand in a 30-year-old man with recurrent pain in the digits. Note progressive arrival of contrast from left to right. In **A**, no vessels are seen. Then, arteries are nicely depicted (**B**). Subsequently, draining veins are observed in addition to the arterial tree (**C**). Other intermediate acquisitions are not shown. In this technique, rapid and continuous acquisition of images prior to, during, and after contrast administration obviates timing adjustments. To capitalize the exquisite high temporal resolution, different strategies are combined for fast imaging such as minimizing the repetition time, using parallel imaging, view sharing, partial Fourier imaging, asymmetric sampling, and zero-filling of k-space [10].

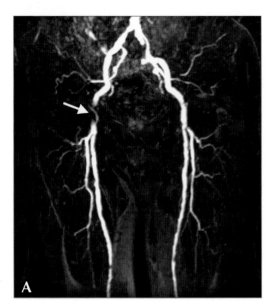

Figure 4-17. Inadequate coverage prescription simulating vessel occlusion. As with any other technique, contrast-enhanced magnetic resonance angiography requires proper coverage of the area of interest [12]. In this case, the more anterior aspect of the proximal right common femoral artery is not seen (*arrow* in **A**)

Continued on the next page

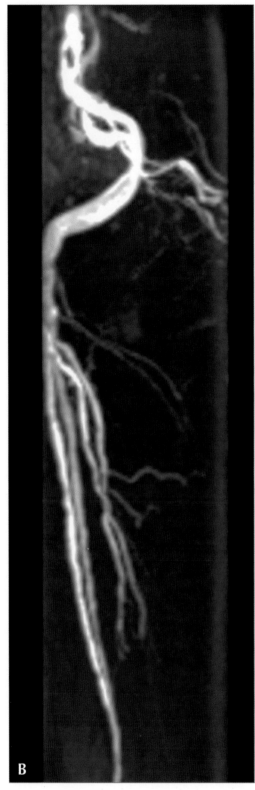

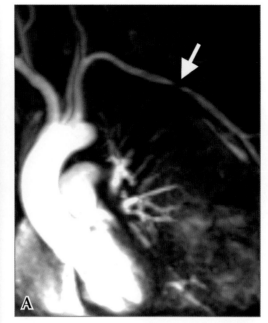

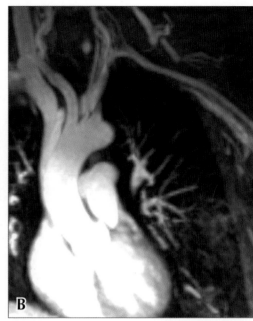

Figure 4-18. Disadvantages of MRI. MR angiography of the thoracic aorta and supra-aortic branches in a 47-year-old woman with asymmetric blood pressure in the upper extremities. **A,** Thin-slab coronal oblique multiplanar reformat of acquisition during first passage of contrast material shows focal stenosis in the distal left subclavian artery (*arrow*). This was not seen in the second-pass acquisition (**B**). Because intravenous contrast material was injected in the left arm in this patient, arterial signal loss resulted from dephasing secondary to the high gadolinium concentration in the adjacent subclavian vein. Intravoxel dephasing is a phenomenon whereby the transverse components of the magnetization from the nuclei within a voxel rotate at different frequencies, resulting in loss of signal. It can be secondary to magnetic field inhomogeneities (*ie,* as in this case with the high adjacent gadolinium concentration) or when nuclei have different velocities in the same voxel (as occurs with turbulent flow in stenotic and poststenotic areas). Because dephasing only occurs during the echo time (TE), this effect can be minimized by using short TEs. Other strategies are to use smaller voxels or a feature available in most scanners called flow compensation. Other limitations of MRI are signal ghosting and signal saturation. The latter refers to a reduction in signal caused by sequential application of excitation pulses to an image slice and was previously discussed.

Figure 4-17. *(Continued)* because it was out of the coronal imaging slab (which becomes more evident in the lateral view of the maximum intensity projection reconstruction, **B**).

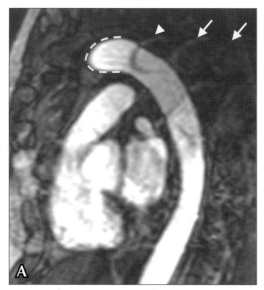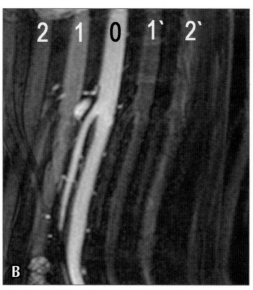

Figure 4-19. Ghosting artifact. **A,** A 58-year-old woman with chest pain in whom examination was done to rule out aortic dissection. Thin-slab oblique maximum intensity projection image shows low-signal structure (*arrowhead*) projected within the lumen of the descending aorta that could be misinterpreted as an intimal flap of dissection. This is a ghosting artifact and can be better appreciated with this different window setting where details extend beyond the aortic boundaries with repetition posteriorly (*arrows*). Note that the shape of the artifact resembles that of the moving structure (*yellow dashed lines*).

B, A 28-year-old woman with suspected mesenteric ischemia. Postcontrast sagittal source from magnetic resonance angiography of the abdominal aorta and mesenteric vessels image shows the unremarkable abdominal aorta (0) and multiple ghosting artifacts (1, 1′, 2, and 2′). These artifacts result from pulsatile motion during image acquisition. When motion is repetitive and periodic (aortic pulsatility, in both these examples), artifacts are located at regular intervals along the phase-encoding axis [16]. Electrocardiogram triggering can alleviate this artifact but is accompanied by at least some time penalty.

REFERENCES

1. Fishman EK, Ney DR, Heath DG, *et al.*: Volume rendering versus maximum intensity projection in CT angiography: what works best, when, and why. *Radiographics* 2006, 26:905–922.

2. Saloner D: The AAPM/RSNA physics tutorial for residents. An introduction to MR angiography. *Radiographics* 1995,15:453–465.

3. Pelc NJ, Sommer FG, Li KC, *et al.*: Quantitative magnetic resonance flow imaging. *Magn Reson Q* 1994,10:125–147.

4. Stemerman DH, Krinsky GA, Lee VS, *et al.*: Thoracic aorta: rapid black-blood MR imaging with half-Fourier rapid acquisition with relaxation enhancement with or without electrocardiographic triggering. *Radiology* 1999, 213:185–191.

5. Finn JP, Nael K, Deshpande V, *et al.*: Cardiac MR imaging: state of the technology. *Radiology* 2006, 241:338–354.

6. Mitchell DG, Cohen M: *MRI Principles*, edn 2. Philadelphia: WB Saunders; 2003.

7. Prince MR, Yucel EK, Kaufman JA, *et al.*: Dynamic gadolinium-enhanced three-dimensional abdominal MR arteriography. *J Magn Reson Imaging* 1993, 3:877–881.

8. Earls JP, Rofsky NM, DeCorato DR, *et al.*: Breath-hold single-dose gadolinium-enhanced three-dimensional MR aortography: usefulness of a timing examination and MR power injector. *Radiology* 1996, 201:705–710.

9. Foo TK, Saranathan M, Prince MR, Chenevert TL: Automated detection of bolus arrival and initiation of data acquisition in fast, three-dimensional, gadolinium-enhanced MR angiography. *Radiology* 1997, 203:275–280.

10. Swan JS, Carroll TJ, Kennell TW, *et al.*: Time-resolved three-dimensional contrast-enhanced MR angiography of the peripheral vessels. *Radiology* 2002, 225:43–52.

11. Maki JH, Prince MR, Chenevert TC: Optimizing three-dimensional gadolinium-enhanced magnetic resonance angiography. Original investigation. *Invest Radiol* 1998, 33:528–537.

12. Lee VS, Martin DJ, Krinsky GA, Rofsky NM: Gadolinium-enhanced MR angiography: artifacts and pitfalls. *AJR Am J Roentgenol* 2000, 175:197–205.

13. Maki JH, Prince MR, Londy FJ, Chenevert TL: The effects of time varying intravascular signal intensity and k-space acquisition order on three-dimensional MR angiography image quality. *J Magn Reson Imaging* 1996, 6:642–651.

14. Lee VS, Flyer MA, Weinreb JC, *et al.*: Image subtraction in gadolinium-enhanced MR imaging. *AJR Am J Roentgenol* 1996, 167:1427–1432.

15. Rofsky NM, Morana G, Adelman MA, *et al.*: Improved gadolinium-enhanced subtraction MR angiography of the femoropopliteal arteries: reintroduction of osseous anatomic landmarks. *AJR Am J Roentgenol* 1999, 173:1009–1011.

16. Zhuo J, Gullapalli RP: AAPM/RSNA physics tutorial for residents: MR artifacts, safety, and quality control. *Radiographics* 2006, 26:275–297.

5

Practical Aspects of CMR Imaging

Kraig V. Kissinger

Cardiovascular magnetic resonance (CMR) imaging is a clinically accepted noninvasive method of evaluating cardiovascular anatomy that measures cardiac volumes and mass to assess function and quantify blood flow in major vessels. CMR presents certain challenges that are usually not present in other MR examinations. A complete understanding of cardiac anatomy and physiology, as well as scan plane selection, is essential for the technologist to perform CMR studies efficiently. The technologist must be intimately familiar with the use of the electrocardiogram gating system, surface coils, and the cardiac-specific software of the MR system.

A solid understanding of the three-dimensional anatomy of the heart and all its variations is crucial for acquiring the views needed for a CMR examination. Knowledge of the array of pulse sequences available for the various parts of a comprehensive CMR study is required. Finally, expertise in overcoming the technical obstacles inherent to cardiac imaging is also necessary.

This chapter concentrates on the issues of successful electrocardiogram gating/triggering, surface coil selection and positioning, normal cardiac anatomy, basic scan planes, and pulse sequence selection and application.

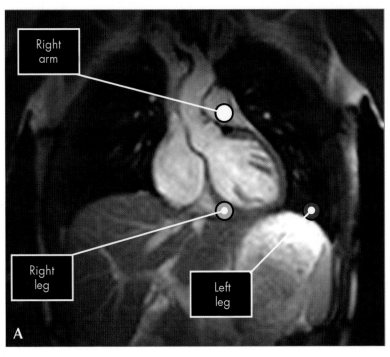

Right arm

Right leg

Left leg

A

Figure 5-1. Successful electrocardiogram (ECG) gating/triggering is essential for all cardiovascular magnetic resonance (CMR) examinations. This requires accurate detection of the QRS complex for every heart beat. The distortion of the ECG signal when the patient is positioned within the CMR scanner is a result of a conductor (blood) moving through a static magnetic field. This phenomenon is known as the magnetohydrodynamic effect and can result in an elevated T wave that can interfere with the proper detection of the QRS complex.

Continued on the next page

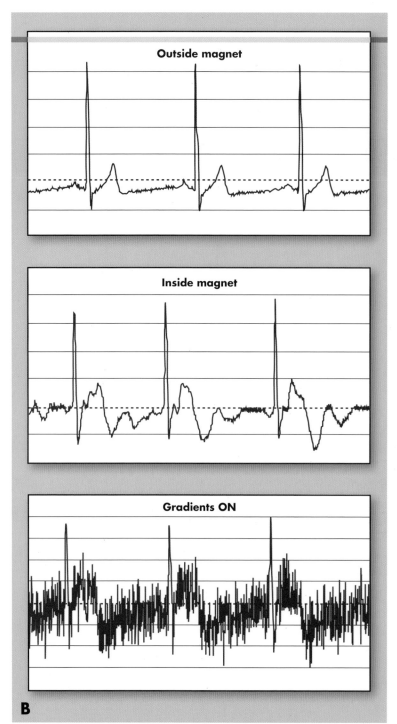

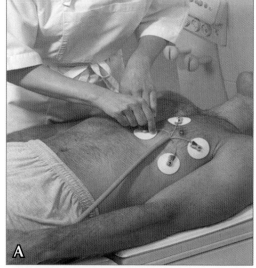

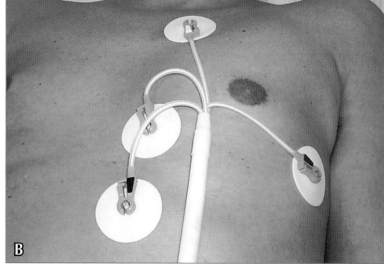

Figure 5-1. *(Continued)* Keeping the leads placed on the same side of the aorta can help to minimize the elevation of the T wave. Cardiovascular magnetic resonance (CMR) system vendors have implemented several techniques to help overcome this problem. The most effective advance has been the implementation of the vector cardiogram, which uses spatial information to minimize the effect of CMR-related distortion of the cardiogram. The first step to a successful CMR examination is adequate ECG detection. Therefore, it is imperative to have an adequate ECG before the examination begins.

Figure 5-2. A reliable electrocardiogram (ECG) for cardiovascular magnetic resonance (CMR) requires the proper preparation of the patient's skin as well as the proper use and placement of electrodes (**A** and **B**). The patient's skin must be clean and dry before the application of electrodes. Hair should be removed if the presence of which will interfere with accurate ECG detection or adherence of the electrodes. Utilization of electrodes designed for the CMR environment is required to minimize the risk of burns to the patient. New or properly stored electrodes must be used to prevent burns resulting from old or "dried out" conductive gel. Lead placement may vary but the basic concept is the same: measurement of the electrical activity of the heart to compensate for cardiac motion during imaging. The CMR system manufacturer will have specific guidelines to be followed by the user for proper use of the ECG system.

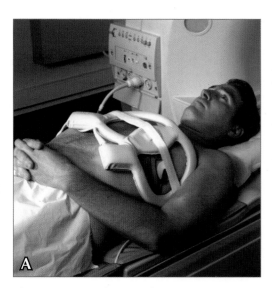

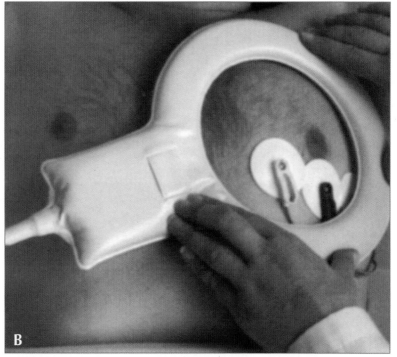

Figure 5-3. Cardiovascular magnetic resonance can be performed with simple surface coils or coil arrays. **A** and **B**, The receiver coil must be placed over the patient's heart as shown according to the manufacturer's directions. Surface coils should be placed accurately over the anatomy to ensure adequate anatomic coverage with sufficient signal for the best image quality. Array coils provide uniform coverage of the entire chest allowing for complete evaluation of thoracic anatomy. Patients must understand that once the receiver coils are positioned they should not be moved, because a change in the position of the coil may lead to poor image quality.

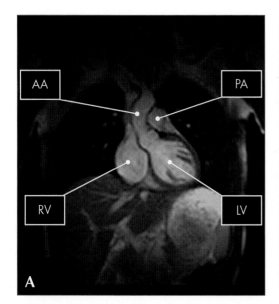

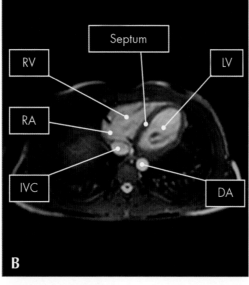

Figure 5-4. **A** and **B**, Selected images in the coronal and axial orientation show much of the basic anatomy with which one must be familiar for planning essential views of cardiac anatomy. In both planes, the position and orientation of the heart is noted. The coronal view demonstrates the left ventricle (LV) and right ventricle (RV), the ascending aorta (AA) and, in cross-section, the pulmonary artery (PA). The axial view shows the LV and RV, right atrium (RA), inferior vena cava (IVC), and descending aorta (DA). Recognition of these structures will allow technologists to begin to plan the basic cardiac views. Note the position of the intraventricular septum on the axial image because this will be important in planning the two-chamber view.

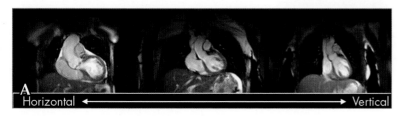

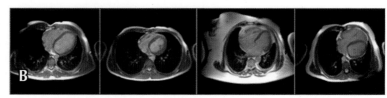

Figure 5-5. The heart's position and orientation can vary greatly from person to person. Body habitus can account for much of this variability. A tall person will tend to have a more vertically oriented heart than a shorter person (**A**). Gender differences also exist. Men tend to have an elongated left ventricle, whereas in women, the left ventricle tends to be more globular. Many other factors determine the shape, size, and orientation of a person's heart (**B**). Understanding these differences will allow the technologist to more easily obtain the views needed for the cardiac magnetic resonance examination.

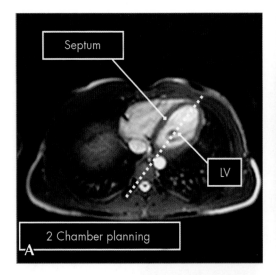

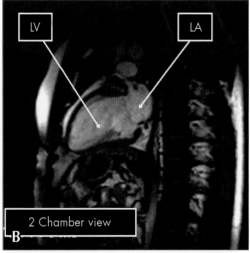

Figure 5-6. The first basic view to be acquired after scout images are obtained is the two-chamber view. This is achieved by planning a single oblique parallel to the intraventricular septum. **A,** The slice plane (*dotted line*) is positioned to intersect the left ventricle (LV) apex and the mitral valve. The resulting image demonstrates the two chambers of the left side of the heart. **B,** The LV and left atrium (LA) are visualized. This scan as well as subsequent scans would typically be a cine acquisition using a steady state free precession sequence to assess cardiac function.

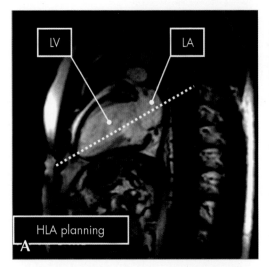

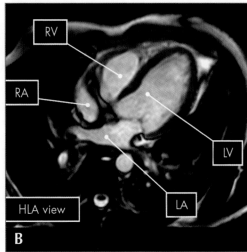

Figure 5-7. The horizontal long-axis (HLA) view is planned perpendicular to the two-chamber view. **A,** The slice plane (*dotted line*) is oriented to intersect the mitral valve and the apex of the left ventricle (LV). This view may, in some people, resemble the four-chamber view, but does not account for rotation of the heart that will be seen in the short-axis view. The LV and right ventricle (RV) should be visualized. The atria may appear foreshortened depending on the position of the heart. **B,** The HLA view demonstrates the atrioventricular grooves that will be important in planning the subsequent short-axis view. LA—left atrium; RA—right atrium.

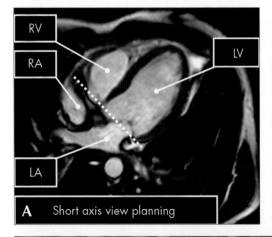

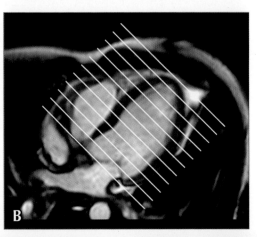

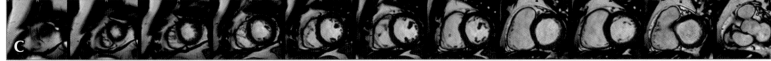

Figure 5-8. The horizontal long-axis view allows for the planning of a short-axis (SA) view that is parallel to the mitral/tricuspid valve plane. By orienting the SA view to intersect the atrioventricular groove on the left and right sides of the heart a true SA can be achieved. **A,** The atrioventricular groove is the landmark for a SA view at the base of the heart (*dotted line*). **B,** For a complete volumetric analysis of the ventricles a stack of slices in this orientation must be acquired. The number of slices required is dependent on the size of the patient's heart. **C,** The stack of SA slices should provide coverage from the atrioventricular groove through the apex of the heart. Quantitative analysis can then be performed using software packages from the magnetic resonance system manufacturer or from independent software developers. LA—left atrium; LV—left ventricle; RA—right atrium; RV—right ventricle.

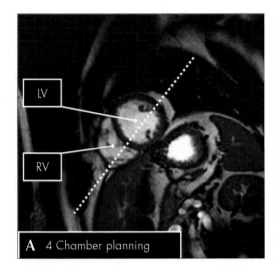

A 4 Chamber planning

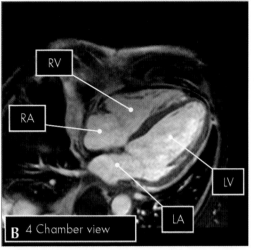

B 4 Chamber view

Figure 5-9. The four-chamber view is planned on a midventricular short-axis view. **A,** The slice plane (*dotted line*) is rotated to bisect the lateral wall of the left ventricle (LV) and the right ventricle (RV) free wall. All four chambers of the heart should be well visualized. **B,** The atria are seen without any foreshortening to allow for accurate assessment of atrial size. LA—left atrium; RA—right atrium.

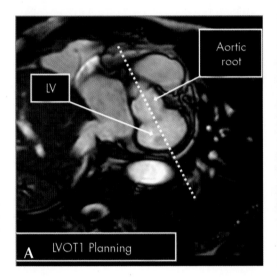

A LVOT1 Planning

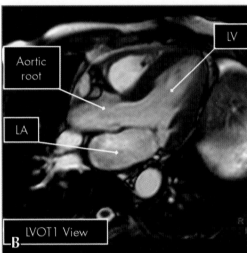

B LVOT1 View

Figure 5-10. The views of the left ventricular outflow tract (LVOT) are used not only for visual assessment of the aortic root and aortic valve but also to acquire two views of the aortic valve to aid in planning a slice parallel to the aortic valve. The LVOT1 view is planned (**A**) on an end-systolic basal short-axis view. It is important to plan the LVOT1 on an end-systolic frame of the short-axis cine because the anatomy of interest moves throughout the cardiac cycle. If the LVOT1 is planned on an end-diastolic frame, it is likely that the aortic root would not be in plane when the aortic valve is open. This would inhibit the assessment of the function of the aortic valve in this view (**B**). The slice plane (*dotted line* in **A**) is oriented along the aortic root parallel to the aortic outflow tract. LA—left atrium; LV—left ventricle.

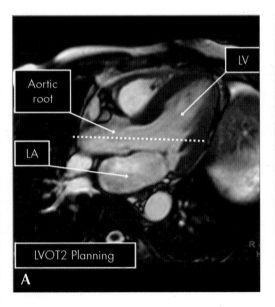

A LVOT2 Planning

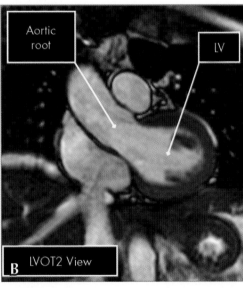

B LVOT2 View

Figure 5-11. The left ventricular outflow tract 2 (LVOT2) view is planned on an end-systolic LVOT1 view. **A,** The slice plane (*dotted line*) is oriented along the aortic root parallel to the aortic outflow tract. **B,** The aortic root, aortic valve, and left ventricle (LV) are seen in this near coronal view. LA—left atrium.

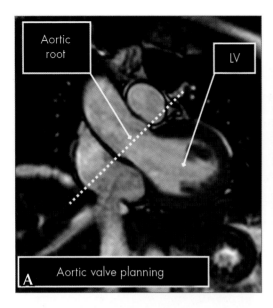

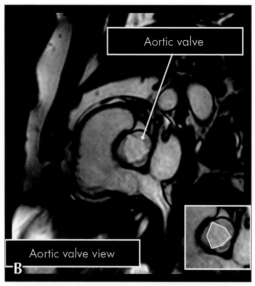

Figure 5-12. A, The aortic valve view is planned on the left ventricular outflow tract 2 view in which the valve leaflets are seen *open*. The slice plane (*dotted line*) is oriented to be parallel to the valve plane. **B,** This cross-section of the aortic valve provides a view in which the valve area can be measured to evaluate for the presence and severity of aortic stenosis (notice the tracing of the borders of the aortic valve on the *inset image*). LV—left ventricle.

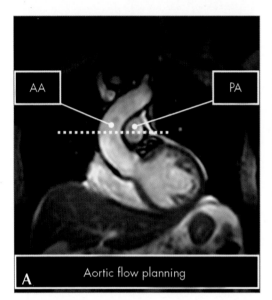

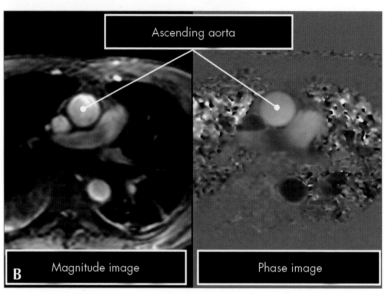

Figure 5-13. A and **B,** Blood flow in the great vessels—ascending aorta (AA) and main pulmonary artery (PA)—is often evaluated as part of the comprehensive assessment of cardiac function. Utilizing a phase contrast gradient echo sequence, volume and velocity of flow can be measured. These measurements provide the data necessary to assess intracardiac shunt as well as calculate aortic, mitral, tricuspid, and pulmonic valve regurgitation. To measure flow in the AA, a simple axial plane is used. The slice plane is prescribed at the level of the bifurcation of the main PA. This can be planned graphically on a coronal view as shown (*dotted line* in **A**). The foot/head offset can be entered manually into the phase contrast scan by locating the bifurcation of the PA on another sequence. Offline analysis of these data shown in the resulting magnitude and phase images are necessary. Magnetic resonance system vendors provide software to analyze quantitative flow data, or third-party software may be used.

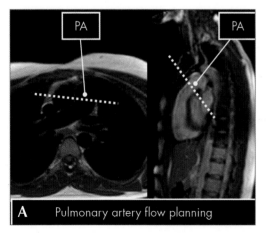

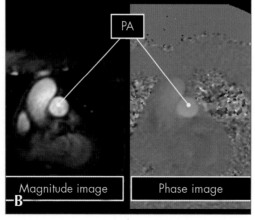

orientation is usually necessary to plan a plane perpendicular to the vessel. **A,** Using an axial and sagittal view, the slice plane (*dotted line*) is graphically prescribed. The view is perpendicular to the vessel proximal to the bifurcation of the main PA, resulting in a circular object for the offline analysis software. Edge detection algorithms used in these software packages normally have greater success in tracking the vessel throughout the cardiac cycle if the plane is perpendicular to the vessel of interest. **B,** The main PA in cross-section is demonstrated on the magnitude and phase images from the resultant scan.

Figure 5-14. The same sequence that is used to assess blood flow in the ascending aorta is also used for measurement through the main pulmonary artery (PA). A double oblique

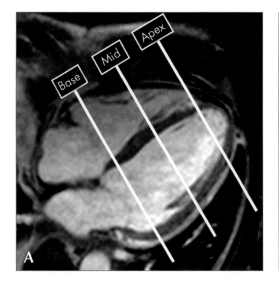

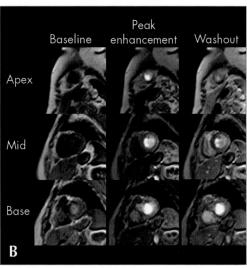

Figure 5-15. A and **B**, A comprehensive cardiovascular magnetic resonance examination may include assessment of myocardial perfusion. An ultra-fast gradient echo sequence is commonly used for these types of scans although other techniques such as echo planar or steady state free precession may be available on some magnetic resonance systems. Regardless of the sequence, myocardial perfusion scans are performed during the intravenous injection of a gadolinium contrast agent. Several slice locations are acquired with each heartbeat during the first pass of the contrast agent. Patients are instructed to suspend respiration at baseline, before the arrival of the contrast, and during the first pass arrival of the contrast. A low dose of contrast (0.05 mmol/kg gadolinium diethyltriaminepentaacetic acid) is typically used for myocardial perfusion imaging, because a higher dose can make quantification difficult. Various software programs are available for analysis of myocardial perfusion scans from magnetic resonance system manufacturers and independent developers.

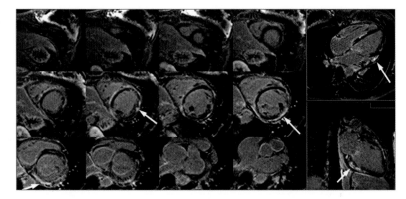

Figure 5-16. After the administration of gadolinium contrast the myocardium can be evaluated for delayed enhancement. The presence of scar or fibrosis (*arrows*) will be visualized after a period of time dependent on the dose and type of contrast material used. The sequence used to visualize the delayed enhancement is an inversion-prepared gradient echo sequence. The inversion time must be set to null the signal from normal myocardium. There are several methods to determine the optimal inversion time for these scans. A formula that factors variables such as heart rate, contrast dose, and delay after contrast administration can be used to give an approximate inversion time. Alternately, short scans using different inversion times can be acquired to give the operator several choices of inversion times. Finally, a sequence acquired before the delayed enhancement scans samples multiple inversion times in one short sequence. Two- or three-dimensional inversion-recovery prepared scans with higher spatial and temporal resolution are then performed using this optimal inversion time to null normal myocardium to visualize the presence or absence of delayed myocardial enhancement in the standard cardiac views.

RECOMMENDED READING

Auckland MRI Research Group. The Cardiac Atlas web site. http://www.atlas.scmr.org.

German Heart Institute web site. http://www.cmr-academy.com.

Society for Cardiovascular Magnetic Resonance web site. http://www.scmr.org.

Higgins CB, de Roos A: *Cardiovascular MRI and MRA.* Philadelphia: Lippincott Williams & Wilkins; 2002.

Manning WJ, Pennell DJ: *Cardiovascular Magnetic Resonance.* New York: Churchill Livingstone Publishers; 2002.

MR Achieva [application guide]. Eindhoven, The Netherlands: Philips Medical Systems; 2005

Sawyer-Glover A, ed.: *Cardiovascular MRI: Update I: SMRT Educational Seminars,* vol. 7; no. 2. Berkeley, CA: Section for Magnetic Resonance Technologists; 2006.

Sawyer-Glover A, ed.: *Cardiovascular MRI: Update II: SMRT Educational Seminars,* vol. 8; no 2. Berkeley, CA: Section for Magnetic Resonance Technologists; 2006.

6

CHAPTER

Left and Right Ventricular Anatomy and Systolic Function

Vikas K. Rathi and Robert W. W. Biederman

Cardiovascular magnetic resonance (CMR) imaging is the gateway to modern cardiovascular medicine. It provides exquisite details of the heart—anatomic and physiologic—which have now taken root in the daily practice of internists, general cardiologists, cardiothoracic surgeons, and vascular surgeons. The role of CMR further extends into the myocardial metabolism by way of MR spectroscopy and also monitoring of drug therapy as well as stem cell implantation [1,2]. On a day-to-day basis, CMR is being used primarily for the evaluation of cardiac anatomy and ventricular function, valvular function, myocardial perfusion, and viability [3]. The well-known attributes of CMR are its high-definition images, practically unlimited field of view, purely noninvasive nature, no radiation exposure to the patient or physician, user independence, and low variability. These characteristics make CMR an ideal choice for routine cardiac imaging and serial studies as well as an effective research tool. The inherent three-dimensional data combined with high spatial and temporal resolution of CMR makes it an ideal choice for the assessment of ventricular volumes, ejection fraction, and mass. Also, its ability to image in virtually any imaging plane makes it an ideal imaging modality for the assessment of right ventricular (RV) function, otherwise difficult on conventional imaging modalities due to its complex anatomy. Because left and right ventricular indices are the mainstay for most cardiovascular applications, the CMR technology has witnessed continued growth and innovations that have led to development of newer faster sequences to acquire the images as well as postprocessing of these images with minimal user interaction. In this chapter, we will explore the uses of CMR focusing on left and right ventricular anatomy and function.

Two conventional imaging planes are used for CMR. The body planes are used for gross anatomy and the cardiac axis planes are used for specific anatomy and ventricular or valvular function. The routine body planes used for cardiac imaging are transaxial, coronal, and sagittal. The common cardiac axis planes used are somewhat similar to echocardiography such as left ventricular outflow view, vertical long-axis view (two-chamber), horizontal long-axis view (four-chamber), and short-axis view. Some double oblique views such as right ventricular outflow view are specific to CMR.

The morphologic left ventricle (LV) is cone shaped, and its basal portion sits to the right and posterior of the chest cavity; the apex is anterior and left. The apex of the LV represents the apex of the heart on chest radiograph, as well as the apical impulse palpated on the chest wall. The inner cavity of the LV is trabeculated mostly at the apex, albeit less prominently compared with the right ventricle (RV). The LV has an inlet through the left atrioventricular canal, which is guarded by the mitral valve and an outlet that is tubular and smooth walled and is guarded by the aortic valve. The LV cavity displays two papillary muscles—the anterolateral and the posteromedial papillary muscles. When viewed from above, the anterolateral papillary muscle is at the two- to three-o'clock position and the posteromedial papillary muscle is at the seven-o'clock position. These papillary muscles are believed to arise from confluence of trabeculations in the LV cavity. Each papillary muscle has at least two heads, and these heads provide attachment to chordae tendinea, which are attached to the commissural margins of the mitral valve leaflets. Each papillary muscle therefore provides anchorage to both mitral leaflets, as well as architectural support to the LV. The walls of the LV are named according to the position they represent in the chest cavity (*see* Figure 7-5) [4]. The LV is separated from the RV by interventricular septum.

The role of the LV is to efficiently pump blood into the systemic circulation, and the capability with which this is performed is evaluated in the form of LV ejection fraction and other matrices related to LV volumes and mass. Each of these parameters is well supported as a prognostic indicator. The role of ejection fraction as a prognostic indicator is the most studied because of the ease of qualitative assessment [5]. It has been well established that ventricular volumes, especially end-systolic volume, serve as excellent prognosticators particularly in valvular heart disease. The role of myocardial mass as an indicator of morbidity and mortality is well established, especially in hypertensive heart disease [6,7]. CMR proves to be the imaging modality of choice to assess these basic measures of LV function due to its inherent accuracy and high reproducibility. The role of CMR for evaluation of more sophisticated LV mechanical metrics extends to mathematical measures such as strain, torsion, wall thickening, and thickness indices.

RIGHT VENTRICLE ANATOMY AND FUNCTION

The RV is triangular and consists of an inlet, an outlet, and the main cavity. The cavity of the RV is walled anteriorly by the free wall, inferiorly by diaphragmatic wall, and posteriorly by the septum. The apex of the RV cavity is formed by the free wall and diaphragmatic wall attachment to the distal portion of the interventricular septum. The inlet of RV is through the tricuspid valve, and the outlet into the pulmonary artery is through the pulmonic valve. The RV cavity is heavily trabeculated with coarse trabeculations. The cavity also houses the papillary muscle and moderator band and in some cases a septoparietal band. The anterior papillary muscle is most prominent and occasionally arises from the septoparietal band. The RV serves as the pumping chamber for pulmonary circulation.

The evaluation of RV function is very challenging with conventional imaging [8]. The wide field of view and three-dimensional nature of CMR imaging coupled with its ability to image in multiple planes make CMR an ideal modality for assessment of RV function.

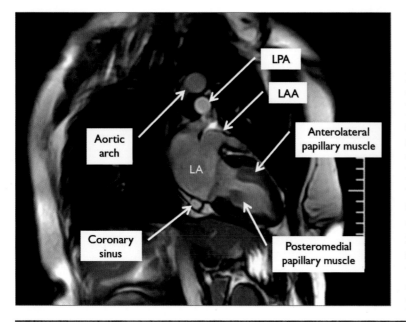

Figure 6-1. Vertical long-axis view (two-chamber) of the left ventricle (LV). This view is obtained by prescribing a slice through the LV apex and mitral valve. Ideally, two consecutive cine slices are obtained to cover the apex. This image is a steady-state free precession (SSFP) cine image in end-systole demonstrating the LV and the left atrium (LA). This view is helpful in evaluating the global LV function in conjunction with the four-chamber view. Also, this view demonstrates the systolic function of the anterior wall, apex, and inferior wall along with the mitral valve apparatus, and the anterolateral and posteromedial papillary muscle, chordae, and mitral leaflets. This view is also ideal for evaluation of left atrial appendage (LAA). The left pulmonary artery (LPA) crosses on top of the LAA and left superior pulmonary vein, and the aortic arch is superior to the LPA. The coronary sinus is seen inferior and posterior to the left atrial appendage.

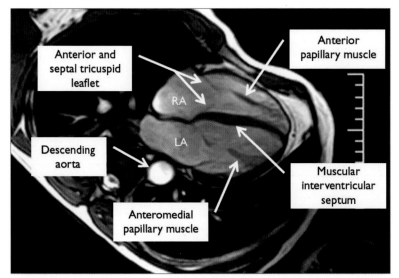

Figure 6-2. Horizontal long-axis view. This is also known as the four-chamber view, and it is obtained by prescribing successive slices on a two-chamber view traversing through the mitral valve and apex or an obliquely oriented horizontal slice over the left ventricle (LV) short-axis view. This image displays both atria and ventricles along with both atrioventricular valves. This view, along with the two-chamber and short-axis views, is used for qualitative assessment of LV and right ventricle (RV) ejection fraction. This view is helpful in demonstrating mitral valvular disease, tricuspid valvular pathology, or papillary muscle dysfunction. The anterolateral papillary muscle of the LV and the anterior papillary muscle of the RV are most readily visualized on this view. Again RV and LV apical function can be evaluated in this view. The right atria (RA) and left atria (LA) with interatrial septum are visualized; therefore, this view is frequently used to demonstrate atrial septal defect with the phase velocity mapping of the atrial septum to demonstrate shunt.

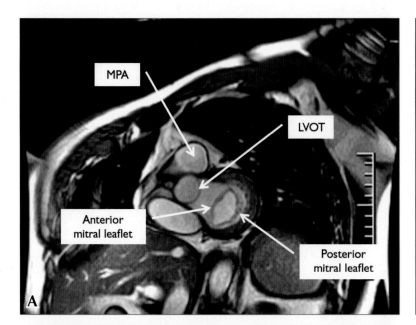

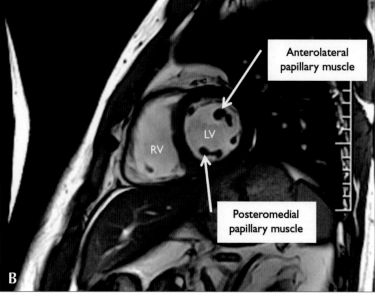

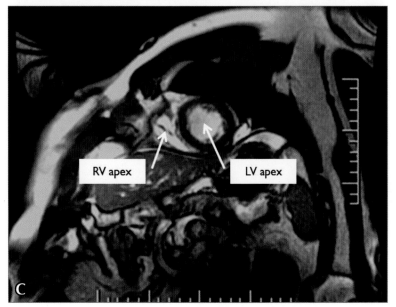

Figure 6-3. Short-axis view of the heart. The basal (A), mid (B), and apical (C) short-axis fast imaging employing steady-state free precession (SSFP) images are shown. These images are acquired from vertical or horizontal long-axis images by prescribing slices from base to apex. The basal slice (A) demonstrates the anterior and the posterior mitral valve leaflets. The left ventricular outflow tract (LVOT) is anterior to the anterior mitral leaflet. This image also demonstrates the main pulmonary artery (MPA) anterior and superior to the LVOT. The mid slices (B) demonstrate the anterolateral and posteromedial papillary muscles. The anterolateral papillary muscle arises at the two- to three-o'clock position, and the posteromedial papillary muscle arises at the seven-o'clock position. The apical slices (C) demonstrate the left ventricle (LV) and right ventricle (RV) apices. The global and regional wall function, ventricular volumes, and mass of the LV and RV are determined using a series of contiguous slices from base to apex. In a normal heart usually eight to 12 slices of 8-mm thickness with 2 mm interslice gap are required for comprehensive qualitative and quantitative biventricular function evaluation.

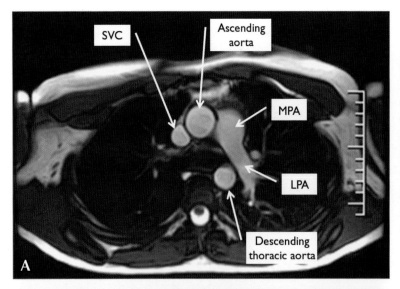

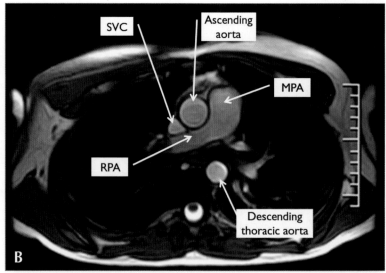

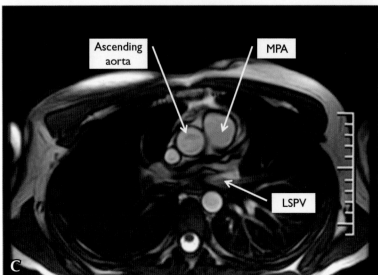

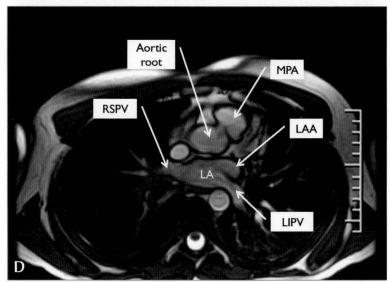

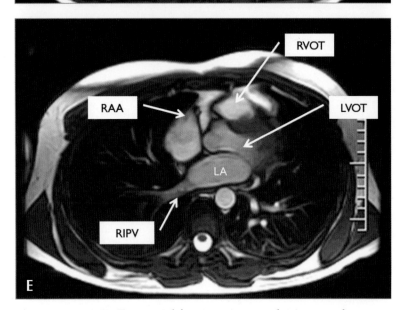

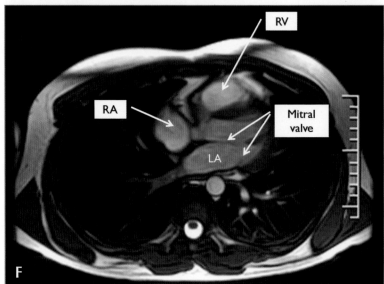

Figure 6-4. A–H, Transaxial fast imaging employing steady-state free precession (SSFP) cine images can be acquired from the level of main pulmonary artery (MPA) to the inferior wall of the left (LV) and right (RV) ventricles. These images are used to display the anatomy of the heart along with the venous and arterial vascular channels connecting the heart. **A** and **B,** These images aid in measurement of the MPA, right and left pulmonary artery (RPA and LPA), and ascending and descending thoracic aorta. These images are helpful in identifying the pulmonary venous return. All the four pulmonary veins—right superior pulmonary vein (RSPV), right inferior pulmonary vein (RIPV), left superior pulmonary vein (LSPV), and left inferior pulmonary vein (LIPV)—are visualized. These images are particularly used for identifying sinus venosus defects in which all the pulmonary venous connections can be visualized along with their relationship with great veins and the interatrial septum.

Continued on the next page

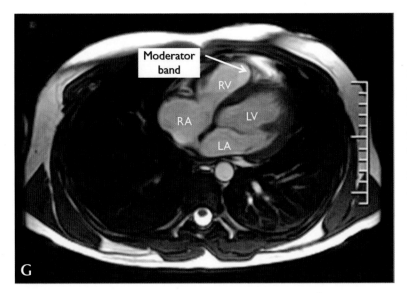

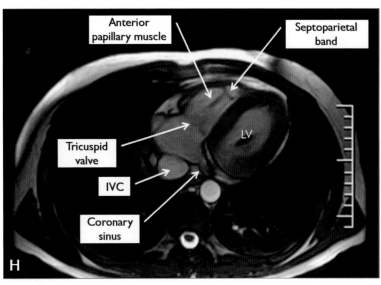

Figure 6-4. *(Continued)* **E–H,** The right ventricular outflow tract (RVOT), as well as the right ventricular free wall function, can be visualized along with the septal wall, lateral wall, and apical wall function of the LV. In the lower slices, the inferior vena cava (IVC) is seen draining into the right atrium (RA). Also, the coronary sinus opening is seen in the RA. In the RV, the moderator band, anterior papillary muscle, and the septoparietal band are visible. The mitral and tricuspid valves are also well visualized. LA—left atrium; LAA—left atrial appendages; LVOT—left ventricular outflow tract; RAA—right atrial appendage; SVC—superior vena cava.

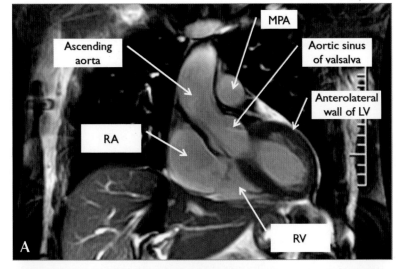

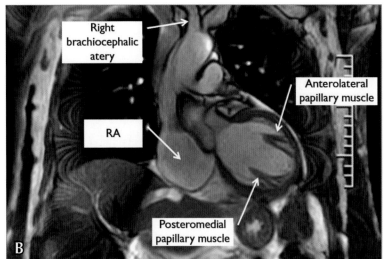

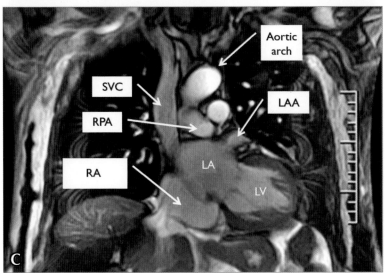

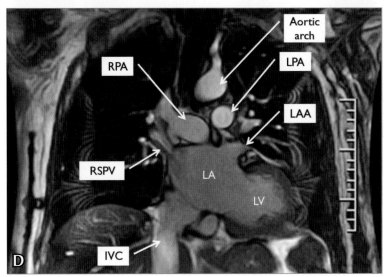

Figure 6-5. A–F, Coronal slices demonstrating the cardiac anatomy. The right ventricle (RV) is best visualized in the anterior coronal slices in which it is seen as a triangular structure (**A**). **A** and **B,** The function of the diaphragmatic wall and the apex of the RV, as well as the infundibulum (not seen in these images), is well visualized. **A–D,** The aortic valve, mitral valve, and the papillary muscle function are also well visualized.

Continued on the next page

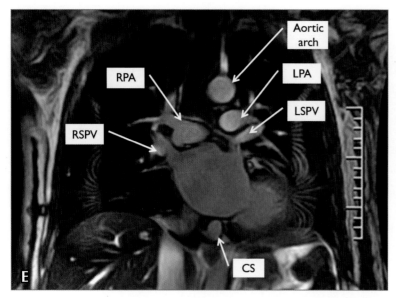

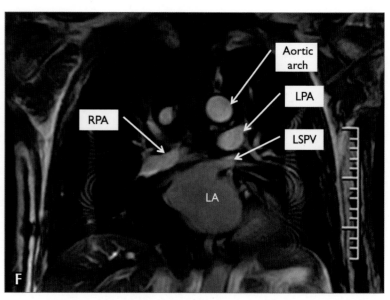

Figure 6-5. *(Continued)* **E** and **F,** The coronal view is complementary to a multiaxial view for evaluation of the pulmonary venous drainage and pulmonary vein anatomy for pre- and postatrial fibrillation ablation procedure. CS—coronary sinus; IVC—inferior vena cava; LAA—left atrial appendage; LA—left atrium; LPA—left pulmonary artery; LSPV—left superior pulmonary vein; LV—left ventricle; MPA—main pulmonary artery; RPA—right pulmonary artery; RSPV—right superior pulmonary vein; SVC—superior vena cava.

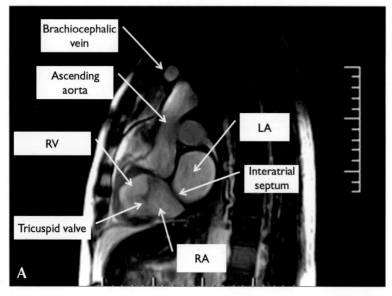

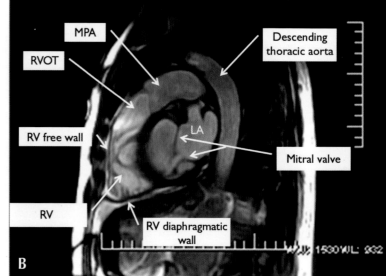

Figure 6-6. **A** and **B,** The sagittal view is used for evaluation of the right ventricular outflow tract (RVOT) function, infundibular function, and the visualization of the mitral valve in oblique plane. The interatrial septum is also seen in this view. MPA—main pulmonary artery; LA—left atrium; RA—right atrium; RV—right ventricle.

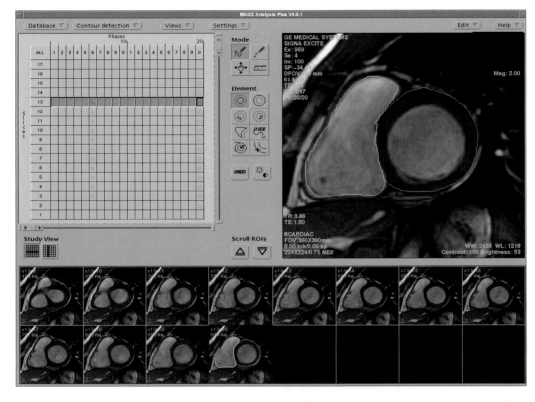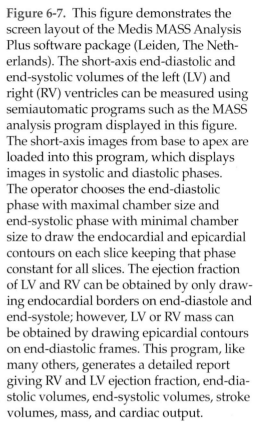

Figure 6-7. This figure demonstrates the screen layout of the Medis MASS Analysis Plus software package (Leiden, The Netherlands). The short-axis end-diastolic and end-systolic volumes of the left (LV) and right (RV) ventricles can be measured using semiautomatic programs such as the MASS analysis program displayed in this figure. The short-axis images from base to apex are loaded into this program, which displays images in systolic and diastolic phases. The operator chooses the end-diastolic phase with maximal chamber size and end-systolic phase with minimal chamber size to draw the endocardial and epicardial contours on each slice keeping that phase constant for all slices. The ejection fraction of LV and RV can be obtained by only drawing endocardial borders on end-diastole and end-systole; however, LV or RV mass can be obtained by drawing epicardial contours on end-diastolic frames. This program, like many others, generates a detailed report giving RV and LV ejection fraction, end-diastolic volumes, end-systolic volumes, stroke volumes, mass, and cardiac output.

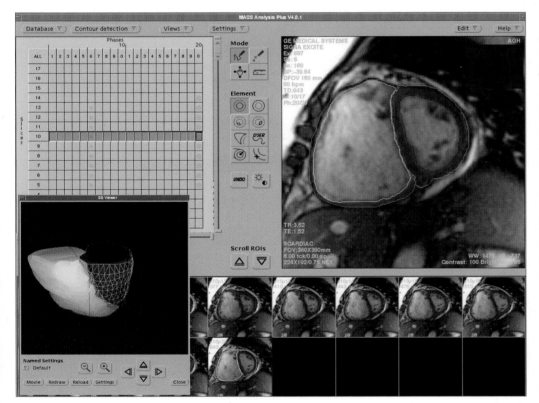

Figure 6-8. This image displays three-dimensional quantification of the left (LV) and right (RV) ventricle volumes and mass using the Medis MASS Analysis Plus (Leiden, The Netherlands) software package on a patient with severe pulmonary hypertension. In the *upper right hand corner*, a midventricular short-axis image in end-diastole is displayed. This image shows markedly dilated RV with D-shaped LV indicative of RV volume overload. The *lower left hand corner* displays a three-dimensional reconstruction image that also demonstrates that the RV is markedly dilated with a normal sized LV. LV and RV parameters are often normalized for the patient's body surface area. The RV indices in this patient were as follows: RV end-diastolic volume index = 185 mL/m²; RV end-systolic volume index = 132 mLm²; RV mass index = 38 g/m²; and three-dimensional RV ejection fraction = 28%. The LV indices were normal as follows: LV end-diastolic volume index = 61 mL/m²; LV end-systolic volume index = 27 mL/m²; LV mass index = 50 g/m²; and three-dimensional LV ejection fraction = 56%.

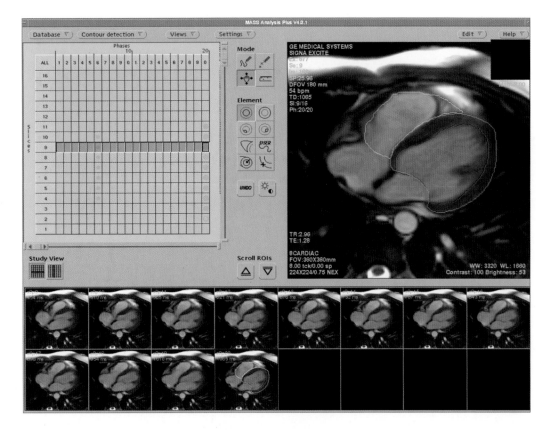

Figure 6-9. Similar to Figure 6-8, the left (LV) and right (RV) ventricle function can also be analyzed on multislice transverse axial images. The transverse axial end-diastolic and end-systolic images from neck to diaphragm are loaded onto this program, which displays images in systolic and diastolic phases. Shown in this image on the *upper right hand corner* is the end-diastolic frame at the level of the LV and RV cavity. This imaging plane is preferred for RV function evaluation because of complete integration of the RV outflow in these slices. However, caution should be exercised while drawing the contours on the lower slice images due to partial volume of the diaphragmatic RV and LV walls to avoid erroneous volume and ejection fraction calculations.

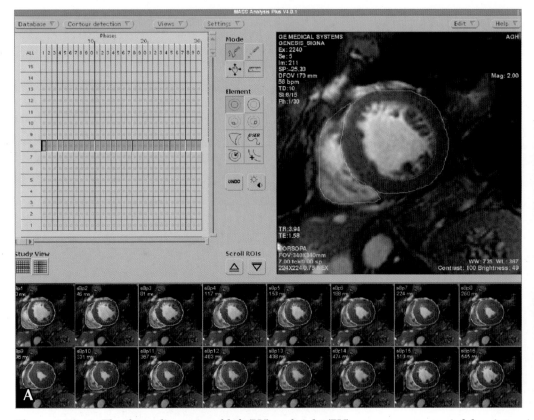

Figure 6-10. A, The three-dimensional left (LV) and right (RV) ventricle volume analysis on the MASS Analysis Plus (Leiden, The Netherlands) software package. The time-resolved three-dimensional LV and RV volume curves are obtained by tracing endocardial borders of all the cardiac phases in a semiautomatic manner. This process is labor-intensive, but gives accurate measure of the LV volumes over each phase of the cardiac cycle. **B,** The program also demonstrates endo- and epicardial surface in three-dimensional cine frames derived from the endo- and epicardial contours.

Continued on the next page

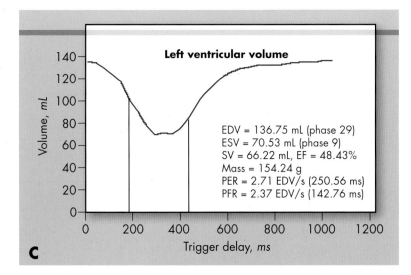

C

Figure 6-10. *(Continued)* The LV three-dimensional time volume curve is also shown (**C**), and temporal analysis can be performed to assess peak ejection and peak filling rates. If the temporal resolution of the cardiac phases is improved to less than 30 ms, the three-dimensional volume and mass analysis can be used for assessment of the LV dyssynchrony using segmental analysis. EDV—end diastolic volume; EF—ejection fraction; ESV—end systolic volume; PER—peak ejection rate; PFR— peak filling rate; SV—stroke volume

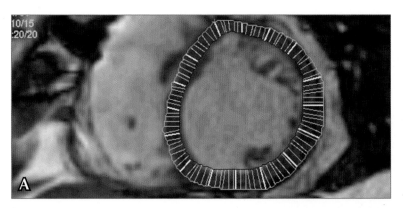

A

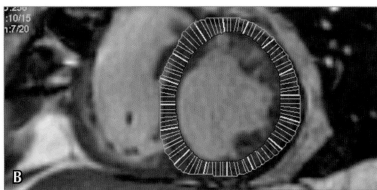

B

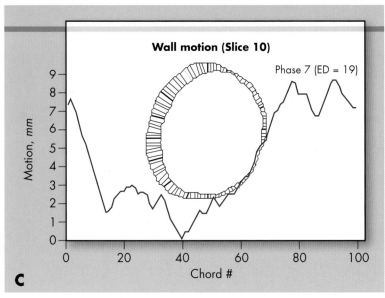

C

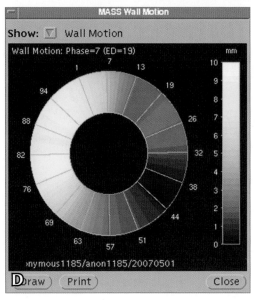

D

Figure 6-11. **A–F**, The centerline method to evaluate left ventricular wall motion and wall thickening. Endocardial and epicardial contours are drawn and the automated program divides the circumference of the myocardium into 100 equal parts as represented by the lines connecting the epi- and endocardial borders. These lines are tracked over the diastolic (**A**) and systolic (**B**) frames to generate the wall motion (**C**) and wall thickening (**E**) graphs and color plots (**D** and **F**).

Continued on the next page

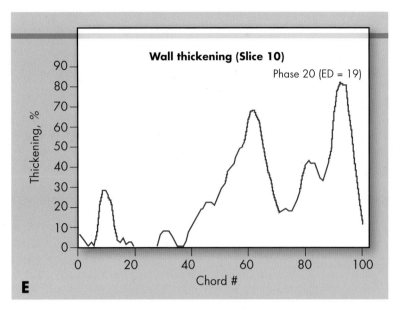

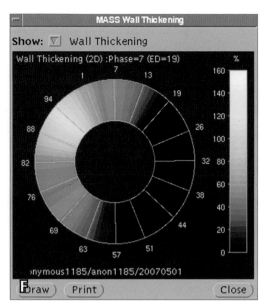

Figure 6-11. *(Continued)* In this case, as seen visually, the anterior wall and the anteroseptal wall display the most wall thickening, which is confirmed on the graphs and color maps where the centerlines 1 through 13 and 76 through 100 display the most dynamic wall motion and thickening, while centerlines 26 through 51 display the worst wall motion, with centerlines 15 through 57 displaying the worst wall thickening. The nonconcordance is explained by tethering, a phenomenon that is best seen by CMR.

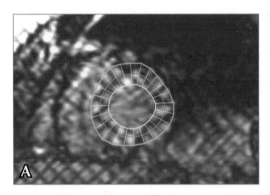

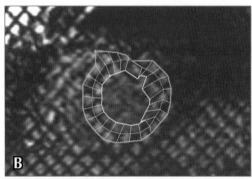

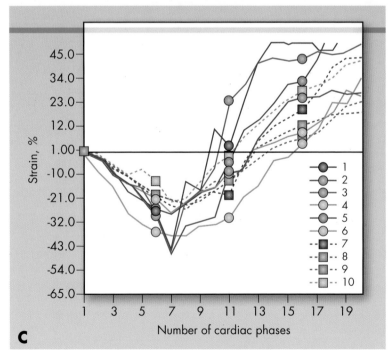

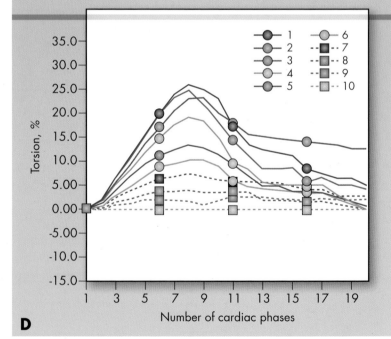

Figure 6-12. Myocardial tissue tagged images on short-axis slices are used for obtaining two- and three-dimensional strain and torsion. The end-systolic (**A**) and end-diastolic (**B**) endocardial and epicardial contours are drawn after loading these images via the HARP (harmonic phase) software package (Diagnosoft, Palo Alto, CA). This software gives phase by phase absolute strain as well as the rotation (torsion and untwisting) in two- and three-dimensional representations. **C**, Absolute three-dimensional strain of base to apical slices. **D**, Relative torsion of the apical slices in relation to the basal slices.

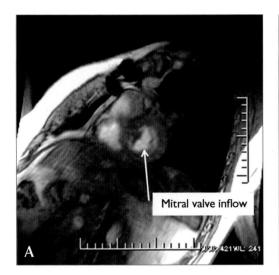

Mitral valve inflow

A

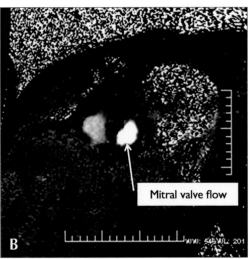

Mitral valve flow

B

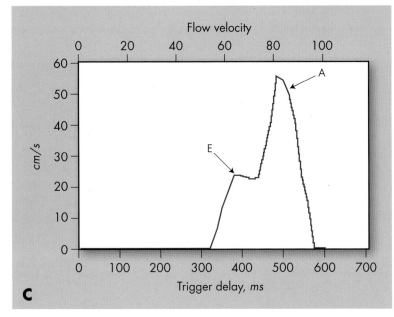

C

Figure 6-13. The diastolic function evaluation is critical for most routine cardiac studies. CMR, just like two-dimensional echocardiography, can evaluate diastolic function of the left or right ventricle. This example displays the evaluation of left ventricular (LV) diastolic function based on the mitral valve flow velocity analysis. **A**, A short-axis magnitude image of the LV base in which mitral valve inflow is clearly visualized. **B**, A phase velocity image at the similar position as the magnitude image and clearly showing mitral valve inflow. On the phase image (**B**), if contours are drawn on the mitral valve inflow, the diastolic flow velocities E and A can be assessed (**C**). In this particular case the E velocity was lower than the A velocity (E:A ratio < 1); therefore, based on these data, the patient had impaired relaxation. Also note that there is E-A fusion, which in this case is probably due to mild tachycardia (heart rate 100 bpm).

REFERENCES

1. Pohost GM, Meduri A, Razmi RM, *et al.*: Cardiac MR spectroscopy in the new millennium. *Rays* 2001, 26:93–107.

2. Kraitchman DL, Heldman AW, Atalar E, *et al.*: In vivo magnetic resonance imaging of mesenchymal stem cells in myocardial infarction. *Circulation* 2003, 107:2290–2293.

3. Rathi VK, Biederman RW: Imaging of ventricular function by cardiovascular magnetic resonance. *Curr Cardiol Rep* 2004, 6:55–61.

4. Bayes de Luna A, Wagner G, Birnbaum Y, *et al.*: A new terminology for left ventricular walls and location of myocardial infarcts that present Q wave based on the standard of cardiac magnetic resonance imaging: a statement for healthcare professionals from a committee appointed by the International Society for Holter and Noninvasive Electrocardiography. *Circulation* 2006, 114:1755–1760.

5. Solomon SD, Anavekar N, Skali H, *et al.*, for the Candesartan in Heart Failure Reduction in Mortality (CHARM) Investigators: Influence of ejection fraction on cardiovascular outcomes in a broad spectrum of heart failure patients. *Circulation* 2005, 112:3738–3744.

6. Devereux RB, Wachtell K, Gerdts E, *et al.*: Prognostic significance of left ventricular mass change during treatment of hypertension. *JAMA* 2004, 292:2350–2356.

7. Verdecchia P, Schillaci G, Borgioni C, *et al.*: Prognostic significance of serial changes in left ventricular mass in essential hypertension. *Circulation* 1998, 97:48–54.

8. Grothues F, Moon JC, Bellenger NG, *et al.*: Interstudy reproducibility of right ventricular volumes, function, and mass with cardiovascular magnetic resonance. *Am Heart J* 2004, 147:218–223.

7 CHAPTER

CMR and Myocardial Infarction

Evan Appelbaum

Prompt restoration of myocardial perfusion is critical to patient survival and long-term prognosis following acute myocardial infarction (MI) [1]. Early reperfusion strategies limit the infarction size and decrease the magnitude of left ventricular (LV) remodeling. Historically, the negative effects of remodeling after MI were detected at the bedside by physical signs of pump failure (*ie*, Killip classification). Adjunctive studies such as electrocardiography (ECG), radionuclide ventriculography, and two-dimensional echocardiography have aided in further defining prognosis after acute MI by identifying patients with adverse remodeling, who are at risk for heart failure, arrhythmia, and sudden death. With the advent of an array of therapeutic strategies that positively alter outcomes after acute MI, there has been a drive to identify high-risk patients as early as possible.

A comprehensive, noninvasive assessment of ventricular structure and function as an adjunct to coronary angiography is thus a desirable method for following patients after acute MI; however, routine echo and nuclear imaging methods have limitations. For instance, two-dimensional echocardiography is limited by the ability to obtain adequate acoustic windows, and nuclear imaging modalities

(single-photon emission computed tomography [SPECT] and positron emission tomography [PET]) fail to define LV mass and structure.

Cardiovascular magnetic resonance (CMR) has rapidly advanced to the forefront of noninvasive cardiac imaging because it accurately defines structure and function with high spatial and temporal resolution in one comprehensive imaging session [2]. Detailed cine images quantitatively measure LV and right ventricular (RV) size and function, including LV ejection fraction, LV mass, and LV and RV volumes. In addition, gadolinium contrast can be used to measure myocardial perfusion and infarction [3,4]. Late gadolinium enhancement (LGE) is a commonly used method of waiting 10 to 20 minutes after administration of the contrast before imaging, to create the greatest contrast between normal, signal-suppressed (dark) myocardium and nonviable infarct tissue, which appears hyperenhanced (bright) [5]. This technique has shown great promise in delineating infarct size, location, and composition (*ie*, homogeneous vs heterogeneous scar) [6,7]. More recently, LGE CMR has proven highly prognostic and may predict those at risk for arrhythmia and sudden death [8,9].

Goals for Noninvasive Imaging in Myocardial Infarction Care

Refining established measures of relevance

Function

Volume

Infarct size

Stunning/viability

Complications (eg, thrombus)

Developing new measures of relevance

Microvascular function/obstruction

Infarct shape and location

Border (peri-infarct) zone

Infarct shrinkage or remodeling

Edema

Benefits of Cardiovascular Magnetic Resonance After Myocardial Infarction

Noninvasive

No ionizing radiation

High spatial and temporal resolution

Comprehensive measurements with superior accuracy and reproducibility

Structure

Function

Infarct scar viability

Perfusion

Edema

Mechanistic probe

Prognostic importance

Figure 7-1. Goals for noninvasive imaging. Noninvasive imaging has historically played a significant role in prognostication following myocardial infarction (MI). Echocardiography is routinely used to confirm the impact of the event on ventricular function, to measure left ventricular ejection fraction (LVEF) and to detect-suspected complications of MI (eg, ventricular thrombus, myocardial rupture, cardiac tamponade, mitral regurgitation). Weeks to months following the index MI, echocardiography, radionuclide myocardial perfusion imaging, or both are used to assess left ventricular (LV) size and function, to detect postinfarct remodeling, and to assist in the prediction of future complications such as arrhythmia, recurrent MI, and sudden death. Currently, LVEF remains the most widely used noninvasive metric. For example, LVEF is an important consideration in targeting patients for medical therapies or devices that may improve longevity, such as angiotensin converting enzyme inhibitors, β blockers, and implantable cardioverter defibrillators.

Research efforts are focused on refining these standard measures both to develop more accurate and reproducible ways to assess LVEF, LV volumes, and LV mass and to establish new ways to more accurately predict outcome or response to therapy at very early stages of recovery (days to weeks post-MI). Infarct size, transmural extent, and residual myocardial viability have shown promise as predictors. In addition, many investigators have linked infarct shape (surface area) and composition (tissue heterogeneity) to post-MI arrhythmia and sudden death. Myocardial microvascular integrity (the degree of persistent microvascular obstruction following reperfusion) has demonstrated powerful, independent prognostic power. Future advances in infarct visualization using higher-resolution techniques will yield a more accurate description of infarct surface area, peri-infarct tissue heterogeneity, and infarct remodeling (involution). Moreover, improved detection of myocardial edema and hemorrhage may allow better insight into the mechanisms influencing prognosis.

Figure 7-2. Benefits of cardiovascular magnetic resonance (CMR). CMR is the most comprehensive noninvasive imaging technique available to assess patients following myocardial infarction. It avoids the potential risks of exposure to ionizing radiation or iodinated contrast, that occur in computed tomography (CT) or nuclear perfusion imaging. CMR maintains high spatial and temporal resolution and can therefore depict myocardial structure and function in great detail. It is a true volumetric technique, avoiding geometric assumptions, and thereby provide superior accuracy and reproducibility. Measures such as ventricular volumes, ejection fraction, ventricular mass, infarct size, and myocardial viability have become standardized with CMR availability at thousands of centers worldwide. Because of these many attributes, CMR imaging has become the gold standard for the determination of both left ventricular ejection fraction (LVEF) and infarct size, two critical measurements for infarct survivors [5,10]. Additionally, CMR imaging has led the research world in the identification of measures such as microvascular obstruction, myocardial viability, peri-infarct tissue heterogeneity, and infarct surface area [7,8,11–13]. It has become a powerful tool in clinical trials: many active research protocols use CMR-derived LV function or infarct size as primary endpoints. Recent safety concerns regarding the association of gadolinium-based MR contrast and nephrogenic systemic fibrosis (NSF) are noteworthy [14–16]. As always, judicious use of exogenous MR contrast should be employed, particularly for those with kidney disease or on dialysis. Modern coronary artery, carotid artery, and aortic stainless steel stents (including drug-coated stents) are safe in magnetic fields of 1.5 to 3.0 Tesla, and are not a contraindication to CMR or MRI in general [17]. The safety of MRI has been demonstrated within hours of stent implantation.

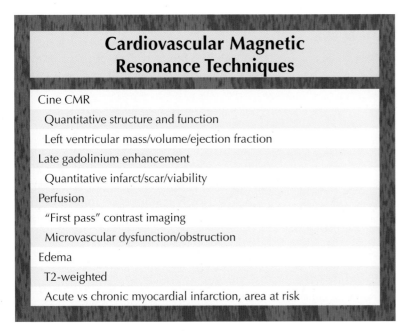

Cardiovascular Magnetic Resonance Techniques

Cine CMR

  Quantitative structure and function

  Left ventricular mass/volume/ejection fraction

Late gadolinium enhancement

  Quantitative infarct/scar/viability

Perfusion

  "First pass" contrast imaging

  Microvascular dysfunction/obstruction

Edema

  T2-weighted

  Acute vs chronic myocardial infarction, area at risk

Figure 7-3. Cardiovascular magnetic resonance (CMR) imaging techniques. The comprehensive CMR examination following myocardial infarction (MI) includes multiple sequences and techniques. A comprehensive CMR scan may be accomplished in 45 minutes. Some components require no contrast, but others (*eg,* late gadolinium enhancement [LGE] infarct imaging) depend on contrast for an adequate contrast-to-noise ratio. Generally, after a three-plane scout image is obtained, a breath-hold sequence using steady-state free precession without exogenous contrast is used for cine ventricular function and serves as the basis for a volumetric assessment of ventricular volumes, ejection fraction, and mass. These data are acquired in short-axis stack and long-axis orientations. This technique also allows for direct assessment (either qualitative or quantitative) of regional systolic function in the standard 17-segment model. Before the addition of exogenous contrast, myocardial edema can be assessed using a T2-weighted, breath-hold sequence in the same short-axis stack orientation as the cine images (for slice matching). Regional and global myocardial edema can then be calculated and related to functional measures. Next, the intravenous injection of 0.05 to 0.1 mmol per kilogram of gadolinium diethylenetriamine penta-acetic acid (DTPA) allows for first-pass measurement of myocardial perfusion. This can be accomplished at rest or with vasodilator stress to assess persistent perfusion deficits following reperfused MI. Three to five short-axis slices (matching basal, middle, and apical cine slices) are obtained with a sustained breath-hold (15–20 seconds on average). If resting images are performed within the first few days of successful percutaneous coronary intervention (*ie,* when the epicardial vessel is known to be patent), then any resting perfusion defect in the infarct territory is likely to be persistent microvascular dysfunction, as the epicardial vessel is known to be patent. Semiquantitative measures of myocardial perfusion can be measured by plotting myocardial signal intensity over time. Immediately following myocardial perfusion imaging, the remaining CMR contrast is given, to a total dose of 0.2 mmol per kilogram. LGE images (allowing time for contrast equilibration) are obtained 10 to 20 minutes later (allowing time for contrast equilibration) and are used to measure infarct size. They are taken in the same short-axis stack orientation as the cine images (slices matched for comparison) and are again obtained with a breath-hold. Areas of LGE depict an irreversible injury, and quantification of these areas can accurately reveal how much infarct size.

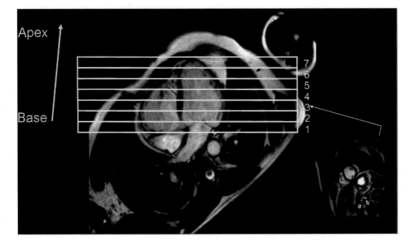

Figure 7-4. Cardiovascular magnetic resonance (CMR) anatomy. CMR imaging accurately defines cardiac anatomy, structure, and function. The operator can obtain images in any plane desired, but most commonly obtains echocardiographic and nuclear cardiology views. A four-chamber still frame from a cine image is chosen to determine the true short axis of the left ventricle (LV). Then, the LV is segmented or sliced (the "bread loaf") into a stack of contiguous short-axis slices for volumetric assessment. At the bottom right, one sample image of a short-axis, end-diastolic frame at mid-ventricle is depicted. This stack of short-axis cines is then analyzed using summation of discs to determine measures such as LV ejection fraction, LV volumes, and LV mass. Other orientations such as two-chamber, horizontal long-axis, and LV outflow tract views also are routinely used.

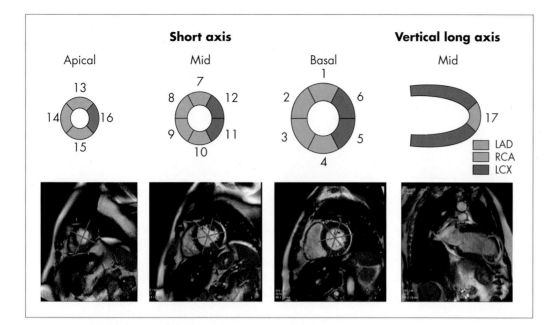

Short axis

Apical   Mid   Basal

Vertical long axis

Mid

LAD
RCA
LCX

Figure 7-5. Cardiovascular magnetic resonance (CMR) anatomy 17-segment model. The standard 17-segment model is used to locate and describe regional ventricular systolic function during assessment following myocardial infarction. As shown here, the distal/apical, middle, and basal portions of the left ventricle can be segmented by this convention; in the long axis, the true apex can be evaluated. One can then qualitatively describe regional kinesis of each segment (*ie*, normokinetic, hypokinetic, akinetic, dyskinetic). A more quantitative assessment can be provided by calculation of regional motion or thickening using a center-line method. LAD—left anterior descending artery; LCX—left circumflex coronary artery; RCA—right coronary artery.

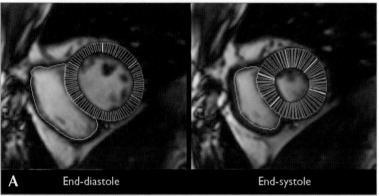

A   End-diastole   End-systole

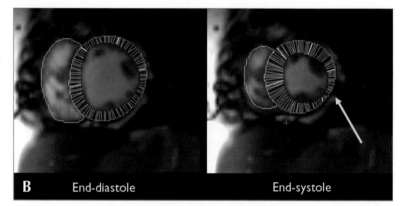

B   End-diastole   End-systole

Figure 7-6. **A** and **B**, Regional left ventricular thickening. Quantitative regional function can be easily measured using end-diastolic (ED) and end-systolic (ES) frames, as shown here. The degree of absolute segment thickening from ED to ES along a centerline (measured in millimeters or centimeters) by region is often termed *motion*. A relative measure (a ratio of motion in a region of interest to the maximal motion of a remote, noninfarcted region) is called *thickening* or *percent thickening*. **A**, This example of normal regional systolic function is midventricular. **B**, A patient with a lateral myocardial infarction demonstrates ED relative thinning and abnormal systolic function in the ES frame (*arrow*). This is an area of hypokinesis with minimal thickening of the chords in the lateral wall.

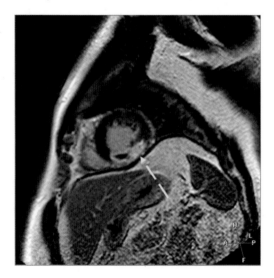

Figure 7-7. Cardiovascular magnetic resonance (CMR) with late gadolinium enhancement (LGE). LGE uses the addition of an extracellular CMR agent, often gadolinium diethylenetriamine penta-acetic acid, and has been shown to depict myocardial necrosis and scarring following myocardial infarction. The most common approach is to use a breath-hold, inversion recovery sequence. Imaging 10 to 20 minutes following injection of 0.1 to 0.2 mmol/kg of contrast depicts nonviable muscle as hyperenhanced (bright white, *arrow*). Areas of microvascular obstruction can be detected on LGE images and will appear hypoenhanced (dark black) within the surrounding zone of bright, infarcted myocardium.

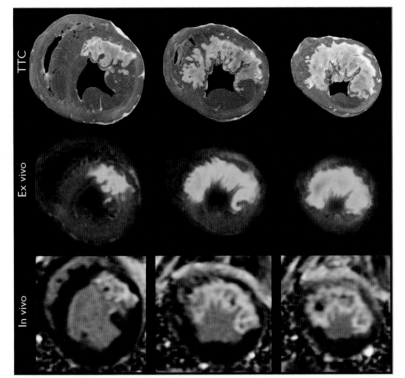

Figure 7-8. Irreversible injury, nonviable tissue. Several animal studies have demonstrated that hyperenhancement on late gadolinium enhancement (LGE) imaging represents only nonviable tissue [5]. Shown here is a near-perfect match between nonviable tissue demonstrated by triphenyltetrazolium chloride (TTC) staining at necropsy in a canine model of a left anterior descending artery infarct and LGE images of the same slices. The concept that LGE depicts only nonviable myocardium has been challenged, as uniformly reproducible data has indicated that LGE volume decreases from the acute phase (first few weeks after myocardial infarction) to the chronic phase (weeks to months later). Currently, most data support the nonviability principle and suggest that time-related infarct changes are due to infarct shrinkage (involution) and remodeling rather than resolution of myocardial edema (overestimation of baseline infarct size). Therefore, LGE does not include surrounding areas of edema or dysfunctional but viable myocardium and allows for a true viability assessment [6]. (*From* Hsu and Glover [5]; with permission.)

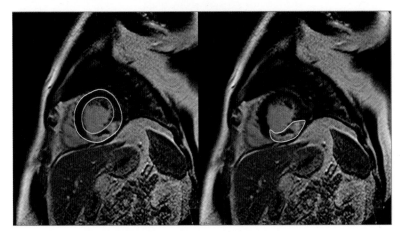

Figure 7-9. Quantification of myocardial infarction by cardiovascular magnetic resonance (CMR). Because of the high spatial resolution and the inherent volumetric technique of CMR imaging using late gadolinium enhancement (LGE), infarct size can readily be quantified. Moreover, CMR LGE technique has now become the gold standard for measurement of infarct size. After the acquisition of an entire short-axis left ventricular (LV) stack

using LGE, planimetry of LGE-positive (hyperenhanced) areas can be performed. Summing the areas of LGE across the entire LV stack using summation of discs (similar to the measurement of LV ejection fraction), a volume of LGE or infarct volume can be calculated. The volume can then be multiplied by the density of myocardium (1.05 g/mL) to determine absolute infarct weight or size. Infarct size can be normalized to LV volume to mass. The latter method, dividing the infarct size by the myocardial mass, yields the percentage of LV that is infarct. In general, small myocardial infarctions are less than 10% of the LV, intermediate-size infarcts are between 10% and 25%, and large infarcts are greater than 25%. For more reproducible measures of infarct size, thresholding techniques are recommended. These include: 1) 2 SD above the mean signal intensity for normal remote myocardium (above this threshold is infarcted tissue), or 2) half maximum (1/2 max), which depicts infarct as those pixels that are greater than or equal to one half the maximal signal of the brightest pixel in the myocardium. (This method requires that visually some infarct needs to be present to be set as the reference.) Thresholding techniques are suggested when studying therapies that may limit infarct size or affect infarct remodeling over time [6].

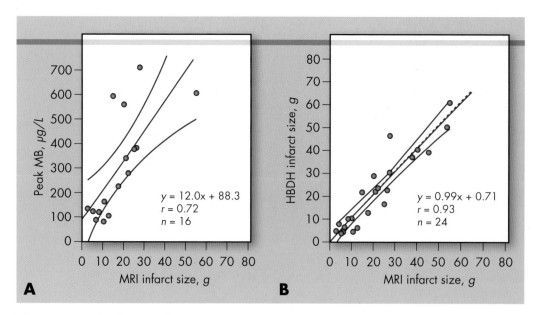

Figure 7-10. Cardiovascular magnetic resonance (CMR) myocardial infarct (MI) size correlates with cardiac enzyme release. In addition to animal-based histology correlation, CMR infarct size has been shown to match well with other standard clinical methods for estimating infarct size. As shown here, CMR infarct size strongly correlates with cardiac enzyme release in the setting of the acute MI. **A,** The linear relationship of infarct size shown by CMR to peak isoenzyme of creatine kinase with muscle and brain subunits (CK-MB) in humans with acute MI demonstrates a good correlation with absolute infarct size. **B,** A human study shows a near-perfect relationship between a quantitative infarct enzyme released in the serum (α-hydroxybutyrate dehydrogenase [HBDH]) and infarct size measured by CMR. Many studies have also shown tight correlations between CMR infarct size and total creatine phosphokinase (CPK) or cardiac troponins. In the author's experience, a peak CPK release of less than 1000 µg/L depicts a small infarct (< 10% LV infarct); 1000 to 3000 µg/L indicates an intermediate-size infarct (10%–25% LV infarct), and more than 3000 µg/L indicates a large infarct (> 25% LV infarct). (*From* Holman *et al.* [18]; with permission.)

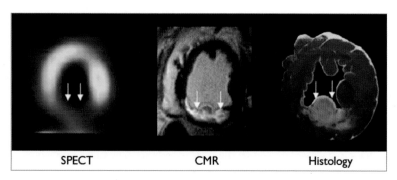

Figure 7-11. Myocardial infarct size on cardiovascular magnetic resonance (CMR) imaging correlates with size on nuclear imaging. Infarct size using late gadolinium enhancement (LGE) CMR correlates well with nuclear myocardial perfusion imaging (thallium or technetium single-photon emission computed tomography [SPECT]). Shown here is a nontransmural inferior myocardial infarction (*arrows*) in a canine model as depicted in a short-axis slice by technetium SPECT, CMR LGE, and triphenyltetrazolium chloride (TTC) staining at necropsy. Visually, there is agreement between methods. However, given the higher spatial resolution of CMR, LGE images more closely resemble the true histologic architecture. On the SPECT image, much of the detail is lost to partial volume effect. This inherent difference leads to SPECT overestimation of infarct size for large infarcts and underestimation of small, subendocardial infarcts (*see* Fig. 7-12). (*From* Wagner *et al.* [19]; with permission.)

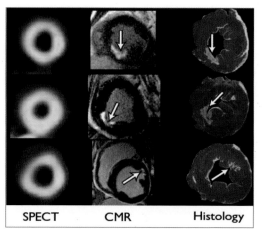

Figure 7-12. Subendocardial myocardial infarction depicted by cardiovascular magnetic resonance (CMR) imaging versus single-photon emission computed tomography (SPECT). Partial volume effect is responsible for false-negative scans using SPECT imaging for small, subendocardial infarctions. In this canine model, all three SPECT images appear normal, whereas the CMR images (with late gadolinium enhancement [LGE]) demonstrate small areas (*arrows*) of subendocardial hyperenhancement that correlate very well with histologic triphenyltetrazolium chloride staining. LGE CMR is a highly sensitive technique that has been shown to be able to detect less than 1 g of infarct tissue. (*From* Wagner *et al.* [19]; with permission.)

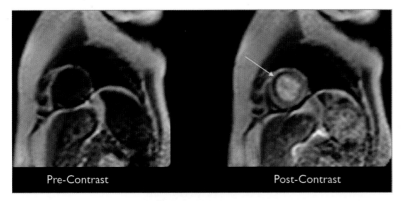

Pre-Contrast   Post-Contrast

Figure 7-13. First-pass myocardial perfusion shown by cardio-vascular magnetic resonance (CMR). Gadolinium-diethylenetri-amine penta-acetic acid is an extracellular contrast agent. Its first pass through the myocardium can reflect its early, intravascular phase. This can be performed at rest, to detect microvascular obstruction, or with vasodilatation, to detect residual ischemia after myocardial infarction. Relative myocardial perfusion can be estimated qualitatively by visual inspection: dark, hypoenhanced areas of attenuated signal reflect hypoperfusion. Semiquantitative perfusion measures require plotting myocardial signal intensity versus time curves and calculating peak enhancement, maximum upslope, or time to peak enhancement. These values may be quoted directly, or often a ratio comparing the segments of interest with a normal, remote segment (so-called relative perfusion) is calculated. Absolute myocardial perfusion and perfusion reserve may be measured.

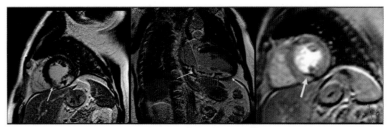

Figure 7-14. Microvascular obstruction (MO) by resting first-pass perfusion (FPP). **Left**, The late gadolinium enhancement (LGE) images show a transmural inferior myocardial infarction (MI). **Right**, Associated MO may be detected on FPP. A few days after reperfusion with successful percutaneous intervention (and assuming the epicardial vessel is patent to the territory of interest), resting FPP can detect persistent MO. Persistent MO is depicted visually by dark areas with (relative hypoenhancement) within the infarct zone. There are no set criteria to define MO by semiquantitative means; some investigators have used a cutoff of less than 50% corrected peak enhancement of a normal, remote territory (for baseline signal-intensity differences by region). Areas of more subtle microvascular dysfunction may escape visual inspection and require definition using semiquantitative or quantitative techniques.

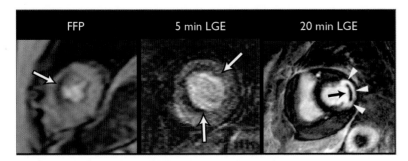

FFP   5 min LGE   20 min LGE

Figure 7-15. Microvascular obstruction (MO) depicted on first-pass perfusion (FPP) versus early and late gadolinium enhancement (LGE). Persistent MO following reperfused myocardial infarction (MI) has been best characterized using FPP. However, some investigators believe that hypoenhancement within the infarct zone ("infarct coring") on LGE imaging may also reflect MO, in the form of a static (single-phase) measurement rather than the dynamic

(cine) measurement seen on FPP. The presence of MO (hypoen-hancement) is most often assessed visually. To quantify MO, either visual planimetry or thresholding (the volume of myocardium within the infarct zone that is less than half the maximum signal intensity that defines infarct/fibrosis) can be used. Some authors have demonstrated that an early LGE infarct image (5 minutes after gadolinium-diethylenetriamine penta-acetic acid injection) may enhance detection of MO by imaging before extravascular equilib-rium is achieved. In this author's experience, however, standard (10–20 min) LGE imaging has an adequate contrast-to-noise ratio for MO assessment. The benefits of measuring MO on LGE images are 1) size and transmural extent of MO may be measured more easily than with lower-resolution FPP images, and 2) MO can be assessed on the same images as infarct size, obviating cumbersome FPP imaging. The downside of measuring MO on LGE images is that these data are derived from a static scan, so subtle differences in myocardial perfusion cannot be fully appreciated.

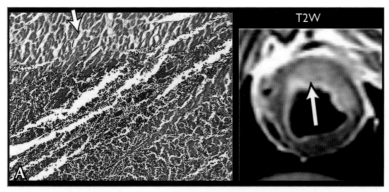

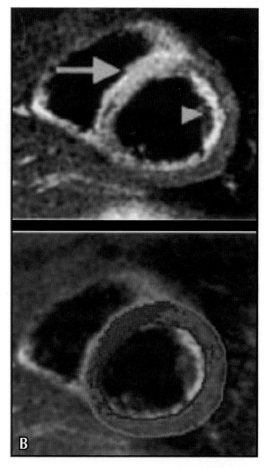

Figure 7-16. T2-weighted images and myocardial edema. **A,** Acute myocardial infarction (MI) produces a heterogeneous environment with components of necrosis, inflammation, and edema. On a microscopic view of myocardial edema following MI, myocardial edema (*arrow*) extends beyond the area of necrosis and encompasses ischemic tissue that is viable [20]. Using T2-weighted imaging (without exogenous contrast), cardiovascular magnetic resonance (CMR) can detect and quantify this area of edema. The edematous tissue is represented by high-signal (bright) myocardium (*arrow*). **B,** Quantification of myocardial edema. Quantification of myocardial edema on T2-weighted CMR can be determined visually (aided by visual references outside of the heart [*eg,* liver, spleen] for relative signal), or the signal intensity (SI) can be measured directly with comparison to normal, remote myocardial regions using thresholding techniques. The most common thresholds are either 2 SD above the mean SI of normal myocardium or half the maximum. These allow more reproducible quantification of edematous tissue. On this image, the *red area* depicts positive edema by half maximum threshold. The amount of edematous tissue is routinely quoted in either grams or milliliters and often is related to left ventricular (LV) volume (similar to infarct size), quoted

as percent LV edema. It has also been shown that T2-weighted CMR assessment of myocardial edema correlates well with the true ischemic area at risk. This metric may be beneficial in estimating the degree of myocardial salvage for a given reperfusion strategy. (*From* Stork *et al.* [20]; with permission.)

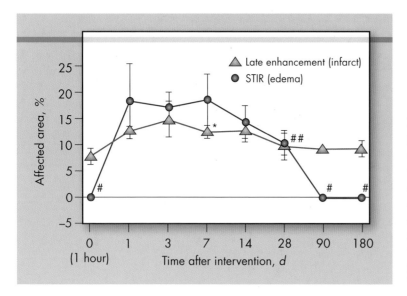

Figure 7-17. Duration of myocardial edema following myocardial infarction. T2-weighted cardiovascular magnetic resonance (CMR) following myocardial infarction can accurately determine the acuity of the event. Myocardial edema arising from ischemia or infarct will diminish or resolve within 3 to 4 weeks after the acute phase. Therefore it is recommended to image patients within a week of their clinical event to detect the maximal extent of edema. Knowledge of this temporal relationship can help determine whether the myocardial infarction is acute or chronic. The short TI inversion recovery (STIR) images on the graph are equivalent to T2-weighted images. (*From* Stork *et al.* [20]; with permission.)

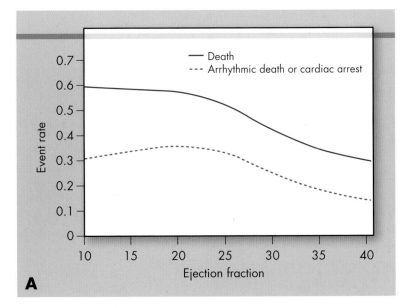

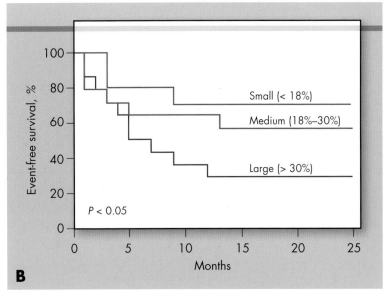

Figure 7-18. **A** and **B**, Left ventricular ejection fraction (LVEF), infarct size, and prognosis. For decades, survivors of myocardial infarction (MI) have been treated based on measurement of post-MI LVEF. **A**, This graph demonstrates the powerful prognostic power of LVEF for overall mortality and arrhythmic death. Data such as these from the Multicenter Unsustained Tachycardia Trial (MUSTT) demonstrate that LVEF best predicts outcomes at lower limits, driven by pump failure and congestive heart failure. As LVEF rises, the mechanism of death shifts towards arrhythmia or sudden death. The current standard of care for treatment of MI has greatly improved outcome. Cardiac failure and low LVEF are increasingly less common, and survivors of MI are more often faced with the risk of sudden death. Therefore, LVEF may not reflect true risk. Increasing data suggest that measures of infarct size and architecture using cardiac magnetic resonance (CMR) may be more important than LVEF [7,11]. (*From* Buxton *et al.* [21]; with permission.) **B**, This graph shows that infarct size on late gadolinium-enhanced CMR (by tertiles of percent left ventricular infarct) has a strong relationship to outcome. (*From* Wu *et al.* [11]; with permission.)

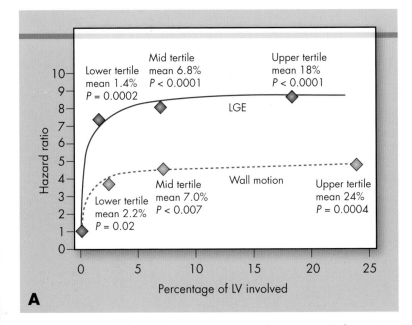

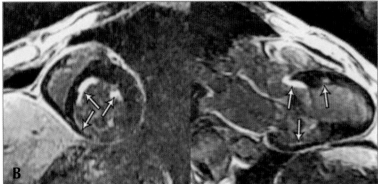

Figure 7-19. **A** and **B**, Infarct presence and outcome. Infarct size has been shown to be a potent predictor of outcome, but even very small infarcts can have devastating consequences. **A**, The presence of scar of any size in subjects with coronary artery disease appears to be a powerful determinant of outcome, even more so than wall motion or infarct size. **B**, Cardiac magnetic resonance late gadolinium enhancement (LGE) images of two such patients, who suffered sudden death despite very small areas of infarct (*arrows*). LV—left ventricle. (*From* Kwong *et al.* [9]; with permission.)

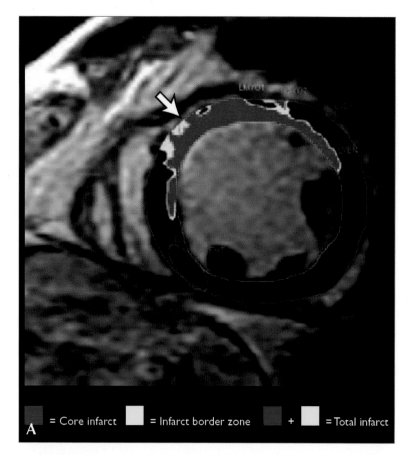

= Core infarct = Infarct border zone + = Total infarct

A

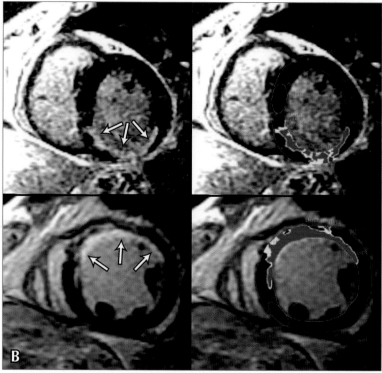

B

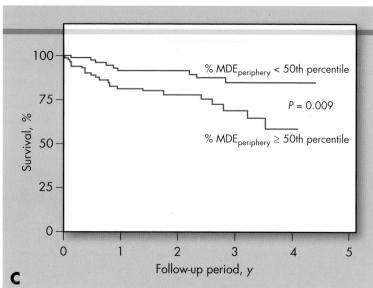

C

Figure 7-20. Infarct architecture: peri-infarct or border zone. In the first year following myocardial infarction, 5% to 10% of survivors will die suddenly. Ventricular tachycardia (VT) is the most common cause of sudden death in these survivors and can occur in those with preserved cardiac function and small areas of ventricular scar. Electrical reentry within scar tissue serves as the basis for VT. Areas at the infarct periphery with a mixture of viable and nonviable "islands" of myocardium appear to be the most likely location for reentrant rhythms to take place. Cardiac magnetic resonance with late gadolinium enhancement (LGE) is able to detect and quantify peri-infarct tissue that is heterogeneous. Myocardium of mixed viability has a signal intensity by LGE that is intermediate between normal muscle and homogeneous scar. **A,** LGE can identify both types of tissue: homogeneous septal/anterior scar ("core infarct") (*red*), with a higher signal intensity, and heterogeneous scar ("border zone") (*yellow*), with intermediate signal intensity. On LGE images, normal tissue appears black (nulled). **B,** Two examples of identification of border zone versus infarct. *Left,* The border zone is identified as bright white on LGE images. The *arrows* show an inferior infarct (*top*) and an anterior infarct (*bottom*). *Right,* Detection of border zone (*yellow*) and core infarct (*red*). Just as with infarct size, border zone may be quantified and reported by either absolute mass (grams), percentage of left ventricle that is border zone (% LV border zone), or relative to the entire sum of the total homogeneous and heterogeneous infarct, calculated as border zone (g) divided by the sum of the border zone (g) plus infarct (g) times 100 (% infarct that is border zone). The last method corrects for differences solely due to infarct size. **C,** Identification and quantification of peri-infarct tissue heterogeneity in the border zone has shown promise as a determinant of survival following MI. In this study [7], a border zone (% $MDE_{periphery}$) at or above the 50th percentile represented a border zone that comprised at least 25% of the total infarct. MDE—myocardial delayed enhancement. (*From* Yan *et al.* [7]; with permission.)

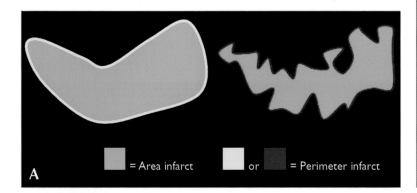

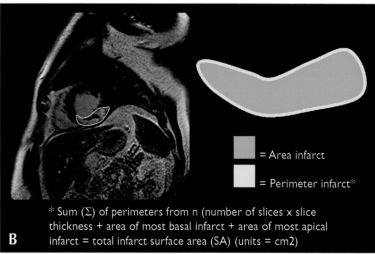

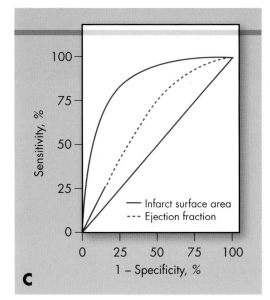

Figure 7-21. Infarct architecture: infarct perimeter and surface area. In addition to the complexity of the peri-infarct zone, core infarct architecture itself may provide insight into arrhythmic potential and outcome. **A,** A three-dimensional infarct of any given size can have an array of shapes, ranging from a very smooth surface to one full of crypts and curves. The area of the infarct size is similar for both the left and right images but the infarct perimeter is much greater with an irregular shape. **B,** Cardiovascular magnetic resonance with late gadolinium enhancement is able to determine and quantify infarct architecture by planimetry. The infarct perimeter (*yellow*) may be easily translated into infarct surface area (*green*) across slices. Directly measuring the surface area or perimeter of an infarct has also been linked to inducibility of ventricular arrhythmias (a surrogate for risk of sudden death). **C,** Receiver operator characteristic curves for infarct surface area versus left ventricular ejection fraction for inducibility of ventricular tachycardia in patients with a prior myocardial infarction suggest that infarct surface area is a better predictor. To what degree infarct size, peri-infarct zone, and infarct architecture interact or act independently in outcome remains to be studied. (Panel **C** *from* Bello *et al.* [13]; with permission.)

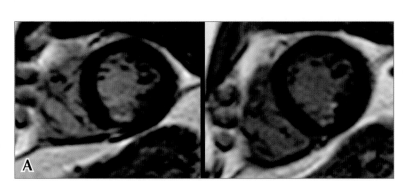

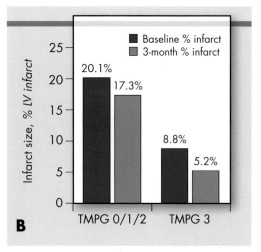

Figure 7-22. A and **B,** Infarct involution and remodeling. Studies using serial cardiovascular magnetic resonance with late gadolinium enhancement (CMR LGE) following acute myocardial infarction (MI) have provided great insight into the process of scar maturation and healing (infarct remodeling). MI size decreases from a maximum found in the acute phase (first few days) to a minimum by 4 to 6 weeks. **A,** At *left* is a small inferior infarct by seen by CMR LGE 3 days after primary percutaneous intervention. At *right* is an LGE image of the same slice 3 months later. Note the significant decrease in the area of LGE over time [6,22,23]. This observation was initially thought to reflect resolu-

tion of myocardial edema, but it is now well established that LGE, at any post-MI stage, reflects nonviable tissue. Therefore, infarct regression over time is a result of tissue involution and remodeling. **B,** What determines the magnitude of infarct remodeling? Microvascular patency following reperfusion is an important determinant of the degree of infarct remodeling. This graph shows a twofold to threefold greater relative decrease in infarct size (% left ventricular [LV] infarct) over 3 months after MI if the microvascular function remains normal, as indicated by TIMI (thrombolysis in MI) myocardial perfusion grade (TMPG) 3, normal angiographic blush [24].

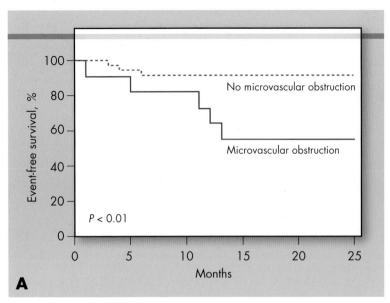

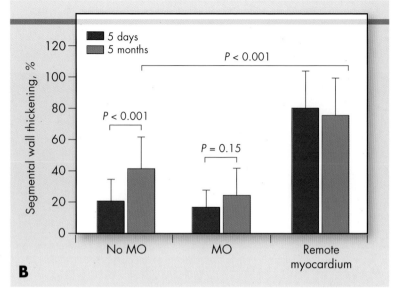

Figure 7-23. A and **B**, Microvascular obstruction (MO) and outcome. Myocardial reperfusion in the setting of acute myocardial infarction (MI) is a complex process that requires not only restoration of flow in large, epicardial coronary arteries but also tissue-level perfusion with patent microvasculature. Coronary angiographic data clearly demonstrate poor outcomes in patients with abnormal myocardial blush despite normal epicardial flow. **A**, Persistent MO within days of reperfused MI can be detected by cardiovascular magnetic resonance using either first-pass perfusion or late gadolinium enhancement techniques. The presence of persistent MO in this population predicts a worse prognosis, independent of left ventricular ejection fraction or infarct size. **B**, Ventricular function and remodeling are directly affected. Dysfunctional myocardial segments without MO show improved segmental wall thickening at follow-up, but function remained impaired compared with remote myocardium. (**A**, *from* Wu *et al.* [11]; with permission. **B**, *from* Baks *et al.* [23]; with permission.)

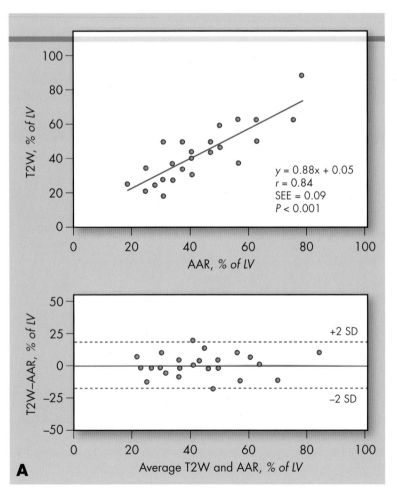

Figure 7-24. Area at risk (AAR) and T2-weighted cardiovascular magnetic resonance (T2W CMR). Myocardial ischemia may result in either myocyte injury with retained viability or myocyte death. Myocardial edema will accompany both processes in the acute phase and therefore reflects the territory or AAR. **A**, T2W CMR shows good correlation with the AAR measured by using injected microspheres in an animal model of left ventricular (LV) infarct and reperfusion. T2W CMR requires no exogenous contrast (gadolinium) and can detect myocardial edema that accurately reflects the AAR.

Continued on the next page

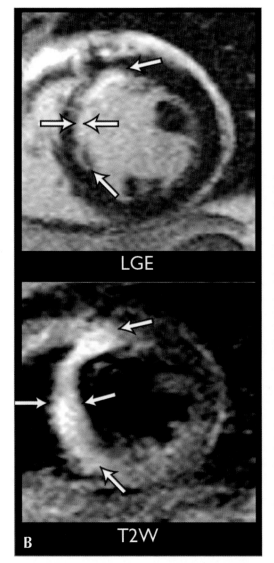

LGE

T2W

B

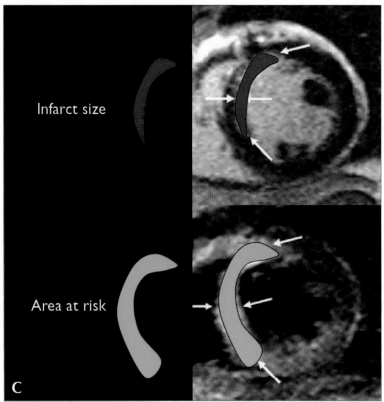

Infarct size

Area at risk

C

Figure 7-24. *(Continued)* **B**, *Top*, a standard short-axis late gadolinium enhancement (LGE) image with an anteroseptal infarct (*bright area, arrows*). *Bottom*, a short-axis T2W edema image of the same slice, with a much larger area of brightness from high T2 signal secondary to edema (*arrows*). **C**, How each area can be quantified: *top*, area of infarct (*red*) shown by LGE; *bottom*, edema (AAR) (*green*). A comparison of the size of the AAR and the infarct may provide understanding of the degree or magnitude of salvage that a particular reperfusion strategy has provided. Quantifying myocardial salvage: T2W CMR detection of myocardial edema may also determine the age of an infarct. As myocardial edema secondary to ischemia completely resolves by 4 weeks after myocardial infarction (MI), the presence of edema suggests a recent infarct. This method is more accurate for determining infarct age than CMR detection of MO, wall thinning, or LGE infarct size. The CMR profile of an acute MI (*left*) and chronic MI (*right*) in the same patient imaged 6 weeks apart. Notice the larger LGE area (*top row*) and even larger area of T2W CMR edema (*middle row*). The *bottom row* shows quantity of edema (*red*) in the acute phase, compared with the smaller infarct size (involution) and absence of edema in the chronic phase. (**A**, *from* Aletras *et al.* [25]; with permission. **B** and **C**, *from* Stork *et al.* [20, 26]; with permission.) SEE—standard error of the estimate.

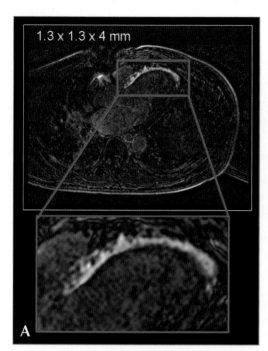
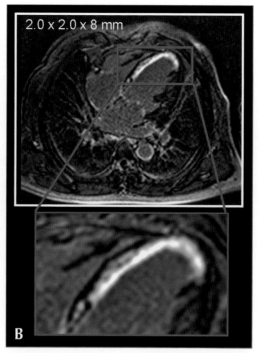

Figure 7-25. A and **B**, Future directions: high-resolution infarct imaging. Despite the advances that cardiovascular magnetic resonance (CMR) has already provided for the assessment of myocardial infarction, this technique continues to grow. Improvements in hardware, higher field strength (3 Tesla and beyond), postprocessing advances, and novel contrast agents have increased the potential for this comprehensive imaging modality. High-resolution infarct imaging remains one of the most exciting areas of research. Measurements such as infarct shape and border zone have microscopic features that are underappreciated by current standards in spatial resolution. High-resolution CMR may significantly limit the negative impact of the partial volume effect, enabling more detailed evaluations of all structures of interest. **A**, An ex vivo (animal) CMR image using late gadolinium enhancement (LGE) with a standard slice thickness (8 mm), depicting a septal infarct *(bottom)*. The arrows at the infarct edges note areas of intermediate signal intensity where architecture remains unclear. By reducing the through-plane spatial resolution (0.5 mm slice thickness), one can see the detail at the infarct edges quite easily, avoiding sample averaging and partial volume effect. **B**, An LGE long-axis view with a septal and apical infarct in a patient with acute myocardial infarction, at high resolution *(top)* and standard resolution *(bottom)*. Note the detail of infarct architecture that is appreciated on the high-resolution image but "smoothed out" on the lower-resolution image because of partial volume averaging. Early evidence shows that higher-resolution imaging may not alter estimation of infarct size but may improve the accuracy of measures of infarct surface area and border zone. The true value of high-resolution infarct imaging remains to be fully appreciated. (*Courtesy of* Dana C. Peters, PhD.)

REFERENCES

1. Gibson CM: Time is myocardium and time is outcomes. *Circulation* 2001, 104:2632–2634.

2. Laddis T, Manning WJ, Danias PG: Cardiac MRI for assessment of myocardial perfusion: current status and future perspectives. *J Nucl Cardiol* 2001, 8:207–214.

3. Van Rossum AC, Visser FC, Van Eenige MJ, *et al.*: Value of gadolinium-diethylene-triamine pentaacetic acid dynamics in magnetic resonance imaging of acute myocardial infarction with occluded and reperfused coronary arteries after thrombolysis. *Am J Cardiol* 1990, 65:845–851.

4. van Dijkman PR, van der Wall EE, de Roos A, *et al.*: Gadolinium-enhanced magnetic resonance imaging in acute myocardial infarction. *Eur J Radiol* 1990, 11:1–9.

5. Hsu JJ, Glover GH: Rapid MRI method for mapping the longitudinal relaxation time. *J Magn Reson* 2006, 181:98–106.

6. Ingkanisorn WP, Rhoads KL, Aletras AH, *et al.*: Gadolinium delayed enhancement cardiovascular magnetic resonance correlates with clinical measures of myocardial infarction. *J Am Coll Cardiol* 2004, 43:2253–2259.

7. Yan AT, Shayne AJ, Brown KA, *et al.*: Characterization of the peri-infarct zone by contrast-enhanced cardiac magnetic resonance imaging is a powerful predictor of post-myocardial infarction mortality. *Circulation* 2006, 114:32–39.

8. Schmidt A, Azevedo CF, Cheng A, *et al.*: Infarct tissue heterogeneity by magnetic resonance imaging identifies enhanced cardiac arrhythmia susceptibility in patients with left ventricular dysfunction. *Circulation* 2007, 115:2006–2014.

9. Kwong RY, Chan AK, Brown KA, *et al.*: Impact of unrecognized myocardial scar detected by cardiac magnetic resonance imaging on event-free survival in patients presenting with signs or symptoms of coronary artery disease. *Circulation* 2006, 113:2733–2743.

10. Salton CJ, Chuang ML, O'Donnell CJ, *et al.*: Gender differences and normal left ventricular anatomy in an adult population free of hypertension. A cardiovascular magnetic resonance study of the Framingham Heart Study Offspring cohort. *J Am Coll Cardiol* 2002, 39:1055–1060.

11. Wu KC, Zerhouni EA, Judd RM, *et al.*: Prognostic significance of microvascular obstruction by magnetic resonance imaging in patients with acute myocardial infarction. *Circulation* 1998, 97:765–772.

12. Kim RJ, Wu E, Rafael A, *et al.*: The use of contrast-enhanced magnetic resonance imaging to identify reversible myocardial dysfunction. *N Engl J Med* 2000, 343:1445–1453.

13. Bello D, Fieno DS, Kim RJ, *et al.*: Infarct morphology identifies patients with substrate for sustained ventricular tachycardia. *J Am Coll Cardiol* 2005, 45:1104–1108.

14. Collidge TA, Thomson PC, Mark PB, *et al.*: Gadolinium-enhanced MR imaging and nephrogenic systemic fibrosis: retrospective study of a renal replacement therapy cohort. *Radiology* 2007, 245:168–175.

15. Sadowski EA, Bennett LK, Chan MR, *et al.*: Nephrogenic systemic fibrosis: risk factors and incidence estimation. *Radiology* 2007, 243:148–157.

16. Kuo PH, Kanal E, Abu-Alfa AK, Cowper SE: Gadolinium-based MR contrast agents and nephrogenic systemic fibrosis. *Radiology* 2007, 242:647–649.

17. Gerber TC, Fasseas P, Lennon RJ, *et al.*: Clinical safety of magnetic resonance imaging early after coronary artery stent placement. *J Am Coll Cardiol* 2003, 42:1295–1298.

18. Holman ER, von Jonbergen HP, van Dijkman PR, *et al.*: Comparison of magnetic resonance imaging studies with enzymatic indexes of myocardial necrosis for quantification of myocardial infarct size. *Am J Cardiol* 1993, 71:1036–1040.

19. Wagner A, Mahrholdt H, Holly TA, *et al.*: Contrast-enhanced MRI and routine single photon emission computed tomography (SPECT) perfusion imaging for detection of subendocardial myocardial infarcts: an imaging study. *Lancet* 2003, 361:374–379.

20. Stork A, Muellerleile K, Bansmann PM, *et al.*: Value of T2-weighted, first-pass and delayed enhancement, and cine CMR to differentiate between acute and chronic myocardial infarction. *Eur Radiol* 2007, 17:610–617.

21. Buxton AE, Lee KL, Hafley GE, *et al.*: Relation of ejection fraction and inducible ventricular tachycardia to mode of death in patients with coronary artery disease: an analysis of patients enrolled in the multicenter unsustained tachycardia trial. *Circulation* 2002, 106:2466–2472.

22. Saeed M, Lee RJ, Weber O, *et al.*: Scarred myocardium imposes additional burden on remote viable myocardium despite a reduction in the extent of area with late contrast MR enhancement. *Eur Radiol* 2006, 16:827–836.

23. Baks T, van Geuns RJ, Biagini E, *et al.*: Effects of primary angioplasty for acute myocardial infarction on early and late infarct size and left ventricular wall characteristics. *J Am Coll Cardiol* 2006, 47:40–44.

24. Appelbaum E, Kirtane AJ, Kissinger KV, *et al.*: Association between TIMI myocardial perfusion grade and cardiovascular magnetic resonance assessment of microvascular obstruction in STEMI. *American Heart Association Scientific Sessions 2005*. Dallas: November 13–16, 2005.

25. Aletras AH, Tilak GS, Natanzon A, *et al.*: Retrospective determination of the area at risk for reperfused acute myocardial infarction with T2-weighted cardiac magnetic resonance imaging: histopathological and displacement encoding with stimulated echoes (DENSE) functional validations. *Circulation* 2006, 113:1865–1870.

26. Stork A, Lund GK, Muellerleile K, *et al.*: Characterization of the peri-infarction zone using T2-weighted MRI and delayed-enhancement MRI in patients with acute myocardial infarction. *Eur Radiol* 2006, 16:2350–2357.

8

Dobutamine Stress Wall Motion CMR Imaging

Robert Manka and Eike Nagel

Cardiovascular magnetic resonance (CMR) offers several methods for the detection of myocardial ischemia, most importantly myocardial perfusion imaging and wall motion imaging at rest and stress. These methods are based on pharmacologic stress. Wall motion imaging with dobutamine has been shown to be superior to wall motion imaging with adenosine [1] and, consequently, this pharmacon is the stressor of choice for wall motion stress imaging. Dobutamine wall motion imaging may be combined with perfusion imaging at the highest stress level. Compared with adenosine, stress dobutamine offers the advantage to induce ischemia, rather than a mere alteration of blood flow, as well as to recruit hibernating myocardium, which may be used for viability imaging. However, wall motion abnormalities occur later, during the ischemic cascade, compared with alterations of blood flow [2].

DOBUTAMINE

Dobutamine is a potent, synthetic catecholamine mainly acting via β1-receptor stimulation, with β2- and α1-receptor stimulation occurring to a much lesser degree. In the low-dose range (5 to 10 μg/kg/min), the positive inotropic effect is most dominant; at higher doses (up to 50 μg/kg/min), a progressive increase of heart rate and blood pressure leads to an increased rate pressure product, which adds to increased oxygen consumption and, thus, may induce myocardial ischemia.

Usually dobutamine is started with 10 μg/kg body weight per minute with 10 μg increments every 3 minutes until target heart rate (220— age × 85%) or peak dose (40 or 50 μg/kg/min) have been reached. If target heart rate is not reached at the peak dobutamine dose, atropine (up to 2 mg) is added.

SAFETY ASPECTS

Because high-dose dobutamine/atropine stress induces myocardial ischemia, side effects have to be expected in a minority of patients. In a routine clinical setting in 1035 consecutive patients, 74 tests had to be stopped because of limiting side effects, including chest pain, dyspnea, and nausea. Atrial fibrillation was provoked in five patients and nonsustained atrial fibrillation was provoked in 16 patients. One patient suffered sustained ventricular tachycardia with successful defibrillation. No cases of death or myocardial infarction occurred [3].

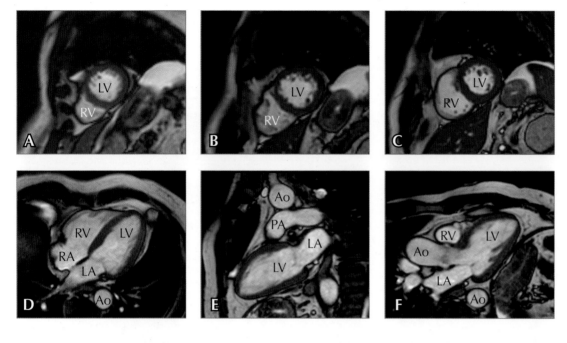

Figure 8-1. Standard views for dobutamine stress CMR. Short-axis views: apical (**A**), mid (**B**), basal (**C**). Long axis views: four-chamber (**D**), two-chamber (**E**), and three-chamber (**F**). Ao—aorta; LA—left atrium; LV—left ventricle; PA—pulmonary artery; RA—right atrium; RV—right ventricle.

Dobutamine and Atropine Contraindications

Dobutamine	Atropine
General contraindications	**Contraindications**
Unstable angina	Narrow-angle glaucoma
Severe arterial hypertension	Myasthenia gravis
Significant aortic stenosis (gradient > 50 mm Hg or area < 1 cm² advanced heart block	Obstructive uropathy
Hypertrophic obstructive cardiomyopathy	
Complex cardiac arrhythmias	
Myocardial inflammation (perimyocarditis)	
Caution	
Co-medication with diuretics (hypokalemia !)	

Figure 8-2. Dobutamine and atropine: contraindications and cautions.

MONITORING

Monitoring needs are similar for the different stressors. Heart rate and rhythm need to be registered throughout the stress examination. Changes of the ST-segment are nondiagnostic as a result of the electrocardiogram wave distortion in the static magnetic field. However, because wall motion abnormalities precede ST-segment changes and the former can readily be detected with CMR, monitoring with rapid cine sequences is effective without a diagnostic electrocardio-gram (*eg*, cine CMR real-time scans can be run repetitively to detect new or worsening wall motion abnormalities at very first occurrence) [4].

Blood pressure monitoring can easily be done with a conventional monitoring system outside the scanner room with an extension line placed through a waveguide in the radiofrequency cage or special CMR-compatible equipment may be used.

Termination Criteria

Target heart rate ([220-age] × 0.85) reached

Hypertension (blood pressure > 240/120 mm Hg)

Systolic blood pressure drop > 40 mm Hg

Intolerable symptoms (chest pain, dypnea, and others)

Significant supraventricular/ventricular arrhythmias

Figure 8-3. Termination criterian for dobutamine stress CMR.

DIAGNOSTIC ACCURACY OF STRESS INDUCIBLE WALL MOTION ABNORMALITIES

Overall, the diagnostic accuracy of dobutamine stress inducible wall motion abnormalities for the detection of significant epicardial coronary disease (> 50% luminal narrowing) has been reported to be approximately 86% (range 83%–90%) [5]. This value has been similar for different patient collectives. In a multicenter study, a mildly lower sensitivity with higher specificity was found [6].

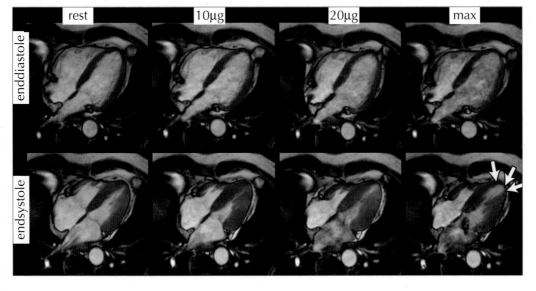

Figure 8-4. Four-chamber dobutamine stress CMR obtained at rest and at low- and peak-dose dobutamine. End-diastolic and end-systolic phases are shown. Note the newly developed wall motion abnormality in the anteroseptal segment and the apex (*arrows*).

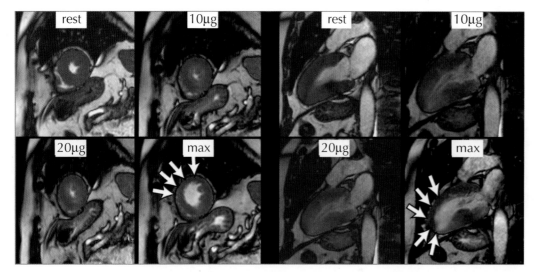

Figure 8-5. Cine images of the dobutamine stress CMR examination (end-systole, mid short-axis and two-chamber view) in a patient with single-vessel disease of the left anterior descending coronary artery. Note the development of akinesia (*arrows*) at peak-dose in anterior and anteroseptal segment and the apex.

Accuracy of Dobutamine Stress Echo and Dobutamine Stress CMR for Identifying Coronary Atherosclerosis

Modality	Study	Patients, *n*	Sensitivity, %	Specificity, %
DSE	Elhendy *et al.* [9]	1446	81	85
	Mädler *et al.* [10]	289	80	80
	Huang *et al.* [11]	93	93	77
	Kertai *et al.* [12]	1877	85	70
	Das *et al.* [13]	530	100	63
Average for all DSE studies			**87**	**75**
DCMR	Sensky *et al.* [14]	6	87	87
	van Rugge *et al.* [15]	39	91	80
	Nagel *et al.* [16]	208	86	86
	Hundley *et al.* [17]	153	83	83
	Paetsch *et al.* [18]	79	89	80
Average for all DCMR studies			**87**	**83**

DCMR=dobutamine stress cardiovascular magnetic resonance
DSE=dobutamine stress echocardiography

Figure 8-6. Accuracy of dobutamine stress echocardiography (DSE) and dobutamine stress CMR (DCMR) for identifying coronary atherosclerosis. (*Adapted from* Mandapaka [7].)

FUNCTIONAL ASSESSMENT OF VIABLE MYOCARDIUM

Low-dose dobutamine stress echocardiography (DSE) plays an established role in the detection of viable myocardium. A potential advantage to the visualization of necrosis as performed with late gadolinium-enhanced CMR is the simulation of the functional status of the myocardium after revascularization [8]. Even though the localization and extent of myocardial infarction can be determined with a much higher precision using late gadolinium-enhanced CMR, the functional status of the remaining viable myocardium can be better assessed with low-dose dobutamine stimulation. Compared with low-dose dobutamine stress echocardiography, CMR has the advantage of better delineation of the endo- and epicardium independent of any imaging windows.

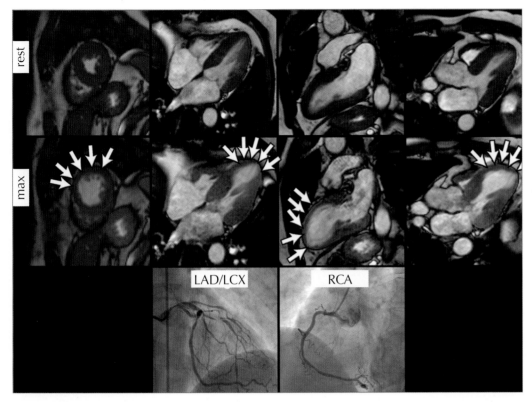

Figure 8-7. Dobutamine stress CMR: example of myocardial ischemia in all standard views (short-axis, four-, two-, and three-chamber views). *Top row*: rest; end-systole; *bottom row*: peak-stress, end-systole.

Coronary angiography demonstrated significant proximal occlusion of the left anterior descending artery (LAD) and significant stenoses of the left circumflex artery (LCX). RCA—right coronary artery.

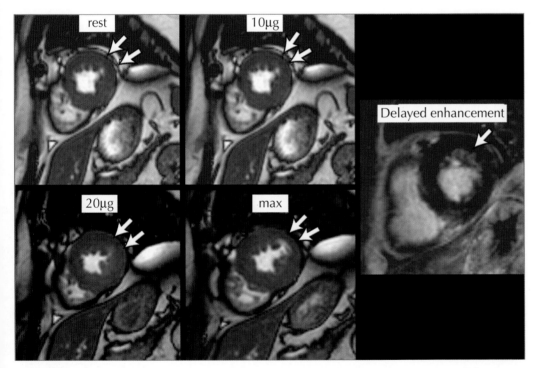

Figure 8-8. Dobutamine stress CMR viability assessment: example of short-axis views (end-systole) showing hypokinesia at rest in the anterolateral segment (*arrows*), with improvement of wall motion under low dose and breakdown of wall motion (akinesia)

under peak-dose dobutamine (biphasic course). Inversion recovery gradient-echo technique revealed delayed enhancement of 25% transmural extent (*arrow*) in the anterolateral segment.

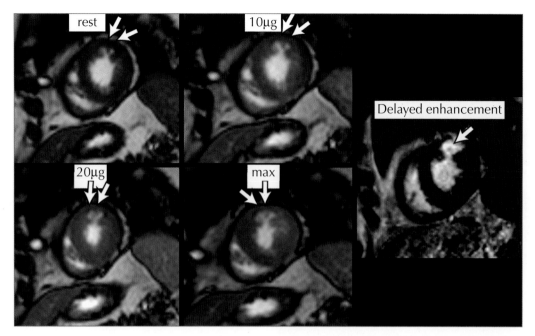

Figure 8-9. Dobutamine stress CMR viability assessment: example of short-axis views (end-systole) showing akinesia at rest in the anterolateral segment (*arrows*), with no improvement of wall motion under low-dose dobutamine (no measurable contractile reserve). Inversion recovery gradient-echo technique revealed late gadolinium enhancement of 100% transmural extent (*arrow*) in the anterolateral segment.

REFERENCES

1. Paetsch I, Jahnke C, Wahl A, *et al.*: Comparison of dobutamine stress magnetic resonance, adenosine stress magnetic resonance, and adenosine stress magnetic resonance perfusion. *Circulation* 2004, 110:835–842.

2. Nesto RW, Kowalchuk GJ: The ischemic cascade: temporal sequence of hemodynamic, electrocardiographic and symptomatic expressions of ischemia. *Am J Cardiol* 1987, 59:23C–30C.

3. Wahl A, Paetsch I, Gollesch A, *et al.*: Safety and feasibility of high-dose dobutamine-atropine stress cardiovascular magnetic resonance for diagnosis of myocardial ischaemia: experience in 1000 consecutive cases. *Eur Heart J* 2004, 25:1230–1236.

4. Nagel E, Lorenz C, Baer F, *et al.*: Stress cardiovascular magnetic resonance: consensus panel report. *J Cardiovasc Magn Reson* 2001, 3:267–281.

5. Hundley WG, Hamilton CA, Thomas MS, *et al.*: Utility of fast cine magnetic resonance imaging and display for the detection of myocardial ischemia in patients not well suited for second harmonic stress echocardiography. *Circulation* 1999, 100:1697–1702.

6. Paetsch I, Jahnke C, Ferrari VA, *et al.*: Determination of interobserver variability for identifying inducible left ventricular wall motion abnormalities during dobutamine stress magnetic resonance imaging. *Eur Heart J* 2006, 27:1459–1464.

7. Mandapaka S, Hundley WG: Dobutamine cardiovascular magnetic resonance: a review. *J Magn Reson Imaging* 2006, 24:499–512.

8. Wellnhofer E, Olariu A, Klein C, *et al.*: Magnetic resonance low-dose dobutamine test is superior to SCAR quantification for the prediction of functional recovery. *Circulation* 2004, 109:2172–2174.

9. Elhendy A, van Domburg RT, Poldermans D, *et al.*: Safety and feasibility of dobutamine-atropine stress echocardiography for the diagnosis of coronary artery disease in diabetic patients unable to perform an exercise stress test. *Diabetes Care* 1998, 21:1777–1781.

10. Mädler CF, Payne N, Wilkenshoff U, *et al.*: Noninvasive diagnosis of coronary artery disease by quantitative stress echocardiography: optimal diagnostic models using off-line Doppler in the MYDISE study. *Eur Heart J* 2003, 24:1538–1593.

11. Huang WC, Chiou KR, Lui CP, *et al.*: Comparison of real-time contrast echocardiography and low-dose dobutamine stress echocardiography in predicting the left ventricular functional recovery in patients after acute myocardial infarction under different therapeutic intervention. *Int J Cardiol* 2005, 104:81–91.

12. Kertai MD, Boersma E, Bax JJ, *et al.*: A meta-analysis comparing the prognostic accuracy of six diagnostic tests for predicting perioperative cardiac risk in patients undergoing major vascular surgery. *Heart* 2003, 89:1327–1334.

13. Das MK, Pellikka PA, Mahoney DW, *et al.*: Assessment of cardiac risk before nonvascular surgery: dobutamine stress echocardiography in 530 patients. *J Am Coll Cardiol* 2000, 35:1647–1653.

14. Sensky PR, Jivan A, Hudson N, *et al.*: Coronary artery disease: combined stress MR imaging protocol: one-stop evaluation of myocardial perfusion and function. *Radiology* 2000, 215:608–614.

15. van Rugge FP, van der Wall EE, Bruschke AV, *et al.*: Magnetic resonance imaging during dobutamine stress for detection and localization of coronary artery disease: quantitative wall motion analysis using a modification of the centerline method. *Circulation* 1994, 90:127–138.

16. Hundley WG, Hamilton CA, Thomas MS, *et al.*: Utility of fast cine magnetic resonance imaging and display for detection of myocardial ischemia in patients not well suited for second harmonic stress echocardiography. *Circulation* 1999, 100:1697–1702.

17. Nagel E, Lehmkuhl HB, Bocksch W, *et al.*: Noninvasive diagnosis of ischemia-induced wall motion abnormalities with the use of high-dose dobutamine stress magnetic resonance imaging: comparison with dobutamine stress echocardiography. *Circulation* 1999, 99:763–770.

18. Paetsch I, Jahnke C, Wahl A, *et al.*: Comparison of dobutamine stress magnetic resonance, adenosine stress magnetic resonance and adenosine stress magnetic resonance perfusion. *Circulation* 2004, 110:835–842.

9

CHAPTER

Myocardial Viability and Fibrosis

Rajiv Agarwal and Scott D. Flamm

In recent years, cardiovascular magnetic resonance (CMR) imaging has come to the forefront for evaluation of myocardial viability. Late gadolinium enhancement (LGE) imaging accurately characterizes a variety of cardiomyopathies and plays an important role in the clinical decision-making process for acute and chronic coronary artery disease. Compared with alternative imaging modalities, the advantages of CMR imaging for assessment of viability include improved spatial and temporal resolution. Improved spatial resolution is particularly important in patients with myocardial infarctions, where the degree of transmurality of infarction must be accurately recognized prior to decisions regarding revascularization. Further, characteristic patterns of LGE are noted in patients with cardiomyopathies, allowing differentiation of ischemic, nonischemic, and inflammatory etiologies, for example. This powerful imaging technique enables physicians to make a specific diagnosis of cardiomyopathy and avoid invasive histologic sampling and biopsies. The most common LGE sequences currently used include inversion-recovery gradient-echo and steady-state free-precession.

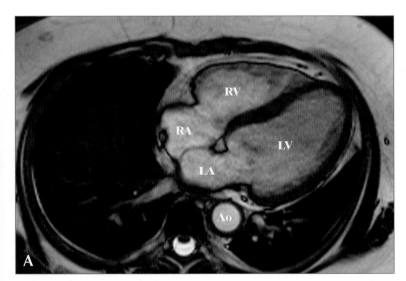
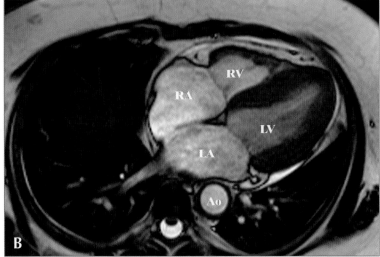

Figure 9-1. **A** and **B**, Normal systolic function of the myocardium. Steady-state free precession cine images of a patient with normal biventricular systolic function. **A** represents end-diastole in the cardiac cycle, whereas **B** represents end-systole. **B**, The myocardium thickens and contracts uniformly. There is basal annuli descent of the mitral and tricuspid valves. The cavities of the left ventricle and right ventricle decrease in volume, whereas the left atria and right atria increase in size. The descending aorta is also visualized. Ao—aorta; LA—left atrium; LV—left ventricle; RA—right atrium; RV—right ventricle.

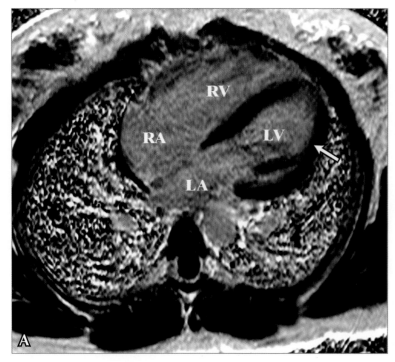

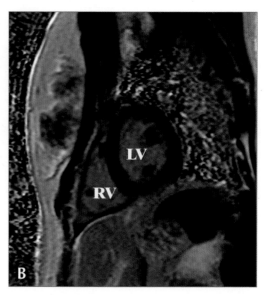

Figure 9-2. A and **B**, Normal late gadolinium enhancement (LGE) images. Shown are LGE images of a patient with uniformly viable myocardium. The optimal time of inversion is selected to null normal viable myocardium, which is black (*arrow*) on LGE sequences. **A** is a horizontal long-axis image, whereas **B** is a short-axis image obtained after alignment using LGE long-axis images. Each image is a phase image obtained during a single breathhold using a phase-sensitive inversion recovery LGE sequence. LV—left ventricle; RV—right ventricle.

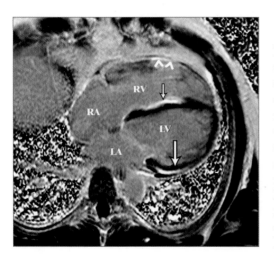

Figure 9-3. Myopericarditis. Late gadolinium enhancement (LGE) image in an axial orientation obtained 15 minutes after administration of gadolinium chelate in a patient with acute onset of congestive heart failure symptoms and clinical suspicion for myocarditis. Both the left ventricle (LV) and right ventricle (RV) are dilated. There are linear areas of hyperenhancement along the epicardial borders of the midinferoseptum (*short arrow*) and the basal to midanterolateral walls (*long arrow*). There is also focal involvement of the RV (*arrows*). This pattern of hyperenhancement is in a noncoronary artery distribution and is atypical for ischemic injury. Though not pathognomonic, in the clinical context, this pattern is highly suspicious for myocarditis. LA—left atrium; RA—right atrium.

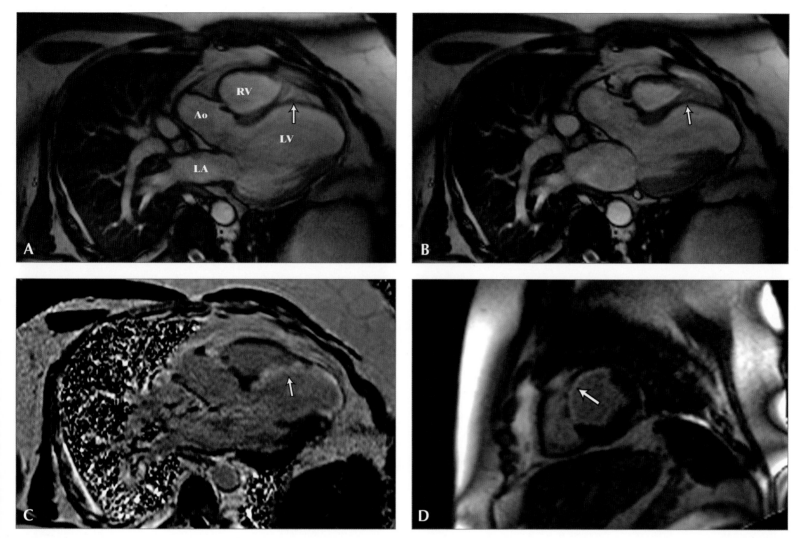

Figure 9-4. Coronary artery disease involving the left anterior descending artery (LAD). These images are taken from a patient with classic LAD distribution infarction. The study was performed to assess viability and suitability of performing bypass grafting of the LAD. The top figures are parasternal long-axis images of end-diastolic (**A**) and end-systolic (**B**) frames. Note that the mid to distal anteroseptal walls (*arrows*) and the entire left ventricular apex are thin and akinetic. The bottom images are late gadolinium enhancement (LGE) images obtained 15 minutes after administration of gadolinium chelate. The bottom left image (**C**) is a phase image (phase-sensitive inversion recovery LGE sequence) that reveals a transmural infarct involving most of the anteroseptal myocardium (*arrow*) and entire apex. A short-axis image (**D**) reveals transmural infarction and nonviability of the anterior and anteroseptal walls (*arrow*).

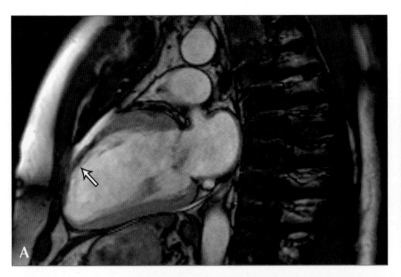

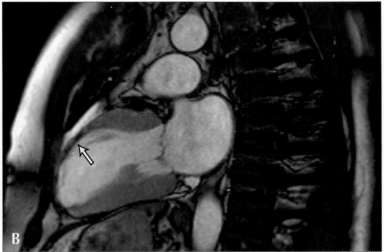

C	Left Ventricle: Normal Values		
Cardiac Measure		Normal Range	Units
Ejection fraction	37	56–78	%
End-diastolic volume	313	77–195	mL
End-systolic volume	197	19–72	mL
Stroke volume	116	51–133	mL
Cardiac output	8.5	2.8–8.8	L/min

Figure 9-5. Coronary artery disease involving the left anterior descending artery. These images are taken from a patient with left anterior descending artery distribution infarction who was evaluated for placement of a defibrillator. The study was performed to assess left ventricular (LV) viability and ejection fraction. Vertical long-axis images of end-diastole (**A**) and end systole (**B**). Note that the mid to distal anterior wall (*arrows*) and the entire LV apex are thin and akinetic. **C**, LV ejection fraction, 37%, obtained after manual tracing of endocardial contours in both end-diastole and systole from a set of contiguous short-axis cine slices encompassing the entire LV. The LV ejection fraction is calculated from a left ventricular an end-diastolic volume of 313 mL and end-systolic volume of 197 mL.

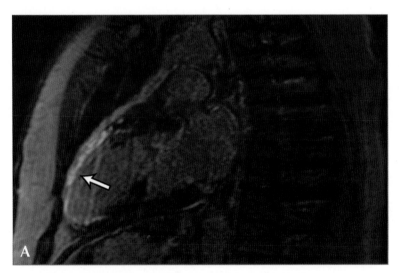

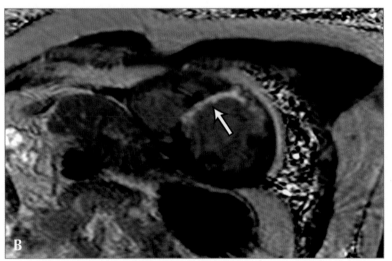

Figure 9-6. Coronary artery disease involving the left anterior descending artery. These late gadolinium enhancement images are from the patient presented in Figure 10-5. **A** is a vertical long axis that shows a transmural infarct involving the mid to distal anterior wall (*arrow*) and the entire apex. A short-axis image (**B**) shows transmural infarction and thus nonviability of the anterior and anteroseptal walls (*arrow*). This patient is not expected to recover function in the left anterior descending artery territory after revascularization.

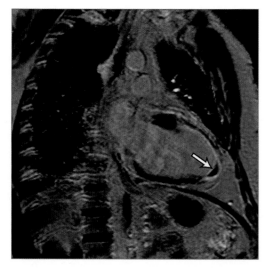

Figure 9-7. Left ventricular apex thrombus. Late gadolinium enhancement image in a vertical long-axis orientation obtained 15 minutes after administration of gadolinium chelate in a patient with new onset left arm numbness. CMR was performed to assess for intracardiac thrombus in this patient because of known coronary artery disease. There is near-transmural to transmural infarction involving the mid to distal anterior wall and the entire apex. Thrombus is identified as a crescent-shaped area (*arrow*) at the left ventricular apex that is completely nulled (dark).

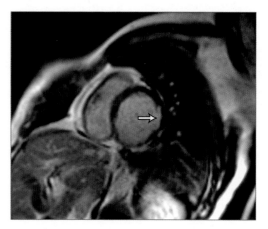

Figure 9-8. Coronary artery disease involving the left circumflex artery. Late gadolinium enhancement (LGE) image taken 15 minutes after administration of gadolinium chelate in a patient with multiple risk factors for coronary artery disease and subacute presentation of angina pectoris. This is a short-axis image revealing near-transmural infarction and thus partial nonviability of the lateral wall (*arrow*). This patient is not expected to recover function in the segment demonstrating near transmural LGE after revascularization.

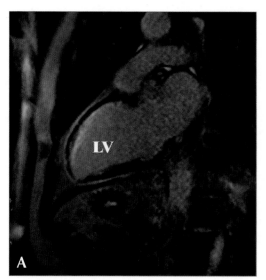

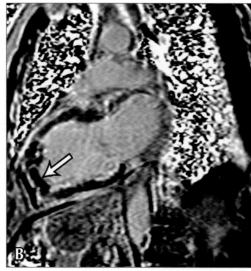

Figures 9-9. **A** and **B**, Pre- and postoperative images of a patient who underwent the Dor procedure for left ventricular (LV) aneurysm repair. Vertical long-axis late gadolinium enhancement (LGE) images taken 15 minutes after administration of gadolinium chelate in a patient with left anterior descending territory infarct and apical aneurysm. **A**, Prior to the Dor procedure, showing extensive LGE hyperenhancement; on cine images the apex was dyskinetic. **B**, Postoperative Dor procedure showing surgical patch repair reconstruction of the LV apex. Note the thrombus (*arrow*) adjacent to the patch. This thrombus is completely nulled at the time of inversion and optimized to null normal viable myocardium.

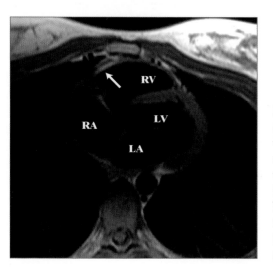

Figure 9-10. Arrhythmogenic right ventricular (RV) cardiomyopathy. T2-weighted turbo spin echo axial image in a patient with a history of nonsustained ventricular tachycardia and syncope. There is high signal intensity fatty infiltration (*arrow*) within the RV myocardium. This region was dyskinetic on cine images and on late gadolinium enhancement images, showing both fatty and fibrous replacement. These findings were consistent with arrhythmogenic right ventricular cardiomyopathy, and the patient subsequently received a cardiac defibrillator. LA—left atrium; LV—left ventricle; RA—right atrium

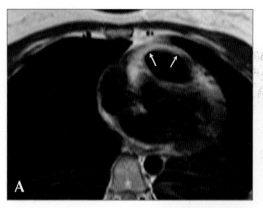
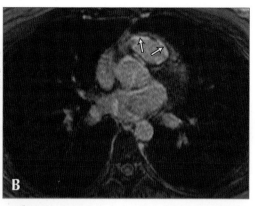

Figure 9-11. **A** and **B,** Arrhythmogenic right ventricular (RV) cardiomyopathy. **A,** A T2-weighted turbo spin echo axial image in a patient with history of nonsustained ventricular tachycardia who had undergone ablation of the right ventricular outflow tract (RVOT). There is high-signal-intensity fatty infiltration (*arrows*) within the RV myocardium. This region is dyskinetic on cine images. **B,** On late gadolinium enhancement (LGE) images, the corresponding RV myocardium is bright (*arrows*), indicating fibrous replacement. These findings would normally be characteristic for arrhythmogenic RV cardiomyopathy; however, in the setting of prior RVOT ablation, the diagnosis is uncertain because LGE scarring may be secondary to the ablation.

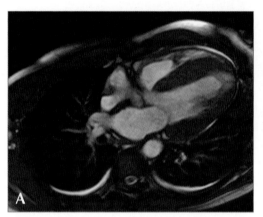
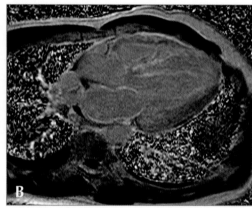

Figure 9-12. Amyloidosis. **A,** Oblique axial steady-state free precession image that shows small pericardial and bilateral pleural effusions. The left ventricular myocardium is thickened and the left atrium is dilated. **B,** Late gadolinium enhancement sequence obtained 15 minutes after administration of gadolinium chelate. Despite varying the times of inversion from 200 to 500 ms, the myocardium could not be nulled. These findings are characteristic of cardiac amyloidosis.

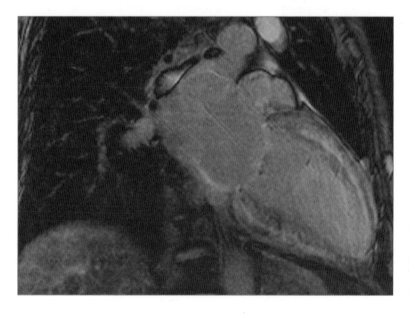

Figure 9-13. Amyloidosis. A vertical long-axis late gadolinium enhancement image obtained 15 minutes after administration of gadolinium chelate. The left ventricular myocardium could not be nulled despite a wide variation in times of inversion. The left atrium is dilated. These findings are characteristic of cardiac amyloidosis.

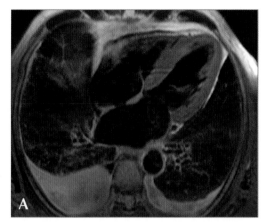
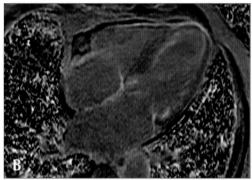

Figure 9-14. Amyloidosis. **A**, Axial T2 turbo spin echo sequence with fat saturation revealing moderate size (*right*) and small (*left*) pleural effusions. Also, the left ventricular (LV) and right ventricular myocardium are thickened, and both atria are dilated. **B**, Corresponding late gadolinium enhancement image obtained 15 minutes after administration of gadolinium chelate. The LV myocardium could not be nulled throughout a range of times of inversion. These findings were consistent with cardiac amyloidosis.

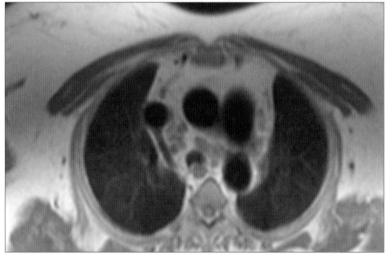
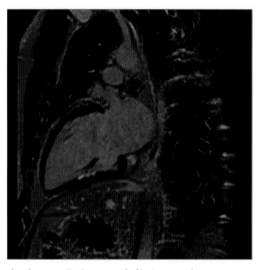

Figure 9-15. Sarcoidosis. These images were obtained from a young woman with biopsy-proven sarcoidosis who presented with palpitations and nonsustained pulmonary ventricular tachycardia of left ventricular etiology. Coronary angiography was normal. **A**, Ultrafast, single-shot, spin echo image showing extensive mediastinal lymphadenopathy and increased signal intensity in the lungs. **B**, Late gadolinium enhancement sequence performed 15 minutes after administration of gadolinium chelate. There is a focal linear area of subendocardial scar that correlated with the origin of the ectopic beats. Despite intensive antiarrhythmic and immunosuppressive therapies, the patient required implantation of a cardiac defibrillator.

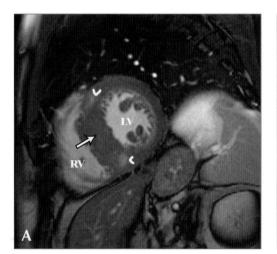
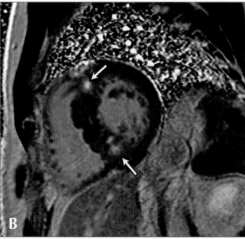

interventricular septum (*arrow*) is markedly thickened. The rest of the myocardium is of normal thickness. There is increased signal intensity (*arrows*) at the anterior and inferior left and right ventricular insertion points. **B**, Late gadolinium hyperenhancement (LGE) image of the same patient in a similar orientation obtained 15 minutes after the administration of gadolinium chelate. Hyperenhancement (*arrows*), consistent with interstitial fibrosis, is noted at the anterior and inferior left and right ventricular (LV and RV) insertion points. This LGE pattern of hyperenhancement is typical for hypertrophic cardiomyopathy.

Figure 9-16. **A** and **B**, Hypertrophic cardiomyopathy. These images were obtained in a patient with a recent syncopal episode and family history of sudden death. **A**, Post–gadolinium chelate steady-state free precession image in the short-axis orientation. The

RECOMMENDED READING

1. Kim RJ, Wu E, Rafael A, *et al.:* The use of contrast-enhanced magnetic resonance imaging to identify reversible myocardial dysfunction. *N Engl J Med* 2000, 343:1488—1490.

2. Shan K, Constantine G, Sivananthan M, Flamm SD: Role of cardiac magnetic resonance imaging in the assessment of myocardial viability. *Circulation* 2004, 109:1328—1334.

3. Lim RP, Srichai MB, Lee VS: Non-ischemic causes of delayed myocardial hyperenhancement on MRI. *AJR Am J Roentgenol* 2007, 188:1675—1681.

4. Mahrholdt H, Wagner A, Judd RM, *et al.:* Delayed enhancement cardiovascular magnetic resonance assessment of non-ischaemic cardiomyopathies. *Eur Heart J* 2005, 26:2601—2602.

5. Hunold P, Schlosser T, Barkhausen J, *et al.:* Myocardial late enhancement in contrast-enhanced cardiac MRI: distinction between infarction scar and non-infarction-related disease. *Am J Roentgenol* 2005, 184:1420—1426.

10
CHAPTER

Cardiac Masses

Rajan A. G. Patel, Brian J. Schietinger, and Christopher M. Kramer

Cardiac masses may be intracardiac, extracardiac, or both. The most common intracardiac masses are thrombi. Abnormal tissue in or around the heart may represent either benign or malignant tissue. The prevalence of primary cardiac tumors is rare and on the order of 0.001% to 0.3% of all tumors [1–3]. The majority of primary cardiac tumors are benign and myxoma is the most commonly found benign primary cardiac tumor. The majority of malignant cardiac tumors are metastases from other organs. They are encountered 30 to 50 times more frequently than primary cardiac tumors and are encountered in as many as 40% of patients who die from malignancy [4,5]. Lung and breast cancer metastases frequently invade the pericardium and epicardium and are, therefore, thought to spread via the lymphatic system. In contrast, lymphomas and melanoma typically result in myocardial metastasis as a consequence of hematogenous spread. The prevalence of malignant primary cardiac tumors is approximately 25%. The most commonly found malignant primary cardiac tumor is a sarcoma [2]. A description of each type of cardiac mass is beyond the scope of this atlas; however, the reference list provides several excellent resources.

Cardiovascular magnetic resonance (CMR) is particularly useful in the noninvasive assessment of intra- and extracardiac masses because of its three-dimensional tomographic capability, excellent spatial resolution, large field of view, and its ability to discern different tissue types by using various pulse sequences and contrast agents. Furthermore, unlike echocardiography, CMR is not limited by poor acoustic windows in some patients and imaging planes can be readily reproduced during serial imaging to monitor the effect or chemotherapy, radiation, or surgery. Finally, the ability of CMR to discern tissue planes and assess tumor vascularity can be useful in surgical planning. The recently published Appropriateness Criteria for the use of CMR rate the use of this imaging modality for the evaluation of cardiac masses as "appropriate" with a score of 9, the maximum possible [6].

The most commonly used CMR pulse sequences for the assessment of cardiac masses include T1-weighted turbo spin echo (T1-TSE) with and without fat saturation; T2-weighted turbo spin echo (T2-TSE); dynamic or cine imaging with steady-state free procession (SSFP) and/or gradient-echo (GRE) sequences; and first-pass perfusion imaging and late gadolinium-enhanced imaging (LGE), both of which use gadolinium-based contrast agents.

Thrombi appear dark on SSFP imaging without contrast and do not take up contrast during first-pass perfusion imaging. On postcontrast SSFP imaging immediately after the intravenous injection of contrast, thrombi appear black relative to the gray myocardium and bright blood pool. Fluid-filled cysts and lipomas have high signal intensity on T1-TSE images similar to adipose tissue. However, the bright signal of lipomas and lipomatous hypertrophy of the atrial septum will be nulled when using sequences with fat saturation [7]. Pericardial cysts have characteristic high signal intensity on T2-TSE imaging. Turbo spin echo sequences can also provide helpful evidence for the presence of a mass by suggesting cavity distortion or wall thickening [1]. Cine imaging techniques are useful for delineating the anatomy surrounding a mass and the relationships of a mass to the surrounding anatomy (*ie*, a pedunculated myxoma or a metastasis with intramural invasion), assessing functional consequences of a mass, and serially measuring the size of a mass. First-pass perfusion sequences and magnetic resonance angiography provide the physician with vascular relationships. LGE identifies both vascularity and fibrosis/necrosis. Figure 10-1, modified from Luna *et al.* [8] summaries the signal characteristics of various primary cardiac masses.

Characteristics of Various Primary Cardiac Masses

	Location	Population	T1-weighted	T2-weighted	Postcontrast	Cine-MRI	Other Data
Myxoma	Interauricular septum	Female, 30–60 y	Isointense, heterogeneous	Hyperintense, heterogeneous	Low to high enhancement	Low signal	Mean size 5.7 cm, hemorrhage, calcification
Papillary fibroelastoma	Left-sided valves	Elderly, often >80 y	Isointense	Hypointense	Not published	Turbulent flow	Mean size 1 cm
Lipoma	Any	Adults	Hyperintense	Hyperintense	None	—	Suppression with fat saturation techniques
Rhabdomyoma	Left ventricle	Children	Iso- or hyperintense	Slightly hyperintense	Strong	Noncontractile areas	Mean size 4 cm, multiplicity
Fibroma	Left ventricle	Children	Iso- or hyperintense	Hypointense	Variable	—	Mean size 5 cm, calcification
Hemangioma	Any	Variable	Isointense	Hyperintense, heterogeneous	Strong, heterogeneous	—	Small calcifications
Paraganglioma	Left atrium	30–40 y	Iso- or hypointense	Hyperintense	Strong	—	Paraneoplastic catecholamine syndrome
Intravenous leiomyomatosis	Right atrium	Female, 35–50 y	Isointense	Isointense	Heterogeneous	Mobile mass	Origin in IVC
Bronchogenic cyst	Interauricular septum	Adults	Hypointense	Hyperintense	None	—	Differential diagnosis: hydatid cyst
Angiosarcoma	Right atrium	Male, 30–50 y	Isointense, with hyperintense areas	Isointense, heterogeneous	Strong	Hypointense foci	Hemorrhage, possible pericardial origin
Undifferentiated sarcoma	Left atrium	Variable	Isointense	Isointense	Nonspecific	—	Possible percardial origin, infiltrative or mass-like appearance
Rhabdomyosarcoma	Any	Children	Isointense	Isointense, heterogeneous	Central nonenhancing areas	—	Necrosis
Osteosarcoma	Left atrium	Variable	Hyperintense	Hyperintense	Nonspecific	—	Calcifications
Malignant fibrous histiocytoma	Left atrium	Female, 30–40 y	Isointense	Hyperintense, heterogeneous	Nonspecific	—	Pulmonary veins involvement
Leiomyosarcoma	Left atrium	Variable	Isointense	Hyperintense	Nonspecific	—	Pulmonary veins and mitral valve involvement
Fibrosarcoma	Left atrium	Variable	Isointense, heterogeneous	Hyperintense	Central nonenhancing areas	Possible pericardial origin	Necrosis
Liposarcoma	Left atrium	Variable	Not published	Not published	Not published	—	Possible pericardial origin, little intratumoral macroscopic fat
Lymphoma	Right atrium	Immunocompromised patients	Hypo- or isointense	Hyperintense	Variable	—	No necrosis, possible pericardial origin, rare intracavitary

Figure 10-1. Characteristics of various primary cardiac masses. IVC—inferior vena cava.

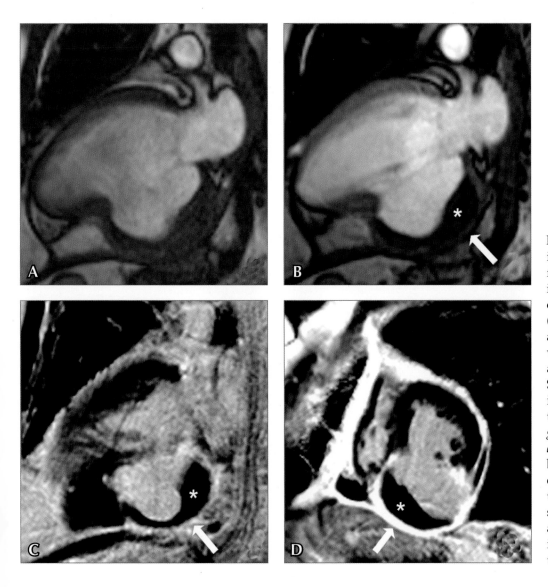

Figure 10-2. Intracardiac thrombus. These images were acquired in a patient referred for a viability study after suffering a large inferior myocardial infarction. The two-chamber steady-state free procession (SSFP) precontrast image demonstrates a large inferior wall aneurysm with a wall that appears relatively thick for an aneurysm (**A**). Two-chamber postcontrast SSFP imaging (**B**) demonstrates a thin wall in the region of the aneurysm that has taken up contrast (**B**, *arrow*) and appears *gray* along with a *dark black* thrombus (**B**, *asterisk*) lining the aneurysm. Two-chamber (**C**) and short-axis (**D**) late gadolinium enhancement images demonstrate that the thrombus (**C** and **D**, *asterisk*) lines and is surrounded by infarcted myocardium (**C** and **D**, *arrow*). A small pericardial effusion is also noted inferior to the apical left ventricle on the two-chamber views.

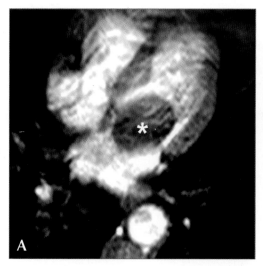
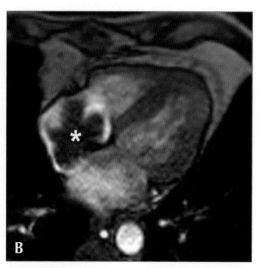

Figure 10-3. Atrial myxoma. Four-chamber long-axis views from two patients demonstrating atrial myxomas (*asterisks*). A pedunculated left atrial myxoma prolapsing across the mitral valve is seen in **A** and a multilobular right atrial myxoma is seen in **B** attached to the fossa ovalis. Both images demonstrate the classic hypointense signal on gradient-echo (GRE) imaging. Myxomas are the most common benign primary cardiac mass. Myxomas are classically attached to the endocardium by a narrow pedicle or stalk. However, broad sites of attachment have been described. The majority of myxomas (75%) are located in the left atrium. The remainder are found in the right atrium,

although there are rare cases of myxomas arising from one of the ventricles [2]. On T1-weighted turbo spin echo images, myxomas may appear to be isointense with myocardium. However, on T2-weighted turbo spin echo images, myxoma tissue may appear brighter than the surrounding myocardium. On both sequences, the appearance is often heterogeneous due to regions of calcification and hemorrhage. Myxomas often have low signal intensity on GRE imaging due to magnetic susceptibility artifact created by the relatively high iron content in these masses. Cystic structures and nonenhancing necrosis may also be appreciated within myxomas [9].

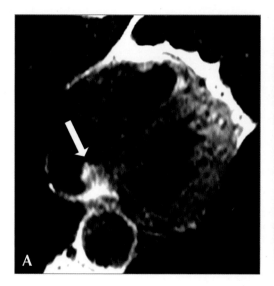
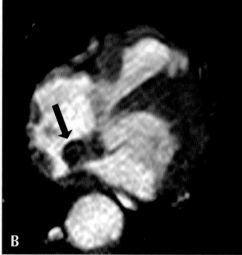

Figure 10-4. Lipoma. Images from a 67-year-old patient referred for further evaluation after a possible right atrial mass noted on transthoracic echocardiography. Right atrial septal hyperintensity (**A**, *arrow*) on an axial T1-weighted black blood turbo spin echo image and hypointensity on an axial T1 fat-saturated gradient-echo image confirm the presence of lipoma (**B**, *arrow*). After myxoma, lipoma is the most frequently observed benign primary cardiac mass. Lipomas are encapsulated masses composed of mature adipose cells. Approximately half of all cardiac lipomas arise from the subendocardium. The remainder arise from the midmyocardium or subepicardium [10].

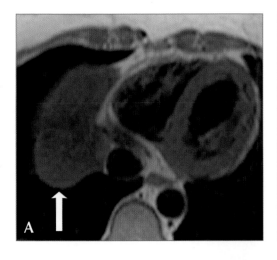
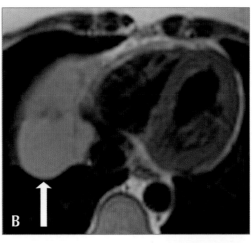

Figure 10-5. Pericardial cyst. A mass (*arrows*) is seen in the right costophrenic angle. Pericardial cysts that contain proteinaceous fluid or hemorrhage may have medium or high signal intensity on T1-weighted turbo spin echo (T1-TSE) imaging (**A**). Cysts containing transudative fluid will have low signal intensity on T1-TSE images. On T2-weighted turbo spin echo imaging (**B**), the mass has the classic bright appearance of a pericardial cyst due to the proteinaceous nature of the fluid [11,12].

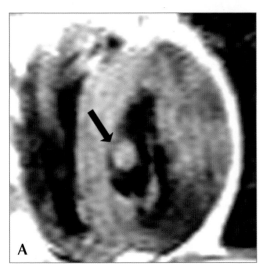
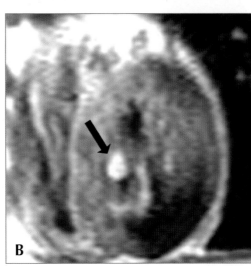

Figure 10-6. Hemangioma. Left ventricular parasagittal short axis demonstrates a mass (*arrows*) on T1 images pre- (**A**) and post-gadolinium (**B**). The postcontrast image illustrates the markedly increased signal from contrast uptake due to hypervascularity of the mass. Postcontrast imaging may have heterogeneous signal due to calcium deposition and septa composed of fibrous, nonvascular tissue within the mass [13]. Cardiac hemangiomas may occur at any location within the myocardium and have also been described within the pericardium [14]. Hemangiomas are classified as capillary, cavernous, or venous based on the size of the vascular components [15]. This mass was removed surgically and proven to be a hemangioma.

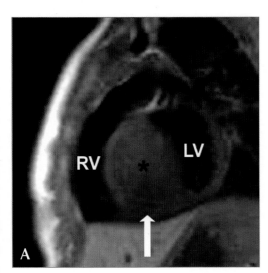
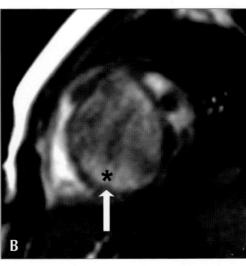
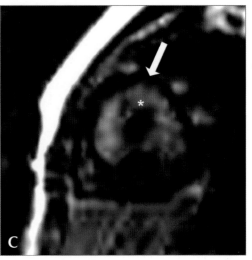

Figure 10-7. Fibroma. In the heart of this child, there is a large mass encased within the interventricular septum. Parasagittal T1-weighted turbo spin echo (**A**) demonstrates that the mass (*asterisk*) is isointense with the normal myocardium. Parasagittal postcontrast steady-state free procession imaging (**B**) demonstrates a "rind-like" border of myocardium (*arrow*) surrounding the contrast containing mass (*asterisk*). Parasagittal late gadolinium enhanced (LGE) imaging (**C**) demonstrates retention of contrast within the fibrotic mass (*asterisk*), a necrotic center without contrast, and a border of normal myocardium without LGE. Among benign primary cardiac masses found in children, fibroma are second in prevalence only to rhabdomyoma [16]. Unlike rhabdomyoma, which are slightly hyperintense on T2-weighted turbo spin echo (T2-TSE), fibroma are classically hypointense on T2-TSE imaging. This is because of the fibrous composition of the fibroma mass and, in some cases, dystrophic calcification [16,17]. LV—left ventricle; RV—right ventricle.

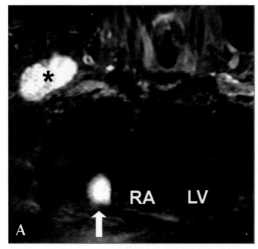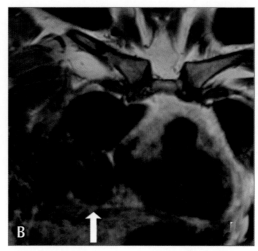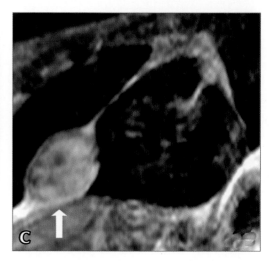

Figure 10-8. Sarcoma. A mass is seen (*arrows*) in the right cardio-phrenic angle, intimately associated with the pericardium along its external surface. This pericardial mass demonstrates the same signal characteristics on STIR (short tau inversion recovery) imaging as a metastatic sarcoma (*asterisk*) noted in the right axilla of this patient (**A**). The pericardial mass measures 5.7 × 5.0 × 5.3 cm. T1-weighted turbo spin echo images acquired in coronal plane at the level of the right atrium (RA) and left ventricle (LV) demonstrate low signal intensity within the mass (**B**). T2-weighted STIR imaging acquired in a parasagittal plane demonstrated high signal intensity (**C**). This mass mildly compresses the right side the heart at the A-V groove. Sarcomas are the most common malignant primary cardiac tumors. Among these, angiosarcomas account for over a third of all cardiac sarcomas. The prevalence of osteosarcomas is approximately 3% to 9% of all cardiac sarcomas, followed by rhabdomyosarcomas, liposarcomas, and leiomyosarcomas. Cardiac sarcomas are aggressive, rapidly invading tumors that generally result in death [2,18].

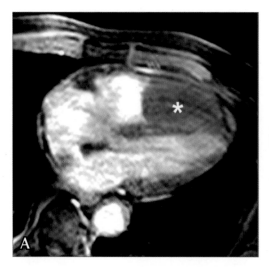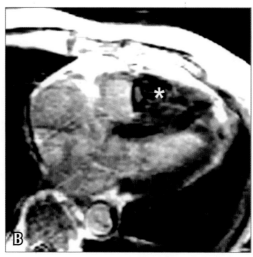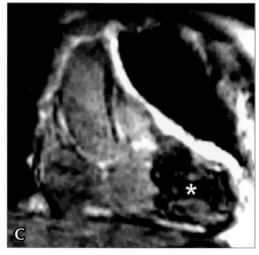

Figure 10-9. Metastatic lung cancer. There is a 6.5 × 3.4 × 6.4 cm mass (*asterisks*) filling the apical half of the right ventricle (RV). This mass extends toward the base of the RV and along the interventricular septum as seen on a T1-weighted gradient-echo four-chamber image with fat saturation (**A**). Four-chamber (**B**) and coronal (**C**) late gadolinium-enhanced (LGE) images demonstrate heterogeneous enhancement of the mass consistent with tumor rather than thrombus. There are regions of fibrosis within the mass. In addition to the mass occupying the apex of the RV, there is a separate mass within the pericardial space at the apex measuring approximately 1 cm in diameter. Metastatic tumors are far more common than primary cardiac neoplasms. Due to the high prevalence of lung cancer, metastases from lung cancer are the most common lesions to migrate to the heart. However, among malignancies, melanoma, lymphoma, and leukemia are much more likely to metastasize to the heart [2]. Cardiac metastases are associated with a poor prognosis regardless of primary tumor type [5]. With the exception of melanoma, metastatic masses in the heart have low signal intensity on T1-weighted turbo spin echo (T1-TSE) and have a relatively higher signal intensity on T2-weighted turbo spin echo. Melanoma appears bright on T1-TSE because of the paramagnetic properties of melanin [19]. Because most metastatic masses are highly vascular, enhancement is noted early following intravenous contrast administration. If the mass contains zones of fibrosis, LGE may also be observed.

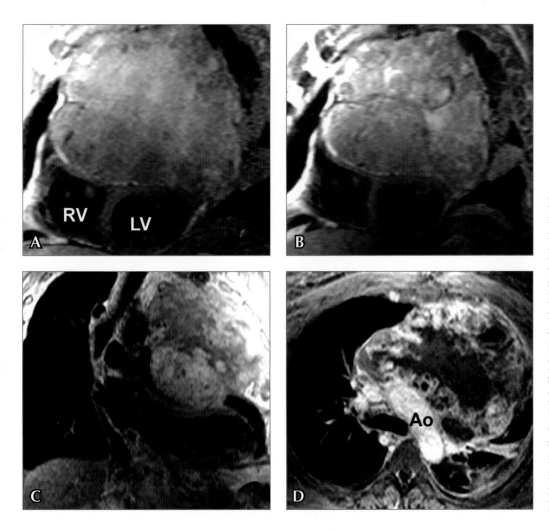

Figure 10-10. Germ cell tumor. A large mass is seen in the anterior, mid to upper mediastinum, left of the midline compressing the right and left ventricles (RV and LV). The mass displaces mediastinal structures posteriorly and to the right. It measures approximately 12 cm craniocaudal × 13.5 cm transverse × 13 cm anterior posterior directions. T1-weighted turbo spin echo parasagittal short axis precontrast (**A**) and T2-weighted turbo spin echo parasagittal short axis (**B**), T1 postcontrast LV two-chamber long axis (**C**) and axial T1 postcontrast imaging (**D**) at the level of the aortic arch (Ao) demonstrate a lobulated contour with a diffusely inhomogeneous signal intensity, including heterogeneous enhancement, central necrosis or cystic change, and possibly hemorrhagic elements.

OTHER MASSES

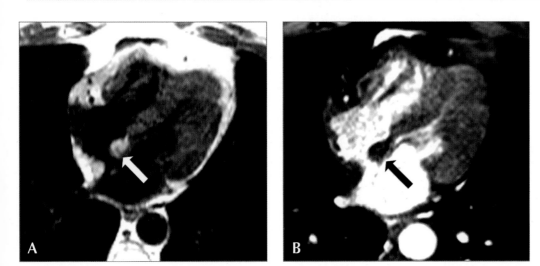

Figure 10-11. Lipomatous hypertrophy of the interatrial septum. CMR performed on a 62-year-old patient with an atrial mass seen on echocardiography. T1-weighted turbo spin echo imaging (**A**) and T1-gradient-echo imaging with fat saturation (**B**) confirms the diagnosis. Lipomatous hypertrophy of the interatrial septum (*arrows*) is defined as adipose tissue within the atrial septum that has a transverse diameter greater than 1 to 1.5 cm [20]. The fossa ovalis is often spared, giving rise to the classical "dumbbell" shaped appearance [21]. Unlike true lipomas, the tissue of lipomatous hypertrophy of the interatrial septum is not encapsulated and consists of both lipoblasts and mature adipose tissue cells [10,20].

REFERENCES

1. Bove C, Kramer C: CMR of cardiac masses. In *Cardiovascular Magnetic Resonance*. Edited by Lardo A, Fayad Z, Chronos N, Fuster V. New York: Martin Dunitz; 2003:253–266.

2. Burke A, Virmani R, eds: *Tumors of the Heart and Great Vessels. Atlas of Tumor Pathology 3rd Series*. Washington, DC: American Registry of Pathology; 1996.

3. Sabatine M, Colucci W, Shoen F: Primary tumors of the heart. In *Heart Disease: A Textbook of Cardiovascular Medicine*. Edited by Zipes D, Libby P, Bonow R, Braunwald E. Philadelphia: Elsevier Saunders; 2005:1741–1755.

4. Abraham KP, Reddy V, Gattuso P: Neoplasms metastatic to the heart: review of 3314 consecutive autopsies. *Am J Cardiovasc Pathol* 1990, 3:195–198.

5. Mukai K, Shinkai T, Tominaga K, Shimosato Y: The incidence of secondary tumors of the heart and pericardium: a 10-year study. *Jpn J Clin Oncol* 1988, 18:195–201.

6. Hendel RC, Patel MR, Kramer CM, *et al.*: ACCF/ACR/SCCT/SCMR/ASNC/NASCI/SCAI/SIR 2006 appropriateness criteria for cardiac computed tomography and cardiac magnetic resonance imaging: a report of the American College of Cardiology Foundation Quality Strategic Directions Committee Appropriateness Criteria Working Group, American College of Radiology, Society of Cardiovascular Computed Tomography, Society for Cardiovascular Magnetic Resonance, American Society of Nuclear Cardiology, North American Society for Cardiac Imaging, Society for Cardiovascular Angiography and Interventions, and Society of Interventional Radiology. *J Am Coll Cardiol* 2006, 48:1475–1497.

7. Dooms GC, Hricak H, Sollitto RA, Higgins CB: Lipomatous tumors and tumors with fatty component: MR imaging potential and comparison of MR and CT results. *Radiology* 1985, 157:479–483.

8. Luna A, Ribes R, Caro P, *et al.*: Evaluation of cardiac tumors with magnetic resonance imaging. *Eur Radiol* 2005, 15:1446–1455.

9. Semelka RC, Shoenut JP, Wilson ME, *et al.*: Cardiac masses: signal intensity features on spin-echo, gradient-echo, gadolinium-enhanced spin-echo, and TurboFLASH images. *J Magn Reson Imaging* 1992, 2:415–420.

10. Hoffmann U, Globits S, Frank H: Cardiac and paracardiac masses. Current opinion on diagnostic evaluation by magnetic resonance imaging. *Eur Heart J* 1998, 19:553–563.

11. Amparo EG, Higgins CB, Farmer D, *et al.*: Gated MRI of cardiac and paracardiac masses: initial experience. *AJR Am J Roentgenol* 1984, 143:1151–1156.

12. Vinee P, Stover B, Sigmund G, *et al.*: MR imaging of the pericardial cyst. *J Magn Reson Imaging* 1992, 2:593–596.

13. Oshima H, Hara M, Kono T, *et al.*: Cardiac hemangioma of the left atrial appendage: CT and MR findings. *J Thorac Imaging* 2003, 18:204–206.

14. Brodwater B, Erasmus J, McAdams HP, Dodd L: Case report. Pericardial hemangioma. *J Comput Assist Tomogr* 1996, 20:954–956.

15. Krombach GA, Saeed M, Higgins C: Cardiac masses. In *Cardiovascular MRI and MRA*. Edited by Higgins CB, de Roos A. Philadelphia: Lippincott Williams & Wilkins; 2003:136–154.

16. Burke AP, Rosado-de-Christenson M, Templeton PA, Virmani R: Cardiac fibroma: clinicopathologic correlates and surgical treatment. *J Thorac Cardiovasc Surg* 1994, 108:862–870.

17. Basso C, Valente M, Poletti A, *et al.*: Surgical pathology of primary cardiac and pericardial tumors. *Eur J Cardiothorac Surg* 1997, 12:730–737.

18. Araoz PA, Eklund HE, Welch TJ, Breen JF: CT and MR imaging of primary cardiac malignancies. *Radiographics* 1999, 19:1421–1434.

19. Enochs WS, Petherick P, Bogdanova A, *et al.*: Paramagnetic metal scavenging by melanin: MR imaging. *Radiology* 1997, 204:417–423.

20. Xanthos T, Giannakopoulos N, Papadimitriou L: Lipomatous hypertrophy of the interatrial septum: a pathological and clinical approach. *Int J Cardiol* 2007, 121:4–8.

21. Araoz PA, Mulvagh SL, Tazelaar HD, *et al.*: CT and MR imaging of benign primary cardiac neoplasms with echocardiographic correlation. *Radiographics* 2000, 20:1303–1319.

11

CHAPTER

Evaluation of Dilated Cardiomyopathy

Sanjay K. Prasad, Rory O'Hanlon, and Ravi Assomull

Dilated Cardiomyopathy	
Definition	Infectious
Dilated cardiomyopathy is a disease of the myocardium that is characterized by dilatation and impaired contraction of the left ventricle or both ventricles	Viral (HIV, Coxsackievirus B, CMV)
Etiology	Rickettsial
Idiopathic	Bacterial (diphtheria)
Familial/genetic	Parasites (Chagas disease, toxoplasma)
Toxic	Fungal
Ethanol	Mycobacterial
Chemotherapeutic agents	Inflammatory
Antiretroviral agents	Collagen vascular disorders (SLE, scleroderma, dermatomyositis)
Lead, cobalt, mercury	Hypersensitivity myocarditis
Chloroquine	Sarcoidosis
Metabolic	Neuromuscular
Endocrine (thyroid, phaeochromocytoma, Cushing's syndrome, diabetes)	Duchenne muscular dystrophy
Nutritional deficiencies (thiamine, selenium, carnitine)	Fascioscapulohumeral muscular dystrophy
Electrolyte disturbance (hypocalcemia, hypophosphatemia)	Erb limb-girdle dystrophy
	Myotonic dystrophy
	Friedreich's ataxia

Figure 11-1. Dilated cardiomyopathy etiology. Dilated cardiomyopathy has a multifactorial etiology and understanding the basis can help guide treatment strategies and enable appropriate risk stratification. CMV—cytomegalovirus; SLE—systemic lupus erythematosus.

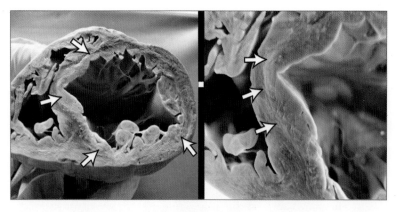

Figure 11-2. Cardiac specimen from a patient with dilated cardiomyopathy corresponding to a CMR short-axis view (*left panel*). Close-up of septum is also shown (*right panel*). The left ventricle (LV) is markedly dilated with global thinning. The interventricular septum is deviated to the right. There is extensive mid-wall fibrosis (*arrows*) with a near circumferential distribution. The pattern of fibrosis does not affect the subendocardium, and this is an important distinguishing feature from LV dysfunction caused by coronary artery disease.

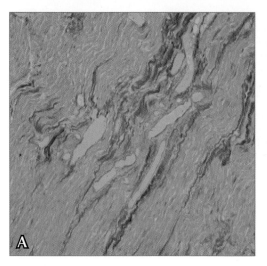
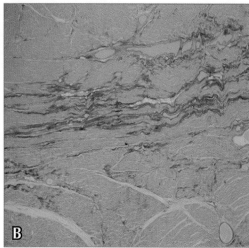

Figure 11-3. Fibrosis in dilated cardiomyopathy. **A** and **B**, Micrograph images from interventricular septum demonstrating replacement fibrosis. There is admixed fibrous tissue (*purple*) and myocytes in this midventricular zone circumferentially. Three main forms of fibrosis are identified in dilated cardiomyopathy—interstitial, replacement, and perivascular. They are particularly associated with advanced stages of the disease process. Typically, replacement fibrosis is seen mainly in the mid-wall and subepicardium. The fibrosis appears to be a common end-result of several different etiologies. CMR is able to detect areas of replacement fibrosis with a spatial resolution of approximately 1 mm (~1 g).

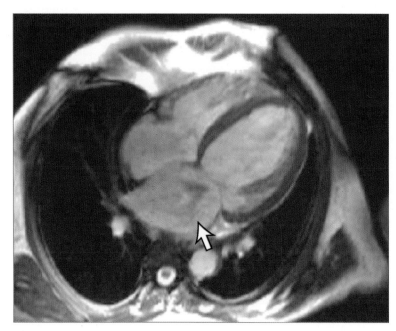

Figure 11-4. Four-chamber gradient echo image of a patient with dilated cardiomyopathy. The left ventricle (LV) is dilated and globular with severe impairment of systolic function. The interventricular septum is deviated toward the right. The left atrium is also enlarged. Function mitral regurgitation can be seen (*arrow*).

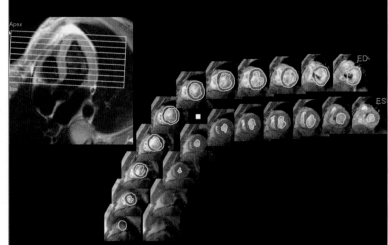

Figure 11-5. Volumetric assessment in dilated cardiomyopathy patients by CMR. Accurate measurement of left ventricle (LV) and right ventricle dimensions and function is important in establishing the diagnosis of dilated cardiomyopathy. A series of sequential short-axis cines is taken from the base to apex, based on long-axis views. LV end-diastolic and systolic endocardial and epicardial borders for each slice are defined manually by planimetry or using contour detection software. Measurements from each slice are summed by the method of disks to derive end-systolic and end-diastolic volumes, overall ejection fraction, and cardiac mass. Reproducibility is high because imaging is volumetric; there is good subendocardial definition, and no geometric assumptions are made.

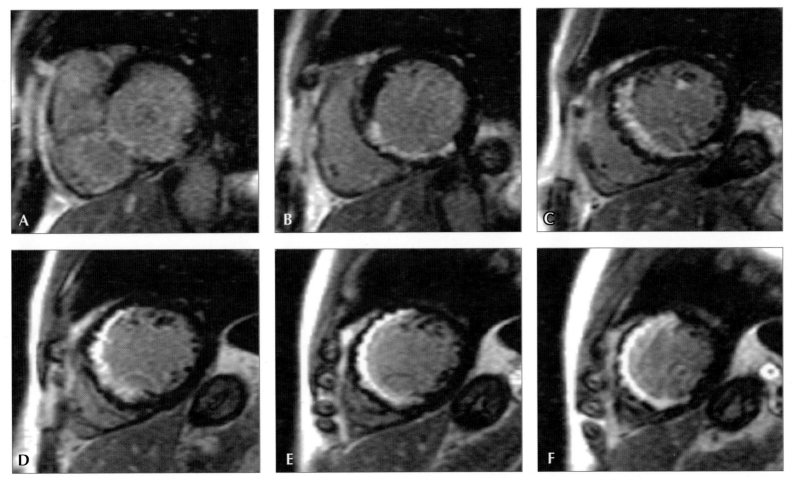

Figure 11-6. A–F, Patterns of fibrosis: myocardial infarction. Short-axis stack after administration of gadolinium-based contrast agent. The gadolinium-based contrast agent has paramagnetic properties that enables in vivo tissue characterization based on the patterns of enhancement. In the infarct setting, the subendocardium is most distal to the epicardial coronary arteries and therefore it is most vulnerable to the effects of ischemia. Fibrosis is always seen in the subendocardium with transmural extension depending on the severity of the ischemic injury. Using T1-weighted inversion-recovery pulse sequences, subendocardial late gadolinium enhancement is seen in this patient in the septal wall, as well as part of the inferior wall. The patient had impaired left ventricular function after a previous infarction.

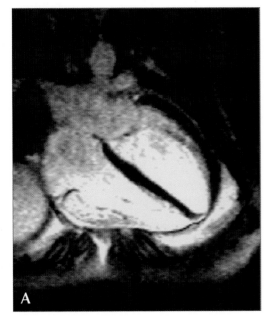
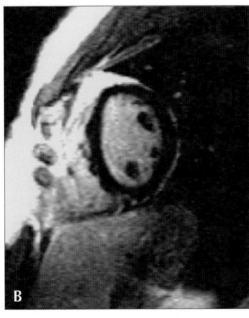

Figure 11-7. A and **B,** Patterns of fibrosis: inversion recovery sequence after administration of gadolinium-based contrast agents in the four-chamber and short-axis views. After the administration of gadolinium-based contrast agents, in patients with dilated cardiomyopathy and unobstructed coronaries, the majority of patients (~60%) do not show late gadolinium enhancement, indicating no detectable replacement fibrosis. This technique is also useful in excluding infarction associated with vessel recanalization or due to embolic phenomenon/spasm as an alternative cause for left ventricular dysfunction. (*Adapted from* McCrohon *et al.* [1].)

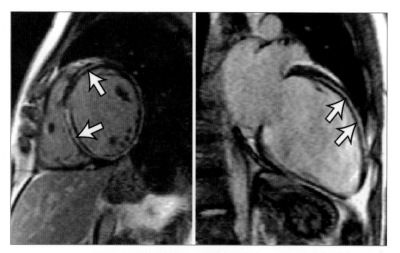

Figure 11-8. Patterns of fibrosis: inversion recovery sequences of the mid-cavity and four-chamber views after administration of gadolinium-based contrast agents. Approximately 30% of patients with dilated cardiomyopathy in several series show a mid-wall or subepicardial pattern of late gadolinium enhancement (LGE) as shown here (*arrows*). Importantly, the subendocardium is not affected, and the pattern of LGE does not accord with the specific territory of a coronary artery supply. This serves as a means of distinguishing an ischemic underlying etiology from a nonischemic dilated cardiomyopathy. The mechanism for fibrosis in this cohort of patients is unclear, but it is thought to reflect a combination of apoptosis, inflammatory changes, and microvascular ischemia. (*Adapted from* McCrohon *et al.* [1].)

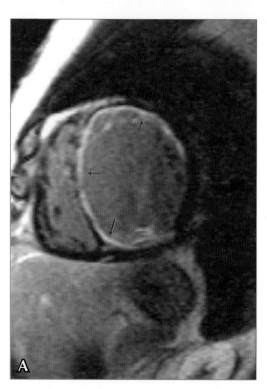

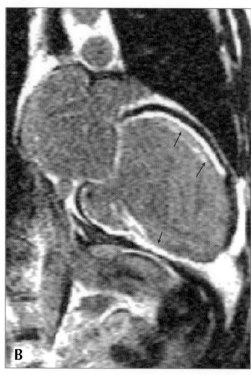

Figure 11-9. **A** and **B**, Patterns of fibrosis: late gadolinium enhancement (LGE) views in the short-axis and vertical long-axis planes after administration of gadolinium-based contrast agents. In approximately 10% to 15% of patients with a diagnostic label of dilated cardiomyopathy based on left ventricular (LV) dysfunction and unobstructed coronaries, a pattern of LGE is seen that is identical to that observed postinfarction. The subendocardium is always affected, and the distribution occurs in a region subtended by a specific coronary artery (or arteries). Mechanisms of infarction in the absence of significant coronary stenoses are recanalization, spasm, or embolic phenomenon. The amount of infarction identified provides a guide to the underlying etiology, whether the infarct is the main causative etiology for the LV dysfunction or if it reflects "bystander" disease particularly in older patients in whom there may be dual pathologies.

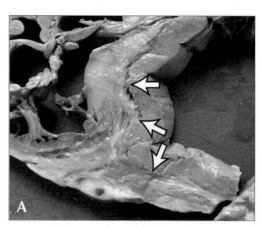

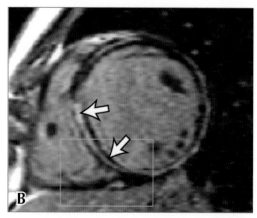

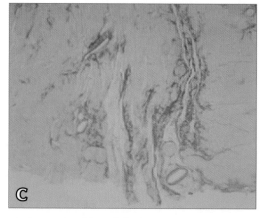

Figure 11-10. In vivo and ex vivo demonstration of fibrosis. Postmortem view of the inferoseptal wall (**A**) and the corresponding in vivo CMR scan (**B**) in a patient with dilated cardiomyopathy. The late gadolinium enhancement short-axis view demonstrates evidence of extensive mid-wall fibrosis (*arrows*) with validation on examination of the ex vivo heart (*arrows*). Histologic examination (**C**) using Sirius Red stain demonstrates replacement fibrosis in an area of LGE. No inflammatory cells were seen. (*Adapted from* Assomull *et al.* [2].)

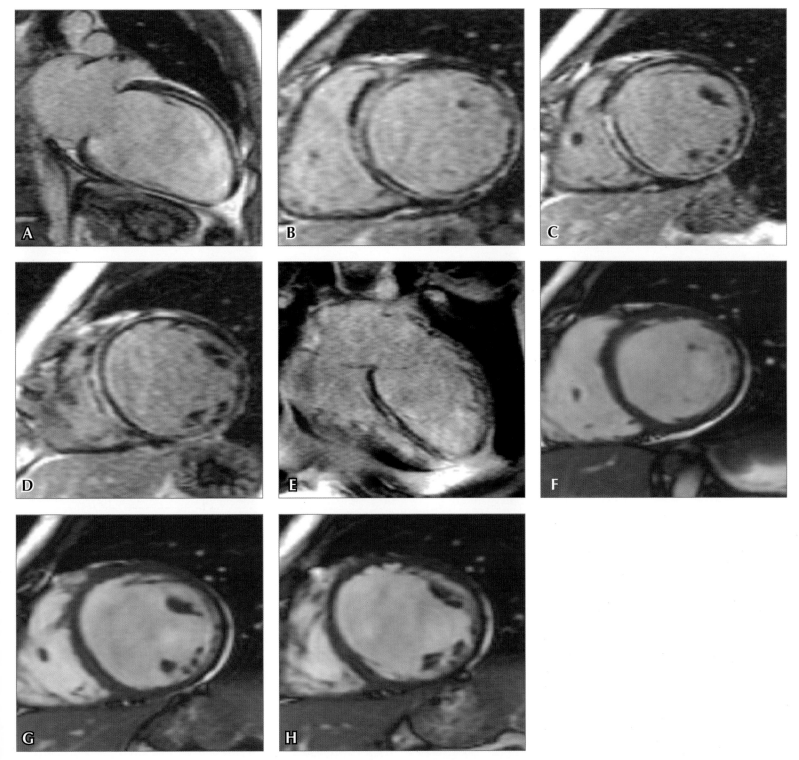

Figure 11-11. **A–H**, Familial dilated cardiomyopathy. Approximately 25% of patients with dilated cardiomyopathy have a familial predisposition. Several underlying mutations have been identified. However, phenotypic expression may be variable and highlights the need for accurate imaging, particularly for screening to enable early detection. In addition to adverse ventricular remodelling, evidence of fibrosis can also be seen reflecting a common pathway with other etiologies of dilated cardiomyopathy. In a cohort of patients, late gadolinium enhancement mid-wall fibrosis may be seen before evidence of left ventricle dilatation so that it is not merely a marker of end-stage disease.

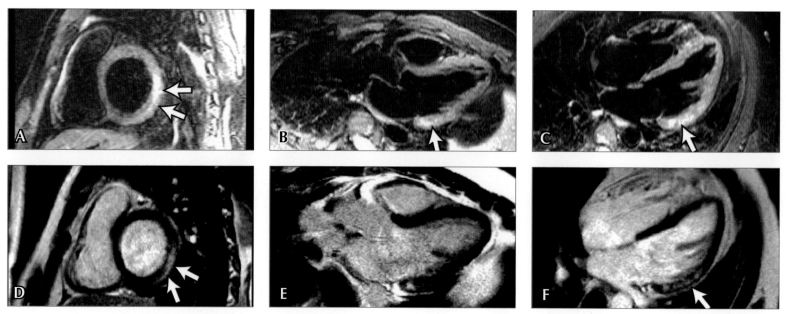

Figure 11-12. Postviral myocarditis. The majority of patients with acute viral myocarditis will recover with normal ventricular function. A proportion will develop dilated cardiomyopathy. In the early phase of the disease process, cine images can detect global and regional wall motion abnormalities. T2-weighted images (**A–C**) can demonstrate global and regional patterns of inflammation and are useful in establishing the diagnosis and following disease activity. In this example, there is increased signal intensity in the lateral wall (*arrows*) indicative of increased myocardial water (*ie*, edema) consistent with myocardial inflammation. Corresponding late gadolinium enhancement (LGE) images (**D–F**) in the acute phase will demonstrate a combination of inflammation and fibrosis in the mid-wall and epicardial layer of the lateral wall (*arrows*). In the chronic phase as inflammation subsides, the LGE pattern reflects predominant fibrosis and it may offer a prognostic guide to functional recovery. In addition, the regional distribution may relate to the underlying viral pathogen. Traditionally, management of these patients has involved endomyocardial biopsies in patients showing clinical deterioration. Apart from its invasive nature, the diagnostic yield is low because the disease process is predominantly left-sided and patchy. By evaluating the whole myocardium with the range of sequences available, CMR may guide appropriate regions for biopsy or, better still, obviate the need for biopsy as well as enabling specific pathogen-targeted treatment strategies in patients who are failing to recover. (*Adapted from* Mahrholdt *et al.* [3].)

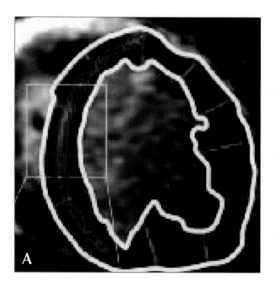
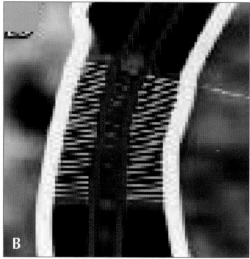

Figure 11-13. Risk stratification: the presence of fibrosis affects myocardial automaticity and provides a mechanism for ventricular re-entry arrhythmias. Therefore, it represents a basis for the occurrence of sudden cardiac death. By planimetry or signal intensity thresholding, the amount of fibrosis can be quantified both in terms of overall amount and segmental transmural extent (**A** and **B**).

Continued on the next page

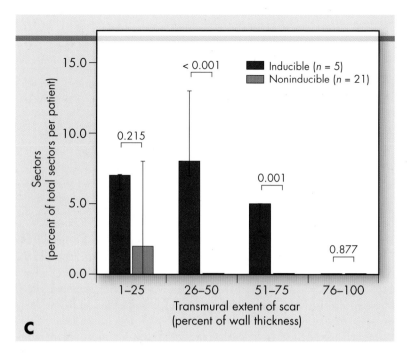

C

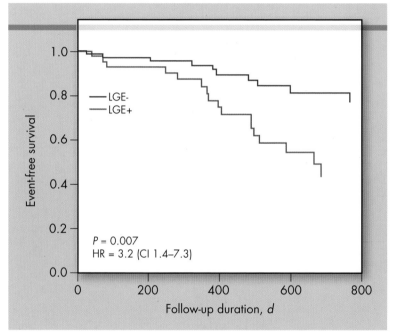

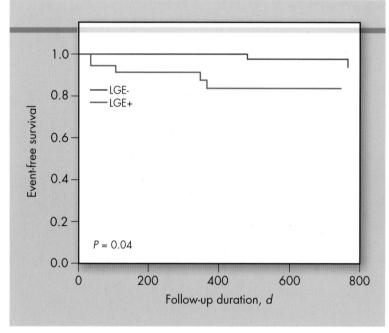

Figure 11-13. *(Continued)* There is close correlation between the likelihood of inducing ventricular tachycardia during an electrophysiological study and mid-wall fibrosis with a transmural extent between 25% to 75% (**C**).

Figure 11-14. Risk stratification: the presence of replacement fibrosis in patients with dilated cardiomyopathy, as detected by CMR, is associated with adverse clinical outcomes. Patients with late gadolinium enhancement (LGE) mid-wall fibrosis have a much higher incidence of the combined end point of all-cause mortality and unplanned cardiac hospitalization compared with those that do not. This finding withstands multivariate analysis to correct for any differences in baseline volumetric parameters, function, or medications. The hazard ratio (HR) for the end point is 3.2. Application of these findings is in risk stratification and potentially guiding device implantation.

Figure 11-15. Risk stratification: patients with late gadolinium enhancement (LGE) mid-wall fibrosis have a higher occurrence of significant arrhythmic events including the combined end point of sudden cardiac death and sustained ventricular tachycardia compared with patients with no detectable fibrosis. Part of the mechanism for this is the occurrence of ventricular re-entry arrhythmias. (*Adapted from* Assomull *et al.* [2].)

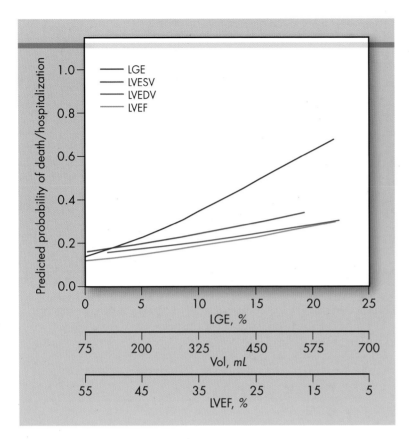

Figure 11-16. Risk stratification: the amount of mid-wall fibrosis in patients with dilated cardiomyopathy correlates with the likelihood of adverse clinical outcomes including the end point of all-cause mortality and unplanned hospitalization. The presence of late gadolinium enhancement (LGE) fibrosis is associated with a greater predisposition to significant arrhythmias. In addition, LGE fibrosis is associated with worse myocardial relaxation. Compared to traditionally used risk stratification measures such as left ventricular ejection fraction (LVEF) and left ventricular end-systolic volume (LVESV), LGE fibrosis may offer better positive predictive values although this will need to be formally assessed in a multicentre trial. LVEDV—left ventricular end-diastolic volume.

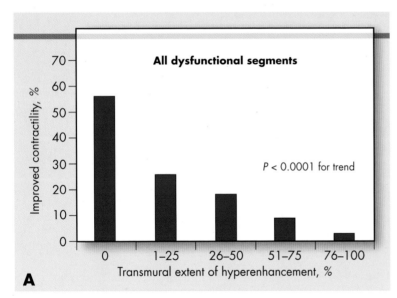

A

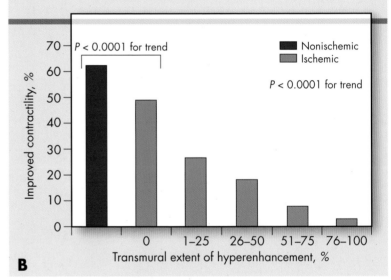

B

Figure 11-17. A and B, Response to therapy. Despite advances in therapy for heart failure, an important cohort of patients is nonresponsive. Mechanisms for this include receptor activity but also the amount of fibrosis. Patients with dilated cardiomyopathy are generally more responsive to treatment than those with underlying coronary artery disease. Despite the presence of fibrosis, dysfunctional segments from patients with nonischemic cardiomyopathy are more likely to improve in contractility than segments from patients with left ventricle dysfunction due to coronary artery disease. Although end-stage ischemic and nonischemic cardiomyopathy may exhibit common features, this finding suggests that there may be important pathophysiologic differences (*Adapted from* Bello *et al.* [4].)

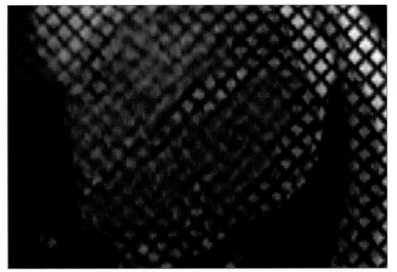

Figure 11-18. Assessment of contractility. Wall motion assessment is important in assessing diastolic dysfunction and mechanical dyssynchrony. Several CMR mechanisms are available to do this. Peak-filling and time-volume curves are useful to measure myocardial relaxation properties. Regional function can be quantified using a technique called CMR *tagging*, in which presaturation tag grids are applied to the myocardium. Their deformation during the cardiac cycle can be used to extrapolate radial, circumferential, and longitudinal strain. Although CMR does not have the temporal resolution of echocardiography, one advantage of CMR, unlike tissue Doppler, is that the exact same section of myocardium is followed throughout the cardiac cycle. Strain rates can be derived from the acquired measurements.

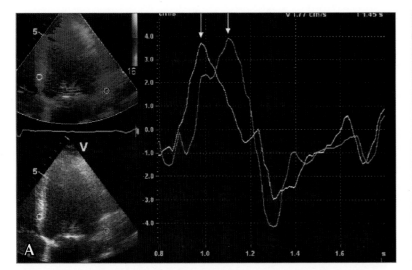

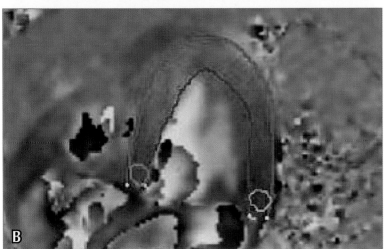

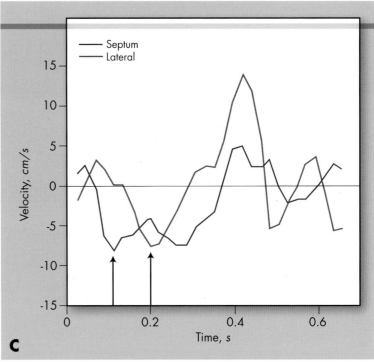

Figure 11-19. A–C, Assessment of dyssynchrony. Using CMR myocardial velocity mapping is an alternative technique used to measure myocardial strain rate and thus regional contractility. There are comparable data between this technique and tissue Doppler in determining myocardial dyssynchrony at the basal septal and lateral walls. When used in conjunction with the late gadolinium enhancement technique, information is also provided to guide lead placement based on the presence, location, and amount of fibrosis. (*Adapted from* Westenberg *et al.* [5].)

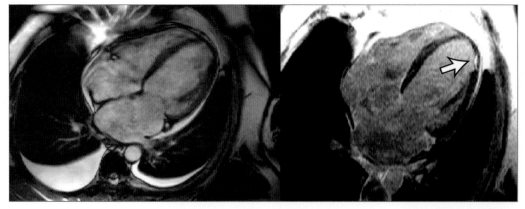

Figure 11-20. Differential diagnosis. Understanding the mechanism for left ventricular (LV) dysfunction is important in guiding treatment strategies. This can be challenging where there may be dual pathologies. This patient presented with an acute coronary syndrome with lateral electrocardiogram changes. His background was notable for vastly excessive alcohol consumption. Echocardiography demonstrated severe LV dysfunction. Radiograph angiography showed only a moderate mid-vessel stenosis in the circumflex vessel with no other evidence of obstruction. This was felt to be out of proportion to the level of LV impairment. CMR showed poor LV function with pleural effusions (*left panel*) and was useful in demonstrating a small apico-lateral wall infarct (*right panel*; *red arrow*) consistent with the electrocardiogram changes but did not account for the poor LV ejection fraction, thus confirming the diagnosis of dilated cardiomyopathy due to heavy alcohol consumption with concurrent "bystander" coronary artery disease.

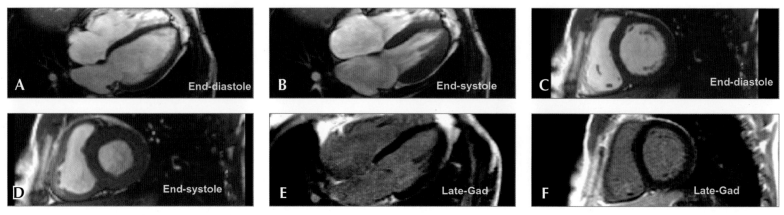

Figure 11-21. Dilated cardiomyopathy versus athletic heart. Distinguishing a heart with dilated cardiomyopathy from an athletic heart in those participating in high level sports is important with an obvious major impact on lifestyle and risk stratification. CMR provides accurate three-dimensional volumetric assessment with the gold standard for dimensions and function. Wall thickness can be measured in all segments. Typically in both cases there may be left ventricular (LV) dilatation, but in the athletic heart, function is usually in the normal range, wall thickness may be mildly elevated (**A–D**), and no mid-wall fibrosis is detectable (**E** and **F**). The diagnosis of athletic heart is usually established in conjunction with a cardiopulmonary exercise test. Where there is diagnostic uncertainty, a repeat scan after 3 months of physical deconditioning is useful; in dilated cardiomyopathy, dimensions and function would remain impaired, whereas in an athletic heart, there would be normalization of LV parameters.

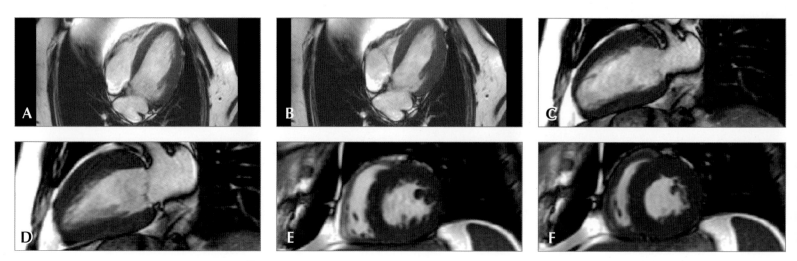

Figure 11-22. Dilated cardiomyopathy versus hypertensive disease. In contrast to dilated cardiomyopathy, hypertensive cardiac disease is characterized by left ventricular (LV) dilatation in conjunction with a concentric pattern of LV wall thickening (**A–F**) in the context of antecedent chronic hypertension. LV systolic function is usually in the normal range until the late stage of the disease process. Mid-wall replacement fibrosis is not seen. Regression of LV hypertrophy is associated with improved clinical outcomes.

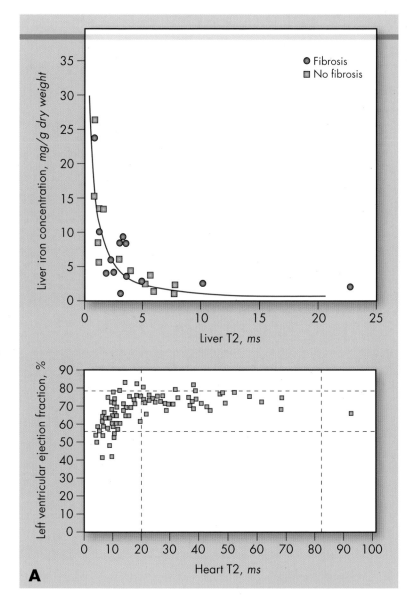

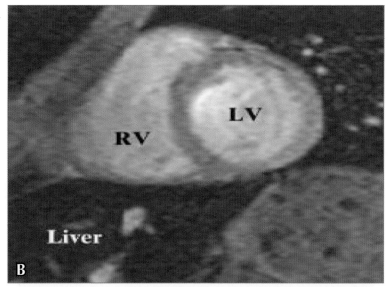

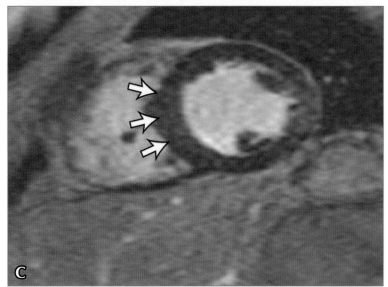

Figure 11-23. Dilated cardiomyopathy versus iron overload cardiomyopathy. In patients with primary hemochromatosis or secondary hemochromatosis conditions (such as transfusion dependent thalassemia major), iron overload may lead to left ventricular (LV) dilatation and functional impairment. Treatment is with chelating agents and traditionally this has been targeted based on liver biopsy iron and serum ferritin levels. This has its limitations. Biopsy carries a tangible risk of complications and serial evaluation is difficult. Serum ferritin levels can also change due to underlying inflammation. An important advance has been the validation of a CMR-based T2* technique that is able to quantify the amount of iron in the heart and liver. It is based on the influence of iron on the signal intensity of T2* scans. This technique can be used for serial evaluation. The liver T2* levels decrease as the liver iron concentration increases (**A**, *top graph*). Myocardial T2* signal intensity (measured in ms) below 20 is associated with a linear reduction in LV ejection fraction (**A**, *bottom graph*). **B**, The liver is dark correlating with a low T2* and high iron overload. By contrast, there is relatively little cardiac iron as shown by the brighter myocardium. **C**, Conversely, this image is a scan from a patient with little liver iron, but excess myocardial iron overload (myocardium hypointense correlating with a low T2*). In the former case, chelation therapy based on liver biopsy would have resulted in excess therapy, whereas in the latter case, the patient would have been undertreated to reduce myocardial loading. This finding further underlines the problems associated with previous practices of guiding chelation therapy using liver biopsies alone. (*Adapted from* Braunwald's Heart Disease [6].)

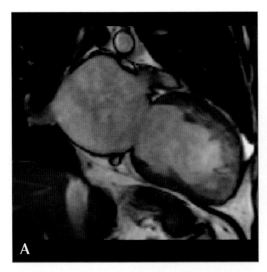

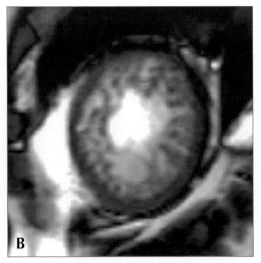

lar recesses, a thinned subepicardial layer. The main regions affected are the apex and lateral LV walls. It is caused by arrest of normal embryogenesis of the endocardium and myocardium. It can occur in isolation or be associated with other congenital defects. It is associated with an increased risk of emboli, and arrhythmias and is thought to have a genetic basis in a subgroup. The apex is an area that can often be difficult to visualize by echocardiography because of near-field signal drop-out. This is not a problem with CMR and as a consequence, it is a condition that is being increasingly recognized. An example is shown in the long-axis (**A**) and short-axis (**B**) planes.

Figure 11-24. Dilated cardiomyopathy versus myocardial noncompaction. Myocardial noncompaction can also result in a dilated left ventricle (LV) with impaired function. It is characterized by a spongy hypertrabeculated subendocardial layer with deep intertrabecu-

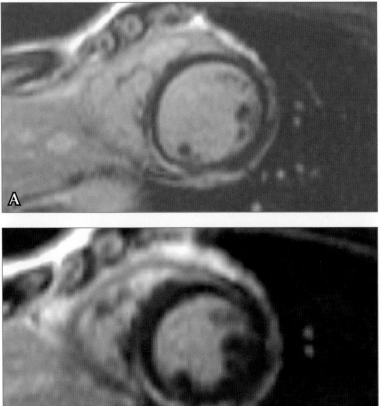

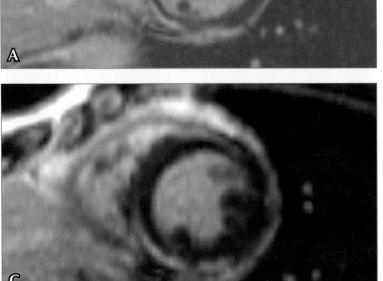

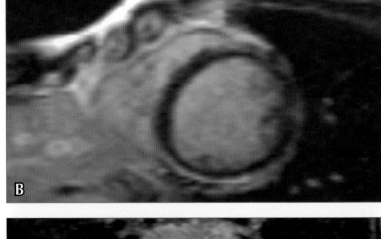

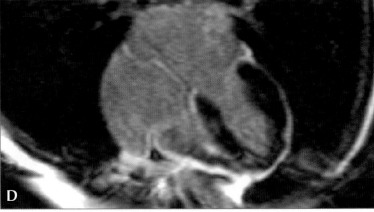

Figure 11-25. Dilated cardiomyopathy versus arrhythmogenic left ventricular (LV) cardiomyopathy. Arrhythmogenic right ventricular (RV) cardiomyopathy is a familial heart muscle disease characterized by progressive fibrofatty replacement of the RV myocardium. Structural abnormalities include myocardial wall thinning, aneurysms, and cavity dilation. LV involvement occurs with disease progression and was present on histology in more than 75% of cases in a multicenter pathologic study. Left-sided arrhythmogenic RV cardiomyopathy has recently been recog- nized on postmortem examination, with fibrofatty infiltration exclusive to the LV and in vivo, although case numbers remain small. Autosomal-dominant arrhythmogenic LV cardiomyopathy caused by a novel frameshift mutation in desmoplakin was described, and findings can be mistaken for a dilated cardiomyopathy. On CMR, there is LV dilatation with an unusual pattern of late gadolinium enhancement that predominantly appears to affect the LV inferior subepicardial wall and RV inferoseptal subendocardial wall (**A–D**).

Role of CMR in Distinguishing Dilated Cardiomyopathy from Left Ventricular Dysfunction due to Coronary Artery Disease

	Sensitivity	Specificity	Accuracy	PPV	NPV
Clinical history of MI	0.49	0.95	0.63	0.95	0.46
Q-wave ECG	0.32	0.95	0.52	0.93	0.39
Wall thickening	0.76	0.79	0.77	0.89	0.6
Regional WMA	0.8	0.53	0.72	0.79	0.56
LGE + WMA	0.8	0.84	0.82	0.92	0.67
LGE + WT	0.8	0.81	0.82	0.92	0.75
LGE	0.98	0.84	0.93	0.93	0.94
LGE (without history of MI)	0.95	0.89	0.93	0.91	0.94
LGE (without Q-wave ECG)	0.96	0.89	0.93	0.93	0.94

Figure 11-26. Role of CMR in distinguishing dilated cardiomyopathy from left ventricular dysfunction caused by coronary artery disease. In patients with heart failure, CMR findings combined with the clinical history and electrocardiogram changes carry a high sensitivity, accuracy, and positive predictive value (PPV) to distinguish between an idiopathic and ischemic etiology. Given that a significant proportion of radiograph angiograms show unobstructed disease, CMR may act as a gatekeeper to angiography with additional prognostic data. ECG—electrocardiogram; LGE—late gadolinium enhancement; MI—myocardial infarction; NPV—negative predictive value; PPV—positive predictive value; WMA—wall motion abnormality; WT—wall thickness. (*Adapted from* Casolo *et al.* [7].)

CMR Protocol

Cine functional images include short axis stack

± T1 for fat replacement/pericardium

± T2 sequence for inflammation/edema

± T2* if iron overload is suspected

Flow maps, if valvular lesion

Late gadolinium enhancement study with

Early images: thrombus detection

Late gadolinium enhancement: infarction/fibrosis

Figure 11-27. CMR protocol. A suggested protocol is shown for a detailed evaluation of the patient with suspected dilated cardiomyopathy. Sequences used will evaluate overall function and dimensions as well as tissue characterization as shown.

Who Should Be Scanned?

Poor transthoracic echo image quality

Patients in whom etiology is unclear from history and initial investigations

DCM vs IHD

Other causes

Assessment of severity

Screening

Guiding treatment strategies

Response to treatment

Risk stratification

Systemic disease process: question cardiac involvement

Combined pathologies

Figure 11-28. When to consider a CMR. A suggested list of when a CMR should be considered in patients with suspected or established dilated cardiomyopathy (DCM). IHD—ischemic heart disease.

REFERENCES

1. McCrohon JA, Moon JC, Prasad SK, *et al.*: Differentiation of heart failure related to dilated cardiomyopathy and coronary artery disease using gadolinium-enhanced cardiovascular magnetic resonance. *Circulation* 2003, 108:54–59.

2. Assomull RG, Prasad SK, Lyne J, *et al.*: Cardiovascular magnetic resonance, fibrosis, and prognosis in dilated cardiomyopathy. *J Am Coll Cardiol* 2006, 48:1977–1985.

3. Mahrholdt H, Goedecke C, Wagner A, *et al.*: Cardiovascular magnetic resonance assessment of human myocarditis: a comparison to histology and molecular pathology. *Circulation* 2004, 109:1250–1258.

4. Bello D, Shah DJ, Farah GM, *et al.*: Gadolinium cardiovascular magnetic resonance predicts reversible myocardial dysfunction and remodeling in patients with heart failure undergoing beta-blocker therapy. *Circulation* 2003, 108:1945–1953.

5. Westenberg JJ, Lamb HJ, van der Geest RJ, *et al.*: Assessment of left ventricular dyssynchrony in patients with conduction delay and idiopathic dilated cardiomyopathy: head-to-head comparison between tissue doppler imaging and velocity-encoded magnetic resonance imaging. *J Am Coll Cardiol* 2006, 47:2042–2048.

6. Libby P, Bonow RO, Mann DL, Zipes DP: *Braunwald's Heart Disease: A Textbook of Cardiovascular Medicine, 8th edition.* Philadelphia:Saunders; 2007.

7. Casolo G, Minneci S, Manta R, *et al.*: Identification of the ischemic etiology of heart failure by cardiovascular magnetic resonance imaging: diagnostic accuracy of late gadolinium enhancement. *Am Heart J* 2006, 151:101–108.

RECOMMENDED READING

Mahrholdt H, Wagner A, Deluigi CC, *et al.*: Presentation, patterns of myocardial damage, and clinical course of viral myocarditis. *Circulation* 2006, 114:1581–1590.

Nazarian S, Bluemke DA, Lardo AC, *et al.*: Magnetic resonance assessment of the substrate for inducible ventricular tachycardia in nonischemic cardiomyopathy. *Circulation* 2005, 112:2821–2825.

Norman M, Simpson M, Mogensen J, *et al.*: Novel mutation in desmoplakin causes arrhythmogenic left ventricular cardiomyopathy. *Circulation* 2005, 112:636–642.

Pennell D: MRI and iron-overload cardiomyopathy in thalassanemia. *Circulation* 2006, 113:43–44.

12

Myocarditis

Oliver Strohm and Matthias G. Friedrich

Diagnosing myocarditis is a challenge to cardiologists, as the symptoms may be nonspecific, and commonly used noninvasive tests have a low sensitivity and specificity for this disease [1-3]. Cardiovascular magnetic resonance (CMR) has evolved into a routine imaging tool for many cardiac diseases. With the use of contrast-enhanced techniques, it also allows for diagnosing inflammatory changes in myocarditis and to follow these patients noninvasively [4-7].

Compared with echocardiography and other imaging modalities, CMR has the advantages of: 1) more robust image quality; 2) large field of view; 3) high spatial and temporal resolution; and 4) excellent reproducibility of measured values. With T1-weighted (pre and post contrast) and T2-weighted images, CMR allows for visualizing all aspects of myocardial inflammation: 1) edema (as seen in the early stages of the disease); 2) contrast accumulation in the early enhancement (as seen in early and chronic stages of the disease); and 3) irreversible damage or fibrosis.

Recent data show that a combined CMR protocol not only can be performed in less than 30 minutes but provides a diagnostic accuracy of more than 80% and thus is more accurate than other tests [1,6.8]. It is by many now considered the preferred first line test in patients with suspected myocarditis [2-3].

This chapter provides clinical cases with suspected or proven myocarditis and demonstrates the capabilities of CMR to provide useful information for diagnostic and therapeutic decision-making.

CASE 1: A 25-YEAR-OLD PATIENT WITH SUSPECTED ACUTE MYOCARDITIS

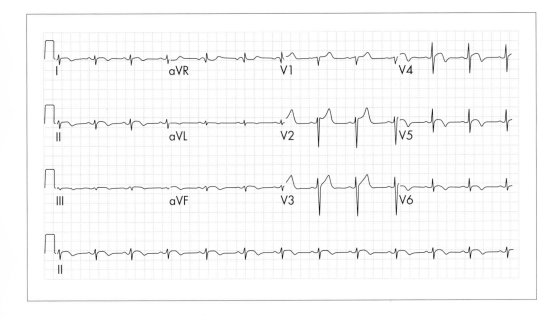

Figure 12-1. 12-Lead electrocardiogram at presentation, demonstrating nonischemic changes in the ST and T segments. Physical examination revealed severe chest pain and shortness of breath (New York Heart Association III), blood pressure 98/58 mm Hg, and heart rate 97 bpm. aVF—augmented voltage, unipolar left leg lead; aVL—augmented voltage, unipolar left arm lead; aVR—augmented voltage, unipolar right arm lead.

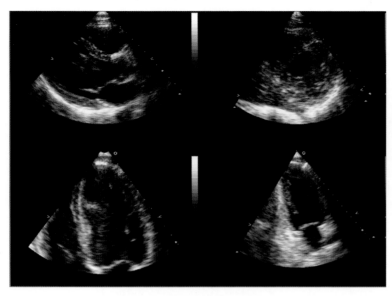

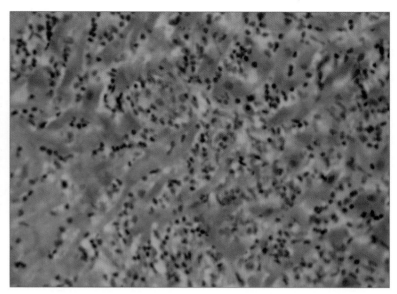

Figure 12-2. Transthoracic echocardiography: Three long axis views (*upper left and lower panels*) and one short axis view (*upper right panel*) are shown. Severely reduced ejection fraction with preserved left ventricular size is demonstrated; valvular function was normal, as was the right ventricular size and function.

Figure 12-3. Endomyocardial biopsy specimen, hematoxylin-eosin staining, magnification 40 × 10. Diffuse severe lymphocytic infiltrates and some myocyte necrosis is noted, consistent with a diagnosis of active lymphocytic myocarditis.

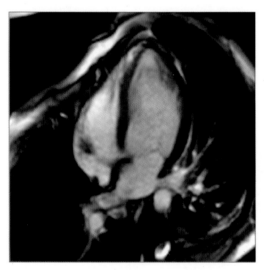

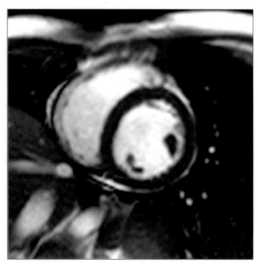

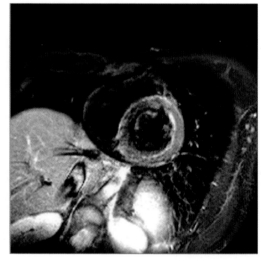

Figure 12-4. CMR cine sequence in four-chamber view orientation as part of a multiple long-axis study is shown. Resolution 192 × 156, echo time 1.1 ms, repetition time 66 ms, slice thickness 8 mm. Normal left ventricular (LV) size and severely reduced ejection fraction (EF) are confirmed. Functional parameters (normal values are shown in parentheses): end-diastolic volume (EDV) 165 mL, end-systolic volume 120 mL, LV stroke volume 45 mL, cardiac output 4.4 L/min, EF 27%, LV EDV index 93 mL (normal 60–120), cardiac index 2.4 L/min/m² (> 2.5), LV mass 99 g (normal 81–165), LV mass index (h) 56 g/m (normal 47–93).

Figure 12-5. CMR cine sequence in multiple short-axis orientation, technical parameters as stated in Figure 12-4. Normal left ventricular size and severely reduced ejection fraction with global hypokinesis are noted.

Figure 12-6. CMR T2-weighted image (STIR) in short-axis orientation at basal level. Diffuse borderline-high myocardial signal ratio is noted (2.1, normal value < 2.0); no effusion is seen. Finding consistent with diffuse myocardial edema of nonischemic origin.

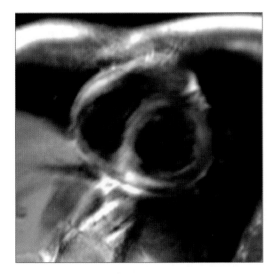

Figure 12-7. CMR T1-weighted short axis (early enhancement) after contrast application (0.1 mmol gadolinium/kg body weight). Globally increased contrast uptake is noted (relative enhancement = 17, normal value < 4.0), consistent with acute inflammation of the myocardium.

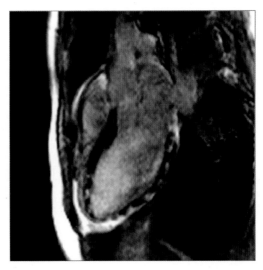

Figure 12-8. CMR late gadolinium enhancement (LGE) image in three-chamber view orientation. Extensive areas of diffuse, non-subendocardial contrast uptake are seen, consistent with non-ischemic scar.

Summary of CMR findings: Extensive LGE in an epicardial distribution, no evidence for ischemic damage. Severely reduced left ventricular (LV) ejection fraction with preserved LV size. Findings consistent with acute myocarditis with some fibrotic changes.

FOLLOW-UP STUDY 1 WEEK AFTER ONSET OF SYMPTOMS

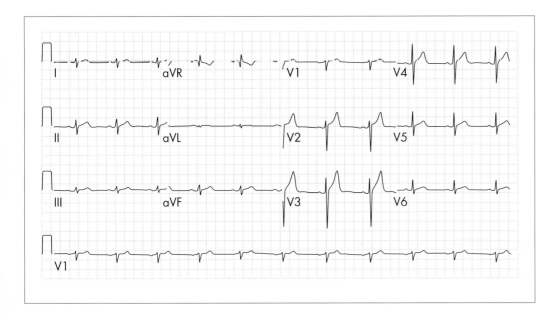

Figure 12-9. 12-Lead electrocardiogram 1 week after onset of symptoms, demonstrating a decrease in the changes of ST and T segments. Physical examination revealed reduced chest pain and shortness of breath compared with initial presentation (now New York Heart Association II–III), blood pressure 108/68 mm Hg, heart rate 85 bpm. No evidence for congestive heart failure on examination. aVF—augmented voltage, unipolar left leg lead; aVL—augmented voltage, unipolar left arm lead; aVR—augmented voltage, unipolar right arm lead.

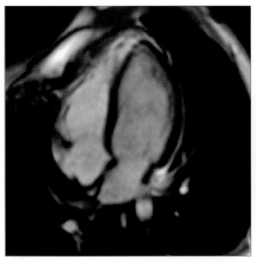

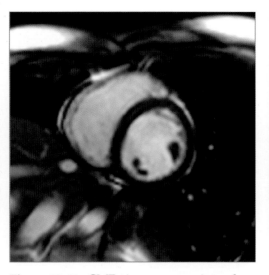

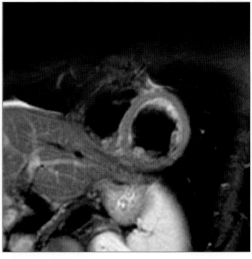

Figure 12-10. CMR cine sequence in four-chamber view orientation as part of a multiple long-axis study is shown. RConstant left ventricular (LV) size to previous study is seen; LV ejection fraction (EF) has normalized. Functional parameters (normal values are shown in parentheses): end-diastolic volume (EDV) 160 mL, end-systolic volume 64 mL, LV stroke volume 96 mL, cardiac output 5.4 L/min, EF 60%, LV EDV index 90 mL (normal 60–120), cardiac index 3.0 L/min/m² (normal >2.5), LV mass 110 g (normal 81–165), LV mass index (h) 62 g/m (normal 47–93).

Figure 12-11. CMR cine sequence in multiple short-axis orientation, technical parameters as stated in Figure 12-10. Normal left ventricular size and normalized reduced ejection fraction with only mild regional hypokinesis are noted.

Figure 12-12. CMR T2-weighted image (STIR) in short-axis orientation at basal level. Diffuse borderline-high myocardial signal ratio is noted (2.0, normal value < 2.0), no effusion is seen. Finding consistent with mild diffuse myocardial edema of a nonischemic origin, as seen in myocarditis.

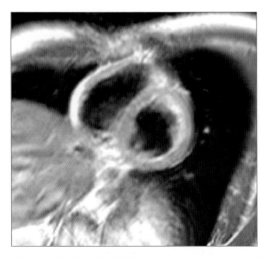

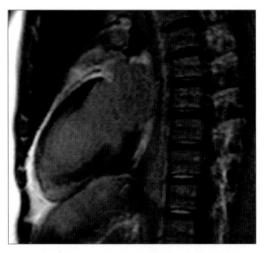

Figure 12-13. CMR T1-weighted short axis (early enhancement) after contrast application (0.1 mmol gadolinium/kg body weight). Globally increased contrast uptake is noted (relative enhancement = 6.4, normal value < 4.0), consistent with acute inflammation of the myocardium. Compared with previous study (*see* Figure 12-7), the inflammation has decreased in intensity.

Figure 12-14. CMR late gadolinium enhancement (LGE) image in two-chamber view orientation. Compared with previous study, the extent of the non-subendocardial contrast uptake has significantly decreased.

Summary of CMR findings: Normalized ejection fraction compared to the first study, reduced early enhancement, and nearly normal cardiac magnetic resonance T2-weighted image (STIR) values. Reduction in the amount of LGE; all findings are consistent with reduced inflammatory activity.

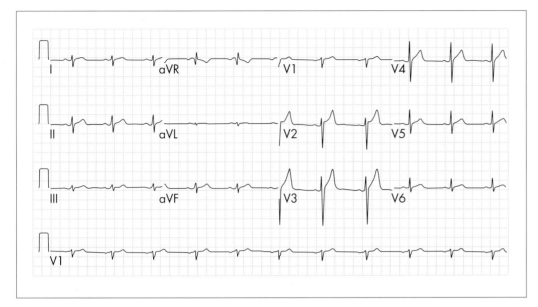

Figure 12-15. 12-Lead electrocardiogram 12 weeks after onset of symptoms, and the changes of ST and T segments are still present. Physical examination revealed no chest pain and only occasional shortness of breath, which had improved significantly compared with initial presentation (now New York Heart Association II), blood pressure 112/64 mm Hg, heart rate 80 bpm. No evidence for congestive heart failure on examination. aVF—augmented voltage, unipolar left leg lead; aVL—augmented voltage, unipolar left arm lead; aVR—augmented voltage, unipolar right arm lead.

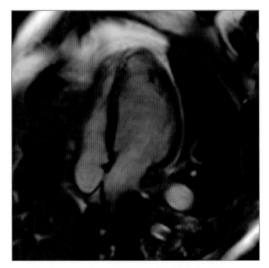

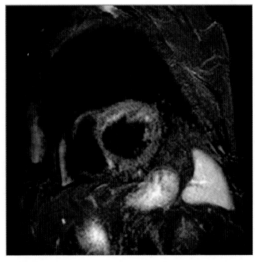

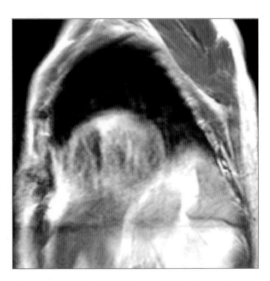

Figure 12-16. CMR cine sequence in four-chamber view orientation as part of a multiple long-axis study is shown. Constant left ventricular (LV) size to previous study is seen, LV ejection fraction (EF) remained normal. Functional parameters (normal values are shown in parentheses): end-diastolic volume (EDV) 160 mL, end-systolic volume 68 mL, LV stroke volume 92 mL, cardiac output 5.9 L/min, EF 58%, LV EDV index 92 mL (normal 60–120), cardiac index 2.7 L/min/m^2 (normal >2.5), LV mass 116 g (normal 81–165), LV mass index (h) 67 g/m (normal 47–93).

Figure 12-17. CMR T2-weighted image (STIR) in short-axis orientation at midventricular level. Normal myocardial signal ratio is noted (1.8, normal value < 2.0), no effusion is seen. Findings are consistent with complete resolving of the previously noted myocardial edema (*see* Figs. 12-6 and 12-12).

Figure 12-18. CMR T1-weighted short axis (early enhancement) after contrast application (0.1 mmol gadolinium/kg body weight). Compared with previous studies (*see* Figs. 12-7 and 12-13), the myocardial contrast uptake is normal in this follow-up study (relative enhancement = 2.6, normal value < 4.0), consistent with resolution of the myocardial inflammation.

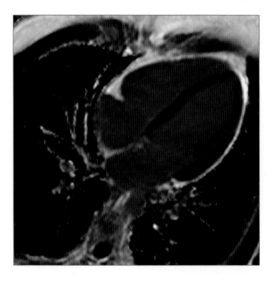

Figure 12-19. CMR late gadolinium enhancement (LGE) image in four-chamber view orientation. Compared with the previous studies, the extent of the non-subendocardial LGE uptake has further decreased.

Summary of CMR findings: Normalized ejection fraction compared to the first two studies, normal early enhancement and nearly normal T2-weighted image (STIR) values. Reduction in the amount of LGE; all findings are consistent with reduced inflammatory activity.

CASE 2: A 35-YEAR-OLD PATIENT WITH ATYPICAL CHEST PAIN

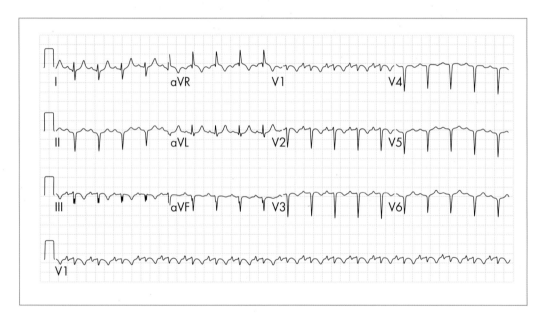

Figure 12-20. 12-Lead electrocardiogram (ECG) at presentation showing sinus tachycardia with unspecific changes in the T-segments. Physical examination revealed chest pain that worsened with positioning; no shortness of breath was reported. Blood pressure 131/74 mm Hg, heart rate 135 bpm. A diagnosis of myocarditis cannot be established with these ECG findings; ischemia is very unlikely. aVF—augmented voltage, unipolar left leg lead; aVL—augmented voltage, unipolar left arm lead; aVR—augmented voltage, unipolar right arm lead.

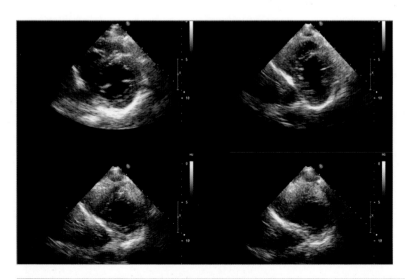

Figure 12-21. Transthoracic echocardiography, four short-axis views are shown. Normal left ventricular size and function are demonstrated; valvular function was normal, as was the right ventricular size and function.

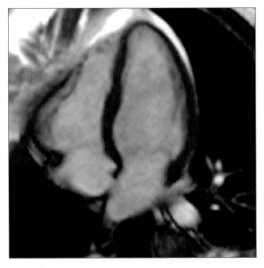

Figure 12-22. CMR cine sequence in four-chamber view orientation as part of a multiple long-axis study is shown. Normal left ventricular (LV) size and normal LV ejection fraction (EF) are confirmed. Functional parameters (normal values are shown in parentheses): end-diastolic volume (EDV) 207 mL, end-systolic volume 73 mL, LV stroke volume 134 mL, cardiac output 9.8 L/min, EF 65%, LV EDV index 116 mL (normal 60–120), cardiac index 4.9 L/min/m² (normal >2.5), LV mass 149 g (normal 81–165), LV mass index (h) 84 g/m (normal 47–93).

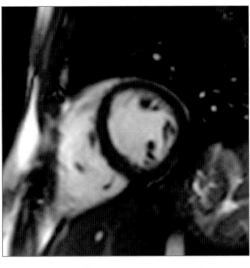

Figure 12-23. CMR cine sequence in multiple short-axis orientation, technical parameters as stated in Figure 12-4. Normal left ventricular size and severely reduced ejection fraction without regional hypokinesis is noted.

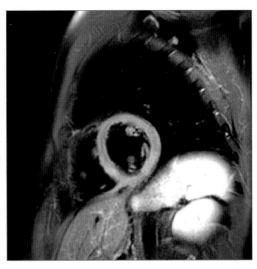

Figure 12-24. CMR T2-weighted image (STIR) in short-axis orientation at basal level. Normal myocardial and pericardial signal ratio is noted (1.6, normal value < 2.0), no effusion is seen. Findings are not consistent with acute myocardial edema or pericarditis.

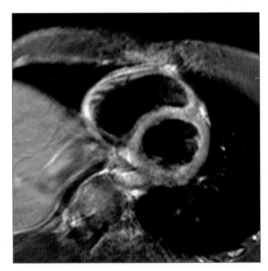

Figure 12-25. CMR T1-weighted short axis (early enhancement) after contrast application (0.1 mmol gadolinium/kg body weight). Normal myocardial contrast uptake is noted (relative enhancement = 3.2, normal value < 4.0), not supportive of a diagnosis of acute inflammation of the myocardium or pericardium.

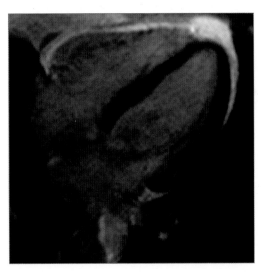

Figure 12-26. CMR late gadolinium enhancement (LGE) image in four-chamber view orientation. No areas of relevant LGE uptake are seen, consistent with the absence of myocardial fibrosis.

Summary of CMR findings: Normal left ventricular size and function; normal T1 and T2 ratios of the myocardium. No evidence for irreversible myocardial injury. This CMR study allows one to exclude an acute myocarditis and/or pericarditis.

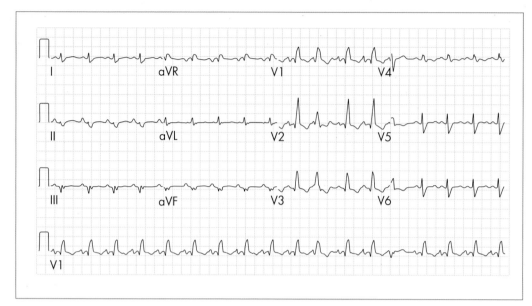

Figure 12-27. 12-Lead electrocardiogram at presentation, showing a right bundle branch block and unspecific changes in the ST and T segments. Physical examination revealed severe shortness of breath (New York Heart Association III), blood pressure 96/58 mm Hg, heart rate 99 bpm. Recently, this patient had suffered from an upper respiratory tract infection, after which his shortness of breath worsened dramatically. He had gained 8 kg over 2 weeks and developed nocturia four to five times per night. aVF—augmented voltage, unipolar left leg lead; aVL—augmented voltage, unipolar left arm lead; aVR—augmented voltage, unipolar right arm lead.

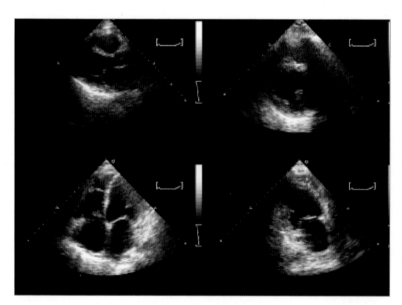

Figure 12-28. Transthoracic echocardiography, three long-axis views and one-short axis view are shown. Moderately enlarged left ventricle with severely reduced ejection fraction is demonstrated, consistent with the previous diagnosis of dilated cardiomyopathy.

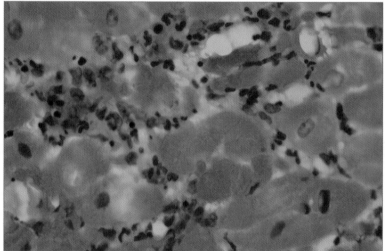

Figure 12-29. Endomyocardial biopsy specimen, hematoxylin-eosin staining staining, magnification 40 × 10. Diffuse lymphocytic infiltrates are noted, consistent with a diagnosis of active lymphocytic myocarditis.

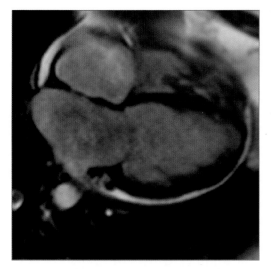

Figure 12-30. CMR cine sequence in four-chamber view orientation as part of a multiple long-axis study is shown. Normal left ventricular (LV) size and severely reduced ejection fraction (EF) are found; there was a trace of pericardial fluid without hemodynamic relevance. Functional parameters (normal values are shown in parentheses): end-diastolic volume (EDV) 247 mL, end-systolic volume 198 mL, LV stroke volume 49 mL, cardiac output 3.5 L/min, EF 20%, LV EDV index 165 mL (normal 60–120), cardiac index 2.1 L/min/m² (normal >2.5), LV mass 102 g (normal 81–165), LV mass index (h) 68 g/m (normal 47–93).

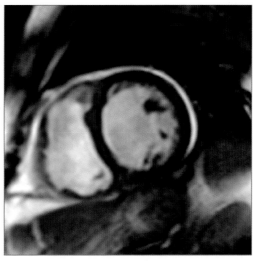

Figure 12-31. CMR cine sequence in multiple short-axis orientation, technical parameters as stated in Figure 12-4. Normal left ventricular size and severely reduced ejection fraction with global hypokinesis are again found.

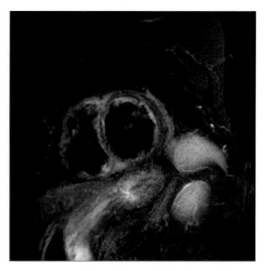

Figure 12-32. CMR T2-weighted image (STIR) in short-axis orientation at mid-ventricular level. Quantitative evaluation showed abnormally high relative signal intensity of the myocardium, when normalized to skeletal muscle (2.6, normal value < 2.0), a small lateral effusion is seen. Finding consistent with diffuse myocardial edema of a nonischemic origin and some pericardial effusion.

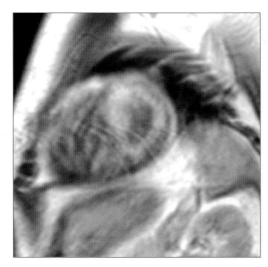

Figure 12-33. CMR T1-weighted short axis (early enhancement) after contrast application (0.1 mmol gadolinium/kg body weight). Image quality is reduced because of the patient's motion and inability to breath regularly; however, evaluation was possible. Globally increased contrast uptake is noted (relative enhancement = 10, normal value < 4.0), consistent with acute inflammation of the myocardium.

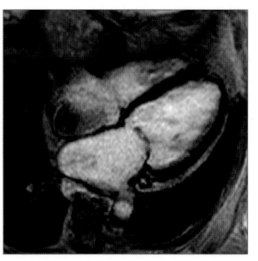

Figure 12-34. CMR late gadolinium enhancement (LGE) image in four-chamber view orientation. No areas of LGE uptake are seen in the myocardium, indicating absence of irreversible myocardial injury/scar tissue.

Summary of CMR findings: Positive early enhancement and positive CMR T2-weighted image (STIR) ratio, allowing for the diagnosis of acute myocarditis. Absence of LGE indicates absence of myocardial fibrosis. Findings are consistent with acute myocarditis without persisting scar.

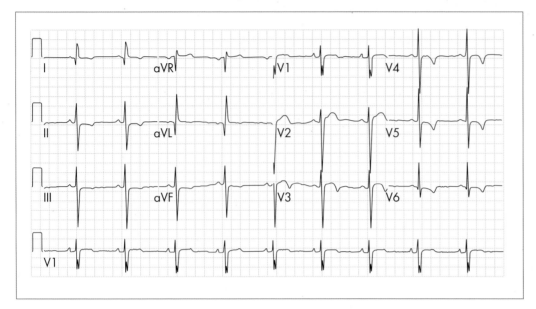

Figure 12-35. 12-Lead electrocardiogram at presentation, demonstrating ST elevation and negative/biphasic T waves. Physical examination revealed chest pain with exertion and shortness of breath (New York Heart Association II), blood pressure 136/82 mm Hg, heart rate 84 bpm. His recent medical history included a mild "flu" within the past 4 weeks, during which the chest pain occurred the first time. aVF—augmented voltage, unipolar left leg lead; aVL—augmented voltage, unipolar left arm lead; aVR—augmented voltage, unipolar right arm lead.

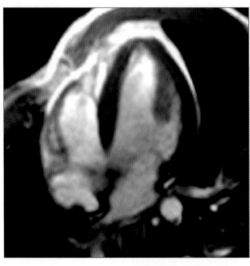

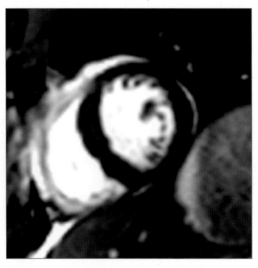

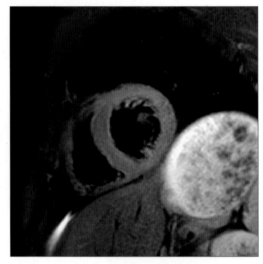

Figure 12-36. CMR cine sequence in four-chamber view orientation as part of a multiple long-axis study is shown. Normal left ventricular (LV) size and severely reduced ejection fraction (EF) are found. Functional parameters (normal values are shown in parentheses): end-diastolic volume (EDV) 139 mL, end-systolic volume 44 mL, LV stroke volume 95 mL, cardiac output 6.1 L/min, EF 68%, LV EDV index 78 mL (normal 60–120), cardiac index 3.2 L/min/m² (normal > 2.5), LV mass 153 g (normal 81–165), LV mass index (h) 86 g/m (normal 47–93).

Figure 12-37. CMR cine sequence in multiple short-axis orientation, technical parameters as stated in Figure 12-4. Normal left ventricular size and severely reduced ejection fraction with global hypokinesis are noted.

Figure 12-38. CMR T2-weighted image (STIR) in short-axis orientation at basal level. Normal myocardial signal ratio is noted (1.7, normal value < 2.0), no effusion is seen. Findings are consistent with absence of a myocardial edema, an acute myocarditis is unlikely.

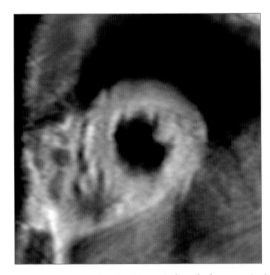

Figure 12-39. CMR T1-weighted short axis (early enhancement) after contrast application (0.1 mmol gadolinium/kg body weight). Globally increased contrast uptake is noted (relative enhancement = 6.3, normal value < 4.0), consistent with acute inflammation of the myocardium.

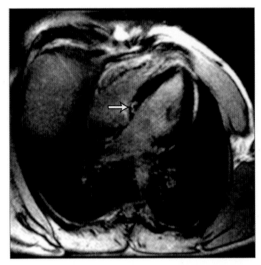

Figure 12-40. CMR late gadolinium enhancement image in four-chamber view orientation. Areas of diffuse, nonsubendocardial contrast uptake are seen, consistent with nonischemic scar.

Summary of CMR findings: Areas of fibrosis in an epicardial distribution, no evidence for ischemic damage. Preserved left ventricular ejection fraction and normal left ventricular size. Negative CMR T2-weighted image (STIR) and positive early enhancement are indicative of a subacute myocarditis. Findings are consistent with an acute myocarditis with some fibrotic changes.

CASE 5: A 65-YEAR-OLD PATIENT WITH VENTRICULAR TACHYCARDIA (EXCLUSION OF CORONARY ARTERY DISEASE)

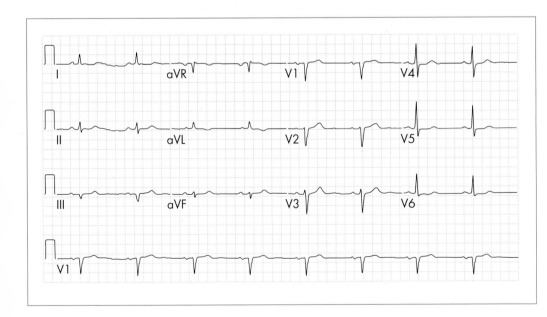

Figure 12-41. 12-Lead electrocardiogram after initial presentation, showing normal sinus rhythm without clear evidence of ischemia or inflammatory changes. Initially, this patient had presented with ventricular tachycardia (280 bpm) and was cardioverted medically; a coexisting coronary artery disease was excluded invasively. Physical examination revealed no signs of congestive heart failure at rest, but shortness of breath on exertion (New York Heart Association III), blood pressure 90/62 mm Hg, heart rate 75 bpm. aVF—augmented voltage, unipolar left leg lead; aVL—augmented voltage, unipolar left arm lead; aVR—augmented voltage, unipolar right arm lead.

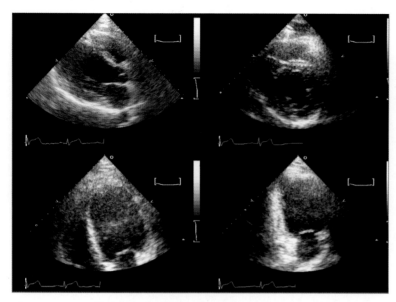

Figure 12-42. Transthoracic echocardiography, three long-axis views and one short-axis view are shown. Mildly reduced ejection fraction with mildly increased left ventricular size is demonstrated.

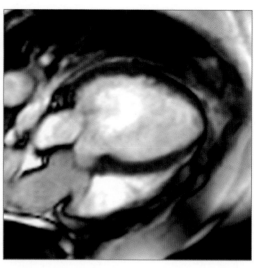

Figure 12-43. CMR cine sequence in two-chamber view orientation as part of a multiple long-axis study is shown. Increased left ventricular (LV) size and moderately reduced ejection fraction (EF) are found. Functional parameters (normal values are shown in parentheses): end-diastolic volume (EDV) 211 mL, end-systolic volume 123 mL, LV stroke volume 88 mL, cardiac output 4.1 L/min, EF 42%, LV EDV index 129 mL (normal 60–120), cardiac index 2.2 L/min/m² (normal > 2.5), LV mass 104 g (normal 81–165), LV mass index (h) 64 g/m (normal 47–93).

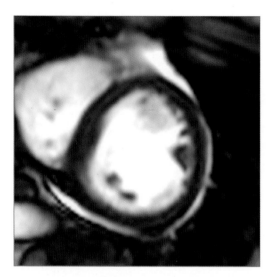

Figure 12-44. CMR cine sequence in multiple short-axis orientation, technical parameters as stated in Figure 12-4. Normal left ventricular size and severely reduced ejection fraction with global hypokinesis are noted.

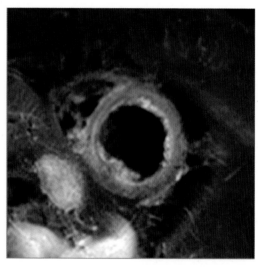

Figure 12-45. CMR T2-weighted image (STIR) in short-axis orientation at basal level. Quantitative evaluation revealed an abnormally high relative signal intensity when normalized to skeletal muscle (2.6, normal value < 2.0); no effusion is seen. Small amount of pericardial fluid is noted. Finding consistent with diffuse myocardial edema of a nonischemic origin.

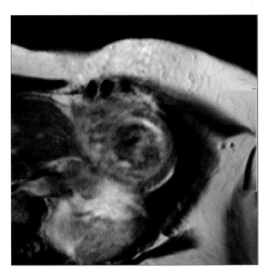

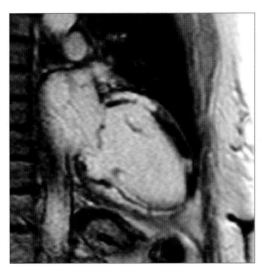

Figure 12-46. CMR T1-weighted short axis (early enhancement) after contrast application (0.1 mmol gadolinium/kg body weight). Globally increased contrast uptake is noted (relative enhancement = 5.8, normal value < 4.0), consistent with acute inflammation of the myocardium.

Figure 12-47. CMR late gadolinium enhancement image in two-chamber view orientation. Extensive areas of diffuse, non-subendocardial LGE uptake are seen, consistent with nonischemic scar formation.

Summary of CMR findings: Extensive LGE in an epicardial distribution, no evidence for ischemic damage. Moderately reduced left ventricular ejection fraction with mildly increased left ventricular size; invasive exclusion of coronary artery disease. Findings are consistent with acute myocarditis with some fibrotic changes.

ACKNOWLEDGMENTS

We want to thank Drs. Pauline Alakija and Debra Isaac for their help with these cases, especially for providing biopsy samples and pictures. Furthermore, we want to thank Dal Disler for his help with the digital echocardiography images.

REFERENCES

1. Liu PP, Yan AT: Cardiovascular magnetic resonance for the diagnosis of acute myocarditis: prospects for detecting myocardial inflammation. *J Am Coll Cardiol* 2005, 45:1823–1825.

2. Skouri HN, Dec GW, Friedrich MG, Cooper LT: Noninvasive imaging in myocarditis. *J Am Coll Cardiol* 2006, 48:2085–2093.

3. Magnani JW, Dec GW: Myocarditis: current trends in diagnosis and treatment. *Circulation* 2006, 113:876-890.

4. Friedrich MG, Strohm O, Schulz-Menger J, *et al.*: Contrast media-enhanced magnetic resonance imaging visualizes myocardial changes in the course of viral myocarditis. *Circulation* 1998, 97:1802–1809.

5. Mahrholdt H, Goedecke C, Wagner A, *et al.*: Cardiovascular magnetic resonance assessment of human myocarditis: a comparison to histology and molecular pathology. *Circulation* 2004,109:1250–1258.

6. Abdel-Aty H, Boye P, Zagrosek A, *et al.*: Diagnostic performance of cardiovascular magnetic resonance in patients with suspected acute myocarditis: comparison of different approaches. *J Am Coll Cardiol* 2005, 45:1815–1822.

7. Wagner A, Schulz-Menger J, Dietz R, Friedrich MG: Long-term follow-up of patients with acute myocarditis by magnetic resonance imaging. New York: Magma; 2003:17–20.

8. Gutberlet M, Spors B, Thoma T, *et al.*: Suspected chronic myocarditis at cardiac MR: diagnostic accuracy and association with immunohistologically detected inflammation and viral persistence. *Radiology* 2008, epub ahead of print.

13

Hypertrophic Cardiomyopathy

Martin S. Maron

Hypertrophic cardiomyopathy (HCM) is the most common genetic cardiomyopathy, with a prevalence of 1:500 [1,2]. HCM is the most common cause of sudden death in young people and can also lead to heart failure symptoms and stroke at any age [1,2]. HCM is inherited as an autosomal dominant disorder; currently, 12 gene mutations of the cardiac sarcomere proteins are responsible for producing the phenotype of left ventricular (LV) hypertrophy [3].

A clinical diagnosis of HCM is established by imaging a hypertrophied but nondilated LV chamber, in the absence of another cardiac or systemic disease (systemic hypertension or aortic valve stenosis, and so forth) [2]. The most common location for LV hypertrophy is the anterior septum [4]. However, because of its genetic etiology, there is substantial heterogeneity in the phenotypic expression, with close to half of HCM patients demonstrating segmental hypertrophy confined to single LV segments, including the LV apex. Therefore, although it is typically asymmetric in distribution, any pattern of LV wall thickening can be seen in HCM [4]. Importantly, maximal LV wall thickness 30 mm or greater (at any location in the LV) was verified as an independent marker for increased risk of sudden cardiac death in HCM [5].

Hypertrophic cardiomyopathy is also characterized by an abnormal histology. Microscopic histology demonstrates the presence of myocyte disarray with increased amounts of interstitial fibrosis. The intramural coronaries are often structurally abnormal, which can result in small vessel ischemia, and, after an extended duration of time, can result in myocardial cell death with areas of replacement fibrosis [6–8].

Left ventricular outflow tract obstruction caused by systolic anterior motion of the mitral valve is present in the majority of HCM patients either at rest or with provocation following exercise [9]. LV outflow obstruction of 30 mm Hg or greater is a mechanism of heart failure symptoms in HCM patients and is an independent predictor of cardiovascular morbidity and mortality [10]. In patients with outflow obstruction and limiting symptoms in whom medical therapy fails (β–blockers, calcium channel blockers, or disopyramide) invasive septal reduction therapy with surgical myectomy (alternatively, alcohol septal ablation) can eliminate or substantially reduce gradients and improve symptoms [2]. Therefore, the identification of LV outflow obstruction is an important part of the evaluation in all HCM patients.

Traditionally, two-dimensional echocardiography was the easiest and most reliable technique for establishing the diagnosis of HCM. Cardiovascular magnetic resonance (CMR) has emerged as a novel, three-dimensional tomographic imaging technique, which provides high spatial and temporal resolution images of the heart, in any plane and without ionizing radiation [11,12]. As a result, CMR is particularly well suited to provide detailed characterization of the HCM phenotype. In this regard, CMR has proven to provide a diagnosis of HCM in cases where the echocardiogram was nondiagnostic [13]. In addition, late gadolinium enhancement (LGE) sequences can provide unique information on tissue characterization, specifically, the identification of myocardial fibrosis/scarring [14]. Although the clinical implications of LGE in HCM are still uncertain, this information may, in the near future, contain important implications for identifying HCM patients at high risk of sudden death and progressive heart failure, including evolution to the end-stage phase of HCM.

The following cases highlight the particular strengths of CMR in providing high-resolution tomographic images of the HCM heart, with implications for diagnosis and management of the HCM patient. In the future, one can expect an expanding role for CMR (in conjunction with two-dimensional echocardiography) in the evaluation of nearly all HCM patients.

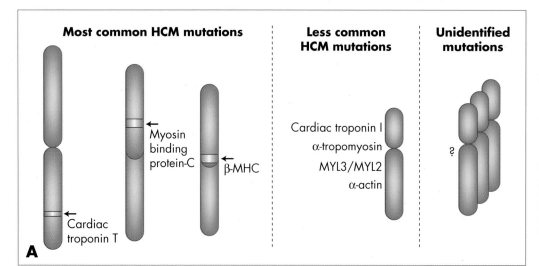

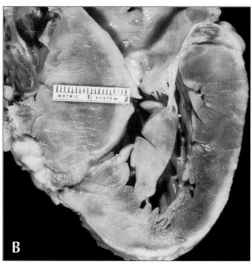

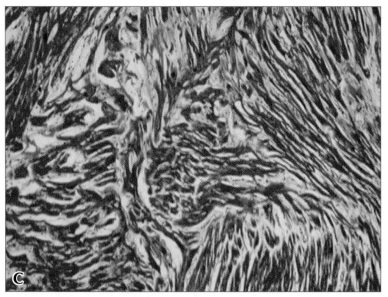

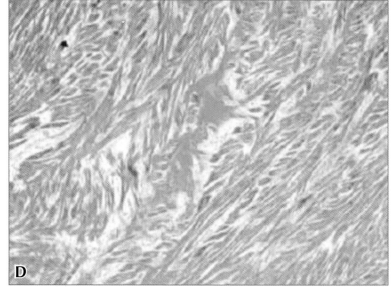

Figure 13-1. Hypertrophic cardiomyopathy (HCM) is caused by mutations in eight different genes that encode cardiac sarcomeric proteins, which perform contractile, structural, and regulatory functions [1–3]. **A,** The three most common disease-causing mutations are β-myosin heavy chain (MHC), cardiac troponin T, and myosin binding protein-C, while a minority of other genes account for a small number of additional HCM cases. In addition, close to half of HCM patients do not carry one of the known genotype mutations, suggesting that a number of disease-causing sarcomere mutations have yet to be identified. However, the diverse phenotypic spectrum of HCM is certainly a result of the genetic cause and likely the contribution from other factors, such as modifier genes and environment [3]. Presently, genetic testing is commercially available and can establish whether patients are carriers of the most common gene mutations for HCM. **B,** Gross pathologic specimen of a young patient who died suddenly from HCM. There is disproportionate hypertrophy of the ventricular septum with respect to the left ventricular (LV) free wall. In addition, other morphologic features of the HCM phenotype are present, including papillary muscle hypertrophy and narrowed LV outflow tract. HCM is also characterized by abnormal histology. **C,** Myocardial fiber disarray is common with cardiac muscle cells arranged in a disorganized pattern. **D,** Masson's trichrome stain demonstrating areas of interstitial fibrosis (*blue*) present between areas of myocyte disarray.

Continued on the next page

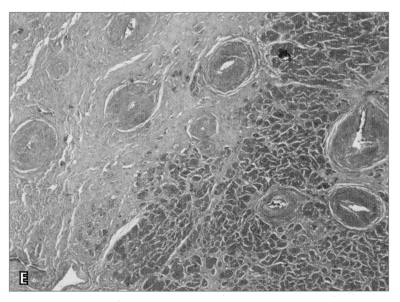

Figure 13-1. *(Continued)* **E**, The intramural coronaries are often structurally abnormal (*ie*, markedly thickened walls and narrowed lumen), which can result in small vessel ischemia, and eventually, myocardial cell death with areas of replacement fibrosis. This abnormal myocardial structure provides a substrate for ventricular arrhythmias and sudden death [4–6].

PATTERN AND DISTRIBUTION OF HYPERTROPHY

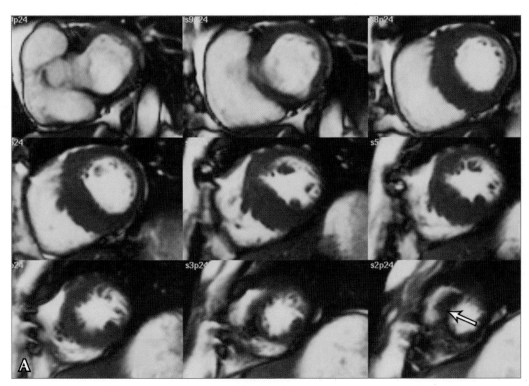

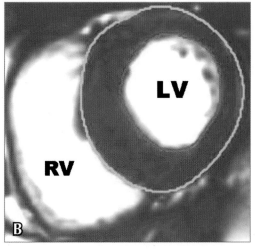

Figure 13-2. **A**, Modern functional cardiovascular magnetic resonance (CMR) imaging sequences (steady-state free precession) generate images with high spatial resolution and sharp contrast between blood (*bright*) and myocardium (*dark*). As a result, endocardial and epicardial borders can be applied to each of these contiguous left ventricular (LV) short-axis images to accurately quantify ventricular parameters such as volume, mass, and ejection fraction. **B**, Represents this technique applied to one of the short-axis slices from **A** [10,12]. In this example, LV septal hypertrophy is present beginning in the most apical slice (**A**, *arrow, lower right corner*) and becoming thickest at the midventricular level. RV—right ventricle.

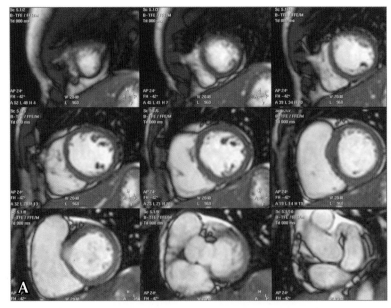

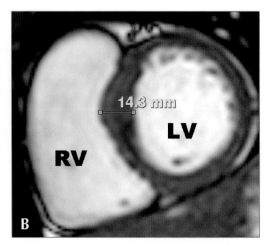

Figure 13-3. **A**, Due to its ability to acquire contiguous tomographic slices, cardiovascular magnetic resonance (CMR) is a technique particularly well suited to evaluate the entire heart and to characterize the pattern and distribution of left ventricular (LV) hypertrophy [10,12]. In select hypertrophic cardiomyopathy (HCM) patients, hypertrophy can be confined to only a focal area of the LV myocardium. By applying thin short-axis slices (6–10 mm) without an interslice gap, CMR is particularly useful at providing a comprehensive display of the entire LV wall thickness from base to apex, allowing for the accurate identification of LV hypertrophy (and, subsequently, a proper diagnosis of HCM). In this HCM patient, a small area of increased LV wall thickness (confined to the basal anterior septum with normal wall thicknesses throughout the entire LV wall) is observed only on one short-axis slice (*outlined in red*). **B**, Enlarged view of outlined image in panel A, which includes a precise measurement of the wall thickness that can subsequently be performed in the area of hypertrophy (> 14 mm in this example). This patient also underwent clinical genotyping and one of the common sarcomeric protein mutations (myosin binding protein-C) known to cause HCM was diagnosed.

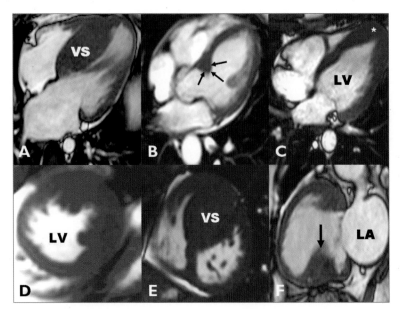

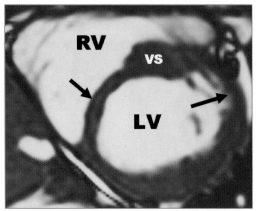

Figure 13-4. Nearly any pattern and distribution of left ventricular (LV) wall thickening can be observed as part of the phenotypic expression of hypertrophic cardiomyopathy (HCM) [4]. Cardiovascular magnetic resonance (CMR) end-diastolic short-axis and long-axis images demonstrating diffuse hypertrophy of the ventricular septum (VS) (**A**); a focal area of hypertrophy sharply confined to the basal anterior septum (*arrows*) (**B**); hypertrophy confined to the LV apex (*asterisk*), consistent with a classification of apical HCM (**C**); hypertrophy localized to the LV free wall with normal ventricular septal wall thickness (**D**); massive asymmetric hypertrophy of the anterior VS (maximal wall thickness of 48 mm) with sparing of hypertrophy in the posterior septum and LV free wall (**E**); hypertrophy confined to a segment of the inferior wall (*arrow*) (**F**). LA—left atrium.

Figure 13-5. Hypertrophic cardiomyopathy (HCM) patient with noncontiguous left ventricular (LV) hypertrophy. Focal segments of LV hypertrophy are separated by areas of normal wall thickness (*arrows*). This type of noncontiguous hypertrophy can be appreciated with cardiovascular magnetic resonance (CMR), and supports the principle that in HCM, only a genetic etiology could produce such a sharply demarcated "patchy" distribution of LV wall thickening. VS—ventricular septum.

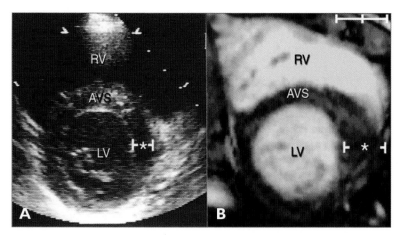

Figure 13-6. Cardiovascular magnetic resonance (CMR) can identify segmental left ventricular (LV) hypertrophy that may not be visualized by echocardiography [13,15]. **A,** A normal two-dimensional echocardiogram of a patient with a family history of hypertrophic cardiomyopathy (HCM). **B,** CMR image of the same patient, which reveals an area of segmental hypertrophy in the anterolateral LV wall (*asterisk*), consistent with a diagnosis of HCM. This case illustrates the phenomenon of lateral ultrasound "drop-out" (*ie,* the anterolateral wall can be a region of the LV difficult to visualize with echocardiography, because of the loss of spatial resolution in the lateral portions of the myocardium, particularly in the epicardial border, on short-axis orientation). As a result, hypertrophy in this region of the LV may not be detected by two-dimensional echocardiography. CMR is not limited by these technical issues and therefore provides a method for identifying hypertrophy in the anterolateral wall. Thus, CMR should be considered in patients suspected of having HCM, particularly when the myocardial borders of this segment of the LV chamber are not well visualized by echocardiography. In one study, CMR identified segmental LV hypertrophy missed by echocardiography in 5% of patients [13]. AVS—aortic valve stenosis; RV—right ventricle.

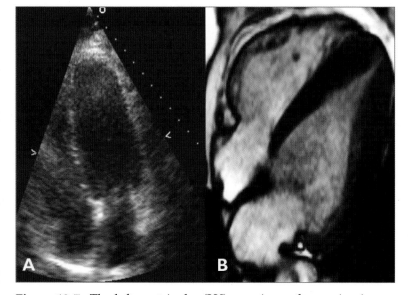

Figure 13-7. The left ventricular (LV) apex is another region in which hypertrophy may be missed by two-dimensional echocardiography [15]. **A,** A patient's abnormal electrocardiogram raised the suspicion of an underlying cardiomyopathy. **Subsequently,** two-dimensional echocardiography was performed, but was considered nondiagnostic. **B,** In the same patient, cardiovascular magnetic resonance (CMR) clearly shows segmental hypertrophy confined to the LV apex, consistent with a diagnosis of apical hypertrophic cardiomyopathy (HCM). CMR is not limited by constraints of thoracic or pulmonary parenchyma in visualizing the LV apex. Therefore, this example (as well as in Fig. 13-6) support the role of CMR in the evaluation of patients in whom HCM is suspected when any LV segment is not well visualized or the echocardiographic study is suboptimal.

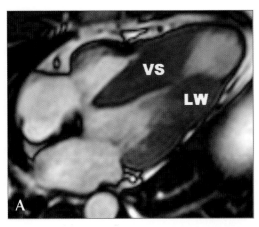
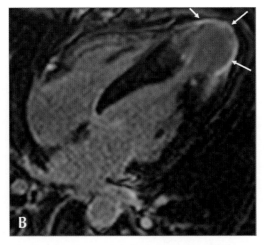

midventricular obstruction because of midsystolic apposition of the hypertrophied ventricular septum (VS) and LV free wall. It was proposed that long-standing increased LV systolic pressures created by midventricular obstruction may contribute to apical aneurysmal formation in select susceptible HCM patients in the absence of coronary artery disease. **A,** HCM patient with an LV apical aneurysm and characteristic midventricular hypertrophy with apposition to the septum and LV free wall in midsystole, creating midventricular obstruction. **B,** Late gadolinium enhanced cardiovascular magnetic resonance of the same patient demonstrates transmural LGE of the apex, representing myocardial fibrosis in this area. LW—lateral wall.

Figure 13-8. Hypertrophic cardiomyopathy (HCM) patients with left ventricular (LV) apical aneurysm represent an important but fairly uncommon subgroup of the HCM disease spectrum. HCM patients with apical aneurysms also commonly demonstrate

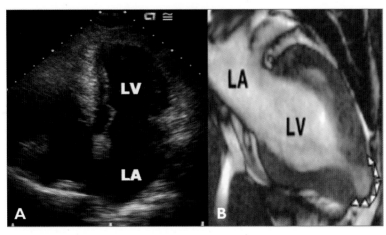
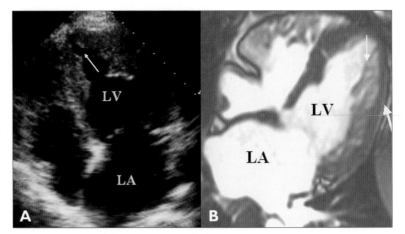

Figure 13-9. Hypertrophic cardiomyopathy (HCM) patients with LV apical aneurysms may have a higher risk of cardiovascular morbidity and mortality (including sudden cardiac death) compared with the general HCM population [16]. In this regard, the heavily scarred apical aneurysm likely provides an additional region of abnormal myocardial substrate (along with an already myopathic ventricle), which may increase the likelihood of the generation of lethal arrhythmias such as ventricular tachycardia/ventricular fibrillation. Therefore, early identification of HCM patients with apical aneurysm is important, and implantable cardioverter defibrillator therapy for primary prevention of sudden death should be considered [16]. However, identification of these patients requires a high index of clinical suspicion. Incidentally, as demonstrated in Figure 13-8, cardiovascular magnetic resonance (CMR) can characterize with great detail LV apical structure and function. **A,** Two-chamber echocardiogram in an HCM patient demonstrating septal hypertophy with no evidence of an LV apical aneurysm. **B,** In the same HCM patient, two-chamber CMR demonstrates a small LV apical aneurysm. This case illustrates that CMR can identify LV apical aneurysms that may be missed by two-dimensional echocardiography, particularly when small in size (≤ 2 cm in diameter). Therefore, CMR should be strongly considered in HCM patients when the LV apex is not well visualized, particularly when there is the presence of midcavitary obstruction. LA—left atrium.

Figure 13-10. Because of its superb spatial resolution, cardiovascular magnetic resonance (CMR) can also provide a detailed characterization of myocardial structure, which may also aid in diagnosis. **A,** A patient with a history of apical hypertrophic cardiomyopathy (HCM). Two-dimensional echocardiographic imaging revealed left ventricular (LV) hypertrophy extending from the mid-LV to apex with normal systolic function. However, the pattern of hypertrophy appeared atypical for apical HCM because it was more irregularly shaped with a "gap" in wall thickening toward the apex (*arrow*). To help clarify the phenotype, the patient underwent CMR. **B,** CMR demonstrates that the LV hypertrophy observed on echocardiography corresponded to areas of extensive LV trabeculations (*ie,* sinusoids). There are two layers of LV myocardium visualized: the endocardium with sinusoids (*ie,* noncompacted, *thin arrow*) and the epicedial layer without sinusoids (*ie,* compacted or "normal," *thick arrow*). These CMR findings were consistent with a diagnosis of LV noncompaction. This case illustrates the role of CMR in characterizing the myocardial phenotype to help clarify (and even alter) the diagnosis. Therefore, CMR should also be considered in clinical situations in which diagnosis remains uncertain with traditional imaging techniques. LA—left atrium.

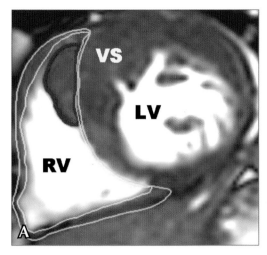

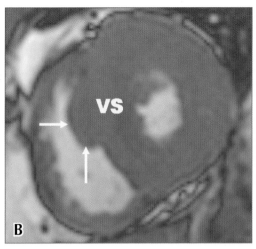

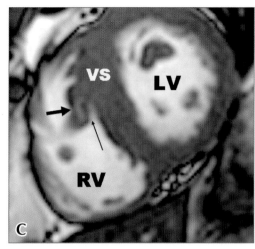

Figure 13-11. When determining where to measure the maximal left ventricular (LV) wall thickness, it is important to be aware that hypertrophic cardiomyopathy (HCM) patients often have prominent and hypertrophied right ventricular (RV) muscular structures, the most common of which is the crista supraventricularis [17]. In some HCM patients, the crista supraventricularis is not only significantly hypertrophied (**A**, *outlined in red*) but, not uncommonly, it inserts from its origin in the RV cavity to directly adjacent to the ventricular septum (VS). As a result, the crista supraventricularis may be inappropriately included in the measurement of septal thickness, resulting in an overestimation of the maximal LV wall thickness and, in rare cases, may even lead to an inappropriate diagnosis of HCM (when included in patients with normal septal thickness but prominent crista supraventricularis). In order to avoid including the crista supraventricularis as part of the septum, close inspection of the cardiovascular magnetic resonance cine images can help clarify this issue. **B**, In end-systole, the crista supraventricularis muscle (*arrows*) appears contiguous with the VS. **C**, In the same patient, in end-diastole, the crista supraventricularis muscle is noted to have moved away from the septum toward the RV cavity (*thick arrow*), with a small area of blood pool noted between the crista and septum (*thin arrow*).

PHENOTYPE CHARACTERIZATION

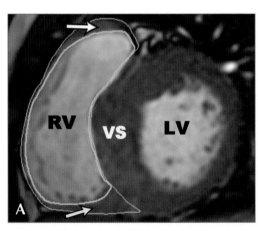

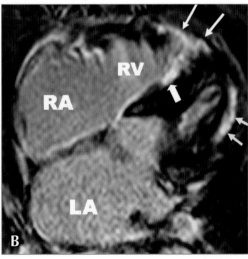

Figure 13-12. Previous assessment of the right ventricle (RV) in hypertrophic cardiomyopathy (HCM) has been difficult, and therefore, it is difficult to determine whether morphologic abnormalities of the RV are present in this disease. However, with the superior spatial resolution and complete volumetric coverage of the entire heart, cardiovascular magnetic resonance (CMR) is a technique particularly compatible for evaluation of the RV. A recent CMR study demonstrated that both RV wall thickness and mass are increased in a substantial proportion of HCM patients [17]. **A**, A basal left ventricular (LV) short-axis image of an HCM patient with increased RV wall thickness in the superior segment (*thick arrow*) and extreme hypertrophy in the inferior segment (*thin arrow*). **B**, In another HCM patient, a four-chamber long-axis image shows late gadolinium enhancement present in the RV wall (*thin white arrows*), the RV side of the ventricular septum (VS) (*thick white arrow*), and LV free wall (*yellow arrows*). This finding supports the idea that a process of abnormal ventricular remodeling (ie, fibrosis) also occurs in the RV in patients with HCM. At present, the clinical significance of RV morphologic abnormalities in HCM remains uncertain, but these observations suggest that the genetic cardiomyopathic process in HCM is more diffuse than previously thought. LA—left atrium; RA—right atrium.

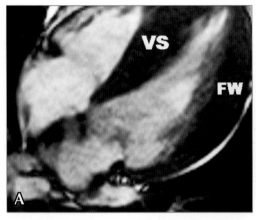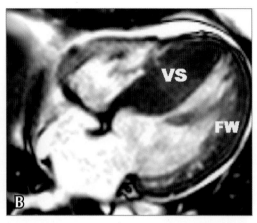

Figure 13-13. Cardiovascular magnetic resonance (CMR) is a tomographic imaging technique with complete volumetric coverage that, as a result, provides an accurate method of calculating total left ventricular (LV) mass. As anticipated, LV mass is significantly greater in hypertrophic cardiomyopathy (HCM) patients compared with controls. However, a significant proportion of HCM patients have a total LV mass that is within normal limits (with only focal region of wall thickening). In addition, disproportionality can be observed between measurements of maximal LV wall thickness and total LV mass, (*ie*, not all HCM patients with

the same maximal LV wall thickness will have the same LV mass) [18]. **A** and **B**, Two HCM patients with an identical maximal LV wall thickness of 28 mm but significantly different LV mass index (**A**, 180 g/m²; **B**, 88 g/m²). The differences in mass are the result of the extension of LV hypertrophy from the septum into the LV free wall (FW) in **A**, whereas hypertrophy is localized only to the ventricular septum in **B**. Although LV mass can be a more robust marker of the extent of hypertrophy, long-term prospective CMR studies are needed before considering LV mass as a risk factor in this disease. VS—ventricular septum.

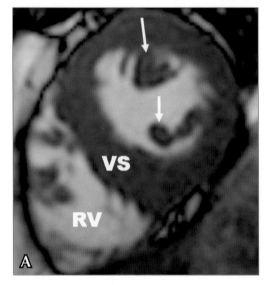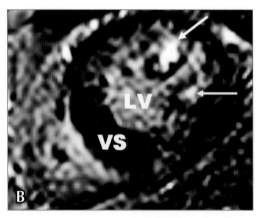

Figure 13-14. Left ventricular (LV) hypertrophy is the predominant diagnostic feature of the hypertrophic cardiomyopathy (HCM) phenotype. Although they are part of the LV chamber, the involvement of the papillary muscles in the cardiomyopathic process in HCM remains uncertain. In this regard, cardiovascular magnetic resonance has recently demonstrated that abnormalities in papillary muscle morphology are common in this disease, including increased number, mass, and fibrosis (*ie*, late gadolinium enhancement (LGE)) [19]. In addition, papillary muscle mass in HCM often contributes substantially to overall LV chamber mass. **A**, HCM patient with substantially increased

papillary muscle mass (*arrows*) even in the presence of normal LV mass (with focal hypertrophy only). This case demonstrates that the papillary muscles may represent a primary morphologic expression of hypertrophy in HCM. **B**, An LGE image demonstrating hyperenhancement confined to both papillary muscles (*arrows*). Although LGE occurs much more commonly in the LV wall in HCM, the presence of fibrosis confined to only the papillary muscles supports the idea that an abnormal process of ventricular remodeling (*ie*, fibrosis) may occur in areas not strictly part of the LV wall in this disease. RV—right ventricle; VS—ventricular septum.

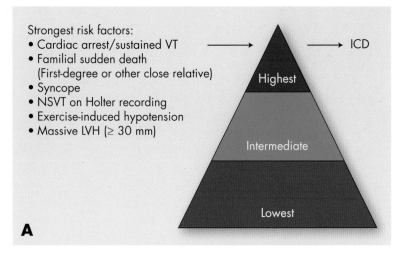

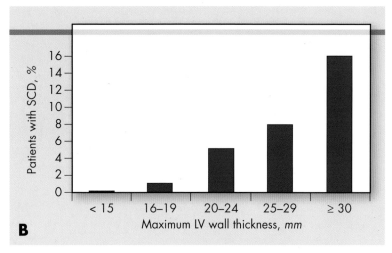

Strongest risk factors:
- Cardiac arrest/sustained VT
- Familial sudden death
  (First-degree or other close relative)
- Syncope
- NSVT on Holter recording
- Exercise-induced hypotension
- Massive LVH (≥ 30 mm)

Figure 13-15. Hypertrophic cardiomyopathy (HCM) is a common cause of sudden cardiac death (SCD) in young patients (< 35 years), including competitive athletes [1]. The mechanism of SCD is ventricular arrhythmias generated from an abnormal myocardial substrate consisting of myocyte disarray, interstitial, and replacement fibrosis [6]. Currently, there are five traditional risk factors that may place an HCM patient into a high-risk category, including: massive left ventricular (LV) hypertrophy (≥ 30 mm), a family history of sudden death from HCM, non-sustained ventricular tachycardia (NSVT) on ambulatory Holter monitoring, and abnormal blood pressure response to exercise and syncope (**A**) [20]. The fifth risk factor, in regard to maximal LV wall thickness, presents a direct, linear relationship between increasing wall thickness and SCD, with massive hypertrophy (≥ 30 mm) being the greatest risk (**B**) [5]. The presence of any one of these risk factors may be enough to warrant consideration for primary prevention of sudden death with an implantable cardioverter defibrillator (ICD) [20]. A history of aborted cardiac arrest or history of sustained ventricular tachycardia are risk factors necessitating ICD implantation for secondary prevention (**A**). LVH—left ventricular hypertrophy; VT—ventricular tachycardia.

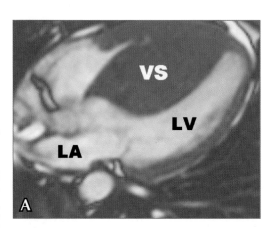

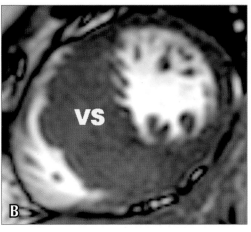

Figure 13-16. A, A 23-year-old in whom hypertrophic cardiomyopathy (HCM) was diagnosed following the detection of a systolic ejection murmur on a routine physical examination. Cardiovascular magnetic resonance (CMR) demonstrates extreme hypertrophy (44 mm) in the ventricular septum (VS) with relative sparing of the left ventricular (LV) free wall. Following CMR, the patient underwent implantation of an implantable cardioverter defibrillator (ICD) for primary prevention of sudden death based solely on the presence of massive LV hypertrophy (with no additional risk factors). Three months after implantation of the ICD, the patient experienced an appropriate shock for ventricular fibrillation. Because of the importance that maximal LV wall thickness conveys in the assessment of an individual patient's risk of sudden death, it is important that accurate measurements of the maximal transdimensional LV wall thickness be reported. In this regard, the current functional CMR imaging sequences produce sharp contrast between the LV cavity blood pool and myocardium, allowing for exceptionally accurate measurements of wall thickness. **B,** A 17-year-old in whom HCM was diagnosed following a syncopal episode while playing competitive football. CMR short-axis image at the midventricular level reveals massive hypertrophy (33 mm) of the VS. As a result of the presence of both syncope and extreme hypertrophy, this patient had an ICD implanted for primary prevention of sudden death. In addition, all HCM patients (regardless of either magnitude of LV wall thickness or the presence of LV outflow obstruction) should be excluded from continued participation in organized competitive sports [21]. LA—left atrium.

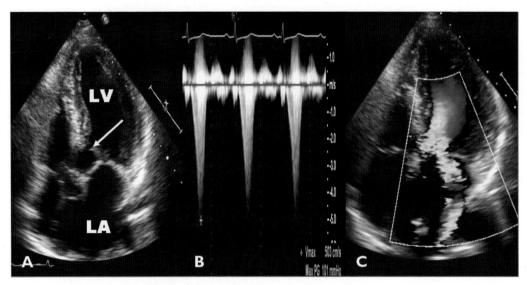

Figure 13-17. Left ventricular (LV) outflow obstruction in hypertrophic cardiomyopathy (HCM) is caused by the systolic anterior motion (SAM) of the mitral valve leaflet making contact with the ventricular septum in midsystole. **A**, A two-dimensional apical five-chamber long-axis view demonstrating SAM-septal contact (*arrow*). SAM-septal contact results in mechanical impedance to LV outflow and the generation of a pressure gradient between the LV cavity and ascending aorta. **B**, This pressure gradient can be quantified by determining the maximal velocity of blood flow through the LV outflow track using Doppler techniques and applying the modified Bernoulli equation to estimate the pressure gradient. **C**, In addition, during obstruction there is inap-

propriate coaptation of the mitral valve leaflets (an interleaflet gap) through which a posteriorly directed mitral regurgitation jet is often produced. A variety of abnormal structural factors within the LV cavity (*ie*, a narrowed outflow diameter, thickened ventricular septum, elongated mitral valve leaflet, and an anteriorly displaced plane of the mitral) can result in the generation of abnormal hemodynamic forces (*ie*, venture and "drag" effect) that draw the mitral valve leaflet toward the ventricular septum. LV outflow obstruction is a dynamic process. Patients without obstruction, under resting conditions, will often develop gradients with provocative maneuvers, such as Valsalva or exercise. LA—left atrium.

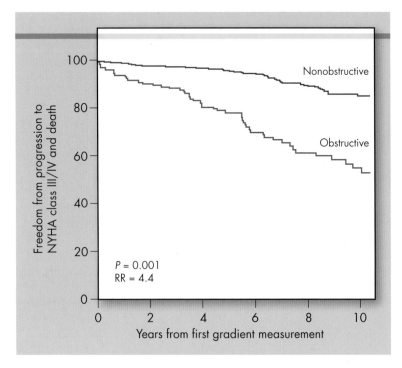

Figure 13-18. A Kaplan-Meier survival estimate demonstrating that LV outflow obstruction of 30 mm Hg or greater (under resting conditions) is an independent predictor of cardiovascular morbidity and mortality [10]. Hypertrophic cardiomyopathy (HCM) patients with left ventricular (LV) outflow obstruction were more than four times more likely to experience progressive heart failure symptoms, heart failure, or stroke death compared with patients without obstruction. Although patients with LV outflow obstruction were more likely to have sudden death compared with patients without obstructions, the positive predictive value (PPV) of obstruction and sudden death remained low (even less compared with the PPV of the other traditional risk factors for sudden death in HCM). Therefore, the presence of LV outflow obstruction alone should not be enough to consider a patient for an implantable cardiodefibrillator for primary prevention. NYHA—New York Heart Association; RR—relative risk.

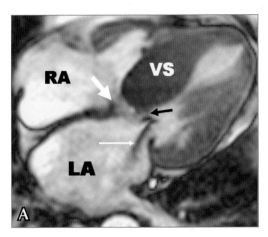 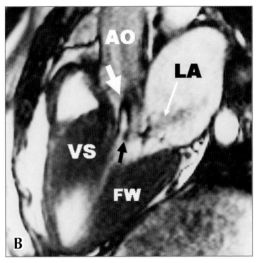

Figure 13-19. Left ventricular (LV) outflow obstruction caused by typical systolic anterior motion (SAM)-septal contact can be visualized on cine cardiovascular magnetic resonance (CMR) images in a number of imaging planes, including: four-chamber long axis, horizontal long axis, or a dedicated LV outflow view. In addition, with routine steady-state free precession cine imaging sequences, a signal void is often visualized in both the LV outflow tract and left atrium (LA), which represents turbulent flow and mitral regurgitation, respectively. Importantly, changes in a variety of the imaging sequence parameters can alter the signal characteristics of the jet. Therefore, one should not rely on the traditional echocardiographic criteria of assessing mitral regurgitation jet severity (such as orifice diameter and amount of the jet) to qualitatively determine the magnitude of mitral regurgitation based on the CMR signal void. In this regard, the application of phase velocity mapping sequences can accurately quantify the amount of mitral regurgitation, which can be expressed as a percentage of the LV volume (regurgitant fraction). Figure shows a midsystolic, four-chamber view (**A**), and, in a different HCM patient, a dedicated LV outflow tract view (**B**), both demonstrating typical SAM-septal contact (*black arrow*) with a posteriorly directed signal void present in the LA, representing mitral regurgitation (*thin white arrow*), and a signal void in the LV outflow representing turbulent flow secondary to obstruction (*thick white arrow*). AO—aorta; FW—free wall; RA—right atrium; VS—ventricular septum.

Late Gadolinium Enhancement

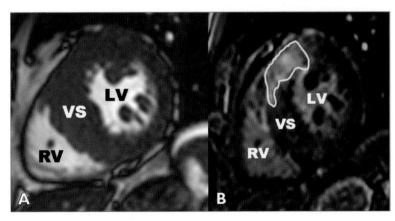

Figure 13-20. One of the most important recent technical advances in cardiovascular magnetic resonance is its ability to provide tissue characterization. Specifically, following the intravenous administration of gadolinium contrast, the application of a segmented inversion-recovery gradient-echo sequence can be used to detect areas of abnormal myocardial structure where gadolinium has deposited [11,12,22]. Specifically, gadolinium will temporarily reside in areas of myocardium with expanded extracellular space, which are represented on late gadolinium enhancement (LGE) as bright (hyperenhancement). The LGE technique proved highly accurate in identifying the presence, extent, and location of previous myocardial infarctions [22]. In addition, it can be applied to patients with hypertrophic cardiomyopathy (HCM) to detect areas of fibrosis/scarring [14,23,24]. **A**, Midventricular left ventricle (LV) short-axis image in an HCM patient prior to the intravenous administration of gadolinium. **B**, In the same patient, following gadolinium injection, LGE image demonstrating a transmural area of hyperenhancement in the anterior septum (*circled in yellow*). Areas of LGE can be planimetered, and the amount can be quantified and expressed as a percentage of the total LV mass. RV—right ventricle; VS—ventricular septum.

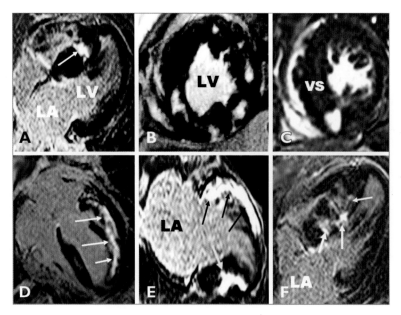

Figure 13-21. Approximately 50% to 80% of hypertrophic cardiomyopathy (HCM) patients demonstrate late gadolinium enhancement (LGE), and when present, the extent of LGE is often substantial, occupying on average, 10% of the overall left ventricular (LV) myocardial volume [14,23]. Importantly, almost any pattern, distribution, and location of LGE can be observed in HCM. In addition, transmural extent of LGE is not uncommon, occurring in half of HCM patients, while LGE confined to only the area of right ventricle (RV) insertion into the septum occurs in 25% of patients. However, as opposed to coronary artery disease, LGE in HCM does not typically correspond to a coronary vascular distribution. **A–F,** LV end-diastolic short- and long-axis LGE cardiovascular magnetic resonance images from six HCM patients showing diverse patterns of LGE. **A,** Focal area of transmural LGE in the anterior septum (*arrow*) and the midventricular level. **B,** Multifocal pattern of LGE predominantly located throughout the entire LV within a midmyocardial distribution. **C,** LGE localized to the insertion site of the RV wall and posterior ventricular septum (VS). **D,** Large area of lateral wall DE extending from base to apex (*arrows*). **E,** Transmural LGE in the anterior wall with a focal area of subepicardial LGE of the inferior wall (*arrows*). **F,** Diffuse area of LGE in the ventricular septum (*arrows*). LA—left atrium.

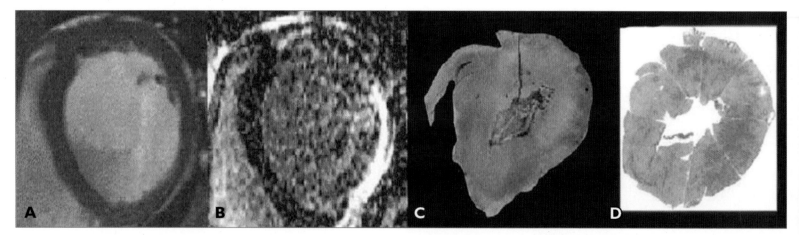

Figure 13-22. A–D, The pathophysiologic basis of late gadolinium enhancement (LGE) in hypertrophic cardiomyopathy (HCM) is still uncertain. However, recently, several case reports have compared in vivo LGE findings of HCM patients with end-stage phase (significantly decreased left ventricular [LV] function) with gross pathology findings following cardiac transplantation [24]. **A,** In an example of one such patient, in vivo end-diastolic LV short-axis image demonstrating dilated LV cavity with significantly decreased systolic function (ejection fraction 12%). **B,** Correspond-ing in vivo LV short axis slice with area of transmural LGE in the anterolateral LV free wall. **C,** Gross specimen of explanted heart with areas of unstained pale myocardium corresponding to the region of LGE. **D,** Histologic section stained with sirius red, with regions of red-stained collagen corresponding to the same areas of LGE. A significant relationship was demonstrated between areas of LGE but not to regions of myocyte disarray. Therefore, in HCM, areas of LGE likely represent myocardial fibrosis characterized by gross or macroscopic scarring.

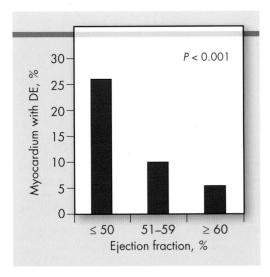

Figure 13-23. The precise clinical implications related to late gadolinium enhancement (LGE) in hypertrophic cardiomyopathy (HCM) are still uncertain. Nevertheless, several cross-sectional studies have demonstrated a relationship between the amount of LGE and left ventricular (LV) ejection fraction. HCM patients with LV ejection fraction of 50% or less (*ie*, end-stage phase) have a significantly greater percentage of LGE than those with mildly decreased or normal systolic function [23]. However, it is currently uncertain whether extensive amounts of LGE in HCM patients with preserved LV function are a marker for increased risk of developing LV systolic function.

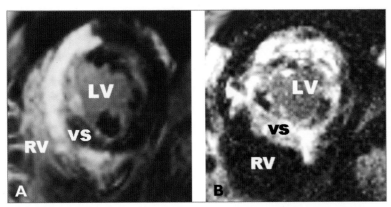

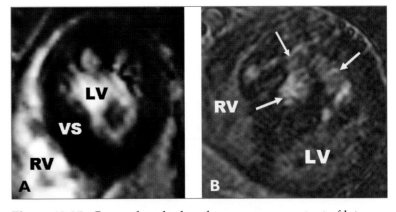

Figure 13-24. The presence of late gadolinium enhancement (LGE) can be unrelated to heart failure symptoms. In fact, a significant portion of hypertrophic cardiomyopathy (HCM) patients with normal left ventricular (LV) function, in whom heart failure symptoms are absent, have extensive (and often transmural) myocardial LGE present. Furthermore, many of these patients appear to experience no adverse consequences from their myocardial fibrosis over many years, causing some uncertainty concerning the ultimate clinical significance of LGE within the broad clinical spectrum of HCM. **A** and **B**, Midventricular short-axis LGE images from two HCM patients, both with extensive LGE, but with significantly different clinical courses. **A**, New York Heart Association (NYHA) functional class III, ejection fraction = 40% and 30% DE in LV. **B**, NYHA functional class I, ejection fraction = 65% and 46% DE in LV. RV—right ventricle; VS—ventricular septum.

Figure 13-25. Currently, whether the presence or extent of late gadolinium enhancement (LGE) is related to an increased risk of sudden death in hypertrophic cardiomyopathy (HCM) is uncertain. HCM is a relatively uncommon disease with a low event rate for sudden death (and cardiovascular magnetic resonance is a new technique). As a result, it will likely require many more years before prospective CMR data are available to help clarify if LGE is an independent predictor of sudden death in HCM. **A**, Left ventricular (LV) short-axis LGE image in a 16-year-old HCM patient with sudden cardiac death in the absence of any traditional risk factors for sudden death and no LGE. **B**, LV short-axis LGE image in a 28-year-old with extensive areas of LGE (*arrows*) in the ventricular septum (VS) (20% of LV mass) who is asymptomatic and has not experienced any arrhythmic complications. As illustrated in this example, prudent restraint is necessary before altering HCM management strategies (*ie*, implantable cardioverter defibrillator therapy for primary prevention of sudden death) based solely on the presence or extent of LGE. RV—right ventricle.

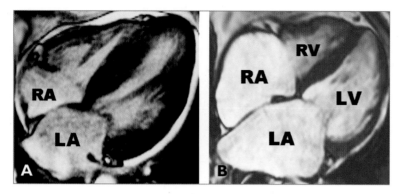

Figure 13-26. An uncommon but important subset of hypertrophic cardiomyopathy (HCM) patients will undergo evolution into the end-stage phase (ES) of this disease. ES is characterized by progressive left ventricular (LV) remodeling with gradual development (over a period of years) from a hypertrophied, nondilated LV cavity with hyperdynamic function (**A**) into systolic dysfunction often with cavity dilation and wall thinning (**B**). The pattern of LV remodeling seen in ES is heterogeneous, with close to half of HCM patients demonstrating either LV cavity dilation or wall thinning [25]. However, not infrequently, some ES patients have persistent hypertrophy without cavity dilation. Therefore, the one common diagnostic feature of ES is the presence of an ejection fraction less than 50%. Importantly, ES patients have an unfavorable clinical course with a high prevalence of sudden death and progressive heart failure symptoms. Therefore, recognition of the ES is important to permit early consideration for necessity of implantable cardioverter defibrillator use and consideration for heart transplantation. In this regard, cardiovascular magnetic resonance (CMR) can be used to reliably detect changes in LV function, wall thickness, and cavity dimensions over time, and therefore should be considered in the routine follow-up imaging among HCM patients in whom ES is suspected. LA—left atrium; RA—right atrium; RV—right ventricle.

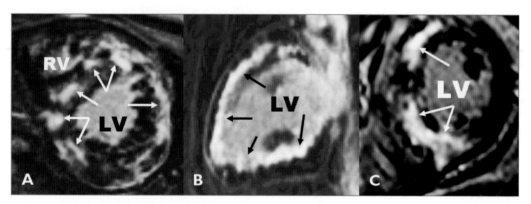

Figure 13-27. Late gadolinium enhancement (LGE) cardiovascular magnetic resonance images among hypertrophic cardiomyopathy (HCM) patients in the end stage (ES) demonstrate substantial amounts of LGE, often occupying more than 25% of the left ventricular (LV) mass, a similar amount of scarring/fibrosis to that produced following a massive anterior wall myocardial infarction [25]. In addition, ES patients have significantly more LGE compared with HCM patients not in the ES (*see* Figure 13-23). **A–C,** Horizontal long-axis and short-axis LGE images from different ES HCM patients demonstrating extensive areas of transmural LGE (*arrows*) in both the septum and LV free wall. RV—right ventricle.

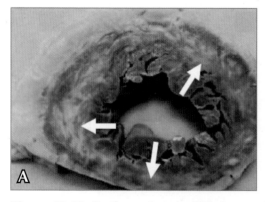
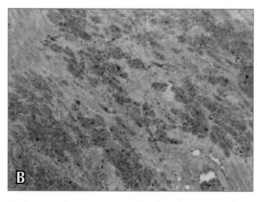

Figure 13-28. In the end stage (ES), late gadolinium enhancement (LGE) corresponds to areas of gross macroscopic myocardial fibrosis [25]. **A,** An explanted heart of a patient with ES hypertrophic cardiomyopathy (HCM) (ejection fraction 40%) but persistent and marked left ventricular (LV) wall thickening in the absence of cavity dilation. Extensive transmural scarring (*arrows*) is present throughout the septum and LV free wall (a similar pattern and distribution of LGE as observed in Figure 13-27A). **B,** Histopathologic examination showed large areas of replacement fibrosis.

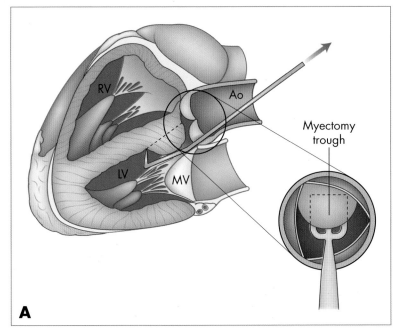

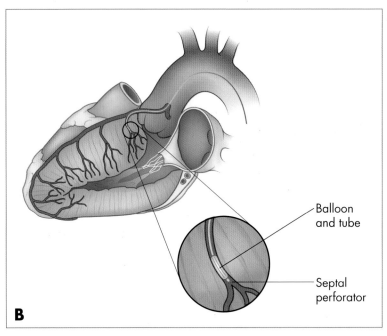

Figure 13-29. Hypertrophic cardiomyopathy (HCM) patients with left ventricular (LV) outflow obstruction gradient of 50 mm Hg or greater at rest or with provocation, who have advanced heart failure symptoms refractory to medical therapy, are candidates for invasive septal reduction therapy to relieve outflow obstruction and to improve limiting symptoms [1,2]. Surgical myectomy is considered the "gold standard" for the treatment of outflow obstruction, providing complete elimination of gradients in the vast majority of patients, resulting in significant long-lasting improvement in symptoms [26]. **A**, During surgical myectomy, the surgeon is provided with direct visualization of the LV outflow and septum, permitting complete resection of muscle extending from the basal to midanterior septum, as well as correction of any valvular or subvalvular anomalies that may be present (*ie*, accessory papillary muscles, anomalous papillary muscle with direct insertion into the mitral valve or mitral valve disease). Alternatively, alcohol septal ablation (ASA) is a catheter-based procedure in which 1 to 2 mL of alcohol are injected into the appropriate septal perforator supplying the basal septum (at the point of systolic anterior motion–septal contact). **B**, This creates a localized myocardial infarction resulting in septal thinning, widening of the LV outflow area, and elimination of obstruction. Short-term follow-up after ASA has demonstrated a decrease in gradients (although less than surgery) with substantial improvement in symptoms [27]. Ao—aorta; MV—mitral valve; RV—right ventricle.

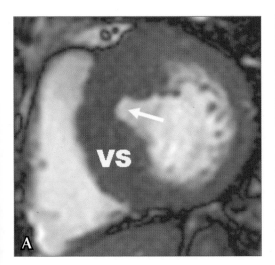

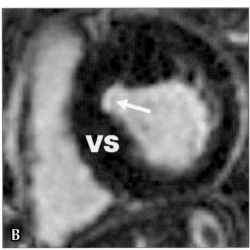

Figure 13-30. Surgical myectomy and alcohol septal ablation produce different effects on the ventricular septum (VS) [28]. **A**, An hypertrophic cardiomyopathy (HCM) patient who underwent surgical myectomy, with a cardiovascular magnetic resonance basal left ventricular (LV) short-axis image demonstrating septal myectomy trough (*arrow*) in the area corresponding to the resection. **B**, In the same HCM patient, a corresponding late gadolinium enhancement image shows the absence of hyperenhancement (*arrow*), confirming that surgical myectomy does not result in the production of an intramyocardial scar.

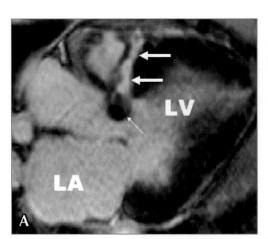

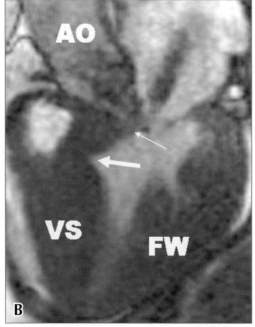

Figure 13-31. Alcohol septal ablation (ASA) produces a localized myocardial infarction resulting in variable amounts and location of tissue necrosis. Late gadolinium enhancement (LGE) can accurately identify and quantify the amount of tissue necrosis following ASA as well as provide important information about the relationship between location of scarring and outflow tract morphology. **A,** LGE image in an hypertrophic cardiomyopathy (HCM) patient who underwent ASA, demonstrating a transmural area of hyperenhancement in the septum (*arrow,* usually located more inferiorly in the septum than the myectomy trough) as a result of myocardial tissue necrosis from the procedure. Generally, the amount of myocardial infarct produced by ASA is not insignificant, totaling, on average, 10% of the total LV mass [28]. In addition, in select patients who undergo ASA, the area of tissue necrosis can spare the basal septum and involve predominantly the right ventricular (RV) side of the ventricular septum (VS) at the midventricular level. In such circumstances, there may be persistence of a left ventricular (LV) outflow gradient. **B,** A long-axis cardiovascular magnetic resonance functional image with corresponding LGE image in an HCM patient who underwent ASA showing a predominant area of hyperenhancement on the RV side of the septum (*thick arrows*) with sparing of myocardial necrosis of the basal septum (*thin arrow*). In such circumstances, the area of septal thinning occurs distal to the area of the basal septum (and systolic anterior motion [SAM]-septal contact) resulting in persistence of an LV outflow tract gradient. In the same HCM patient, a dedicated LV outflow tract view demonstrating thinning of the distal ventricular septum at the location of the alcohol injection (*thick arrow*) without affecting basal septal hypertrophy and as a result persistence of SAM-septal contact (*thin arrow*) with an LV outflow tract gradient. AO—aorta; LA—left atrium; FW—free wall.

REFERENCES

1. Maron BJ: Hypertrophic cardiomyopathy: a systematic review. *JAMA* 2002, 287:1308–1320.

2. Maron BJ, McKenna WJ, Danielson GK, *et al.*: American College of Cardiology/European Society of Cardiology clinical expert consensus document on hypertrophic cardiomyopathy. A report of the American College of Cardiology Foundation Task Force on Clinical Expert Consensus Documents and the European Society of Cardiology Committee for Practice Guidelines. *J Am Coll Cardiol* 2003, 42:1687–713.

3. Seidman JG, Seidman C: The genetic basis for cardiomyopathy: from mutation identification to mechanistic paradigms. *Cell* 2001, 104:557–567.

4. Klues HG, Schiffers A, Maron BJ: Phenotypic spectrum and patterns of left ventricular hypertrophy in hypertrophic cardiomyopathy: morphologic observations and significance as assessed by two-dimensional echocardiography in 600 patients. *J Am Coll Cardiol* 1995, 26:1699–1708.

5. Spirito P, Bellone P, Harris KM, *et al.*: Magnitude of left ventricular hypertrophy and risk of sudden death in hypertrophic cardiomyopathy. *N Engl J Med* 2000, 342:1778–1785.

6. Basso C, Thiene G, Corrado D, *et al.*: Hypertrophic cardiomyopathy and sudden death in the young: pathologic evidence of myocardial ischemia. *Hum Pathol* 2000, 31:988–998.

7. Shirani J, Pick R, Roberts WC, Maron BJ: Morphology and significance of the left ventricular collagen network in young patients with hypertrophic cardiomyopathy and sudden cardiac death. *J Am Coll Cardiol* 2000, 35:36–44.

8. Varnava AM, Elliott PM, Sharma S, *et al.*: Hypertrophic cardiomyopathy: the interrelation of disarray, fibrosis, and small vessel disease. *Heart* 2000, 84:476–482.

9. Maron MS, Olivotto I, Zenovich AG, *et al.*: Hypertrophic cardiomyopathy is predominantly a disease of left ventricular outflow tract obstruction. *Circulation* 2006, 114:2232–2239.

10. Maron MS, Olivotto I, Betocchi S, *et al.*: Effect of left ventricular outflow tract obstruction on clinical outcome in hypertrophic cardiomyopathy. *N Engl J Med* 2003, 348:295–303.

11. Pennell DJ: Cardiovascular magnetic resonance: twenty-first century solutions in cardiology. *Clin Med* 2003, 3:273–278.

12. Lima JA, Desai MY: Cardiovascular magnetic resonance imaging: current and emerging applications. *J Am Coll Cardiol* 2004, 44:1164–1171.

13. Rickers C, Wilke NM, Jerosch-Herold M, Casey SA, *et al.*: Utility of cardiac magnetic resonance imaging in the diagnosis of hypertrophic cardiomyopathy. *Circulation* 2005, 112:855–861.

14. Moon JC, McKenna WJ, McCrohon JA, *et al.*: Toward clinical risk assessment in hypertrophic cardiomyopathy with gadolinium cardiovascular magnetic resonance. *J Am Coll Cardiol* 2003, 41:1561–1567.

15. Moon JC, Fisher NG, McKenna WJ, Pennell DJ: Detection of apical hypertrophic cardiomyopathy by cardiovascular magnetic resonance in patients with non-diagnostic echocardiography. *Heart* 2004, 90:645–649.

16. Maron MS, Bos JM, Ackerman MJ, *et al.*: Left ventricular apical aneurysms: a novel under-recognized subgroup within the hypertrophic cardiomyopathy disease spectrum. *Circulation* 2006, 114(suppl 1):II-439.

17. Maron MS, Hauser TH, Dubrow E, *et al.*: Right ventricular involvement in hypertrophic cardiomyopathy. *Am J Cardiol* 2007, 100:1293-1298.

18. Casolo G, Olivotto I, Rega ML, *et al.*: Relationship of echocardiographic maximum left ventricular wall thickness to cardiac mass assessed by magnetic resonance in hypertrophic cardiomyopathy. *Eur Heart J* 2005, 26:387.

19. Harrigan CJ, Appelbaum E, Gibson CM, *et al.*: Evidence for papillary muscle involvement in hypertrophic cardiomyopathy by cardiac magnetic resonance. *J Cardiovasc Magn Reson* 2007, 9:428.

20. Maron BJ, Estes M, Maron MS, *et al.*: Primary prevention of sudden death as a novel treatment strategy in hypertrophic cardiomyopathy. *Circulation* 2003, 107:2872–2875.

21. Maron BJ, Thompson PD, Ackerman MJ, *et al.*: Recommendations and considerations related to preparticipation screening for cardiovascular abnormalities in competitive athletes: 2007 update: a scientific statement from the American Heart Association council on nutrition, physical activity, and metabolism: endorsed by the American College of Cardiology Foundation. *Circulation* 2007, 115:1643–1655.

22. Kim RJ, Wu E, Rafael A, *et al.*: The use of contrast-enhanced magnetic resonance imaging to identify reversible myocardial dysfunction. *N Engl J Med* 2000, 343:1445–1453.

23. Choudhury L, Mahrholdt H, Wagner A, *et al.*: Myocardial scarring in asymptomatic or mildly symptomatic patients with hypertrophic cardiomyopathy. *J Am Coll Cardiol* 2002, 40:2156–2164.

24. Moon JC, Reed E, Sheppard MN, *et al.*: The histologic basis of late gadolinium enhancement cardiovascular magnetic resonance in hypertrophic cardiomyopathy. *J Am Coll Cardiol* 2004, 43:2260–2264.

25. Harris KM, Spirito P, Maron MS, *et al.*: Prevalence, clinical profile, and significance of left ventricular remodeling in the end-stage phase of hypertrophic cardiomyopathy. *Circulation* 2006, 114:216–225.

26. Maron BJ. Dearani JA. Ommen SR, *et al.*: The case for surgery in obstructive hypertrophic cardiomyopathy. *J Am Coll Cardiol* 2004, 44:2044–2053.

27. Alam M, Dokainish H, Lakkis N. Alcohol septal ablation for hypertrophic obstructive cardiomyopathy: a systematic review of published studies. *Interv Cardiol* 2006, 19:319–327.

28. Valeti US, Nishimura RA, Holmes DR, *et al.*: Comparison of surgical septal myectomy and alcohol septal ablation with cardiac magnetic resonance imaging in patients with hypertrophic obstructive cardiomyopathy. *Cardiology* 2007, 49:350–357.

14

Arrhythmogenic Right Ventricular Cardiomyopathy

Harikrishna Tandri and David A. Bluemke

Arrhythmogenic right ventricular cardiomyopathy (ARVC) is a genetic cardiomyopathy characterized by fibrofatty replacement of the right ventricular (RV) musculature, ventricular arrhythmias, and progressive RV failure [1,2]. This condition accounts for up to 5% of sudden deaths in young individuals less than 35 years of age [3,4]. ARVC rarely manifests before adolescence, and usually presents in the second or third decade of life [1]. Presenting symptoms vary from occasional palpitations, syncope, to sudden death. The diagnosis is based on a set of major and minor criteria proposed by the Task Force of Cardiomyopathies in 1994 [5]. Current structural and functional abnormalities in the RV constitute a criterion for ARVC diagnosis. RV involvement in ARVC can be nonuniform; hence, comprehensive assessment of the RV is desirable. During the past decade, cardiovascular magnetic resonance (CMR) has emerged as a robust tool to evaluate RV structure and function in ARVC [6–12]. The ability to provide tissue characterization noninvasively and to allow quantitative assessment of the RV is ideal for assessment and follow-up evaluation of ARVC. Although CMR has the greatest potential for diagnosis of ARVC, the complex contraction pattern of the thin-walled RV and the normal variation in the presence of epicardial fat pose the greatest challenges for CMR of ARVC. The purpose of this chapter is to discuss the CMR protocol, the CMR abnormalities observed in ARVC, and the challenges that exist in diagnoses of this rare cardiomyopathy.

NORMAL RIGHT VENTRICULAR ANATOMY AND FUNCTION

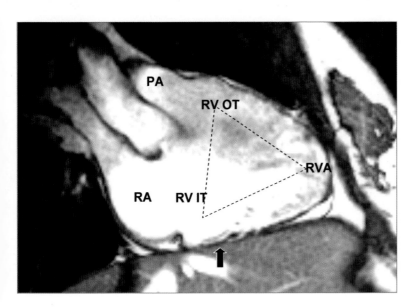

Figure 14-1. Normal long-axis view of the right ventricle (RV) by cardiovascular magnetic resonance (CMR). Bright blood CMR diastolic image of the RV long-axis view (similar to the right anterior oblique view on cine angiography) from a healthy volunteer obtained with steady-state free precession CMR. Cardiac structures visualized in this view include RV, right atrium, RV outflow tract (RVOT), and the pulmonary artery (PA). The RV can be divided anatomically into an RV inflow region (RVIT), the body of the RV, the RVOT, and the apex (RVA). Arrhythmogenic right ventricular cardiomyopathy (ARVC) most commonly affects the subtricuspid region (*arrow*), the apex, and the RVOT. Thus, these three regions are collectively termed *the triangle of dysplasia*.

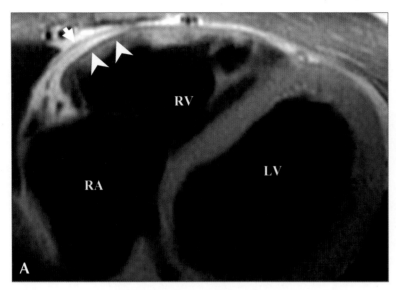

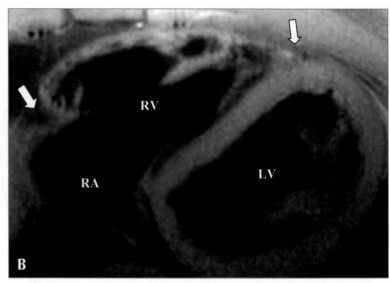

Figure 14-2. Normal axial views of the right ventricle (RV) by cardiovascular magnetic resonance (CMR). **A,** Midventricular axial black blood image of the heart from a healthy volunteer obtained with dual-inversion fast spin-echo pulse sequence. In this image, fat appears as a high-intensity signal, myocardium is gray (intermediate signal), and blood appears black. Cardiac chambers visualized in this view include the RV, right atrium, and left ventricle. The RV free wall is thin and normally measures 3 to 4 mm in thickness. Epicardial fat (*arrow*) overlies the RV free wall and is typically abundant at the apex and at the atrioventricular groove.

A clear line of demarcation (*arrowheads*) is often seen between the RV epicardial fat and the RV myocardium. Disruption of the line of demarcation with hyperintense signals observed within the gray RV myocardium is suggestive of intramyocardial fat infiltration, seen in patients with arrhythmogenic right ventricular cardiomyopathy (ARVC). **B,** The same image from the volunteer obtained with fat suppression. Note that the hyperintense signal in the atrioventricular groove and the RV apex is now replaced by signal void (*arrows*). The RV wall has a uniform contour with absence of intramyocardial signal voids suggestive of fat.

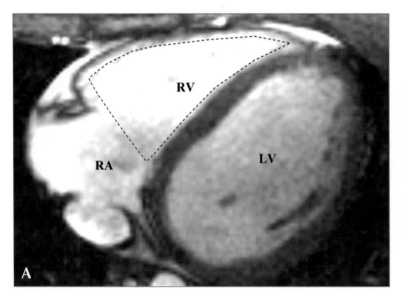

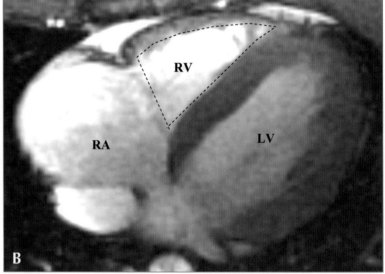

Figure 14-3. Pattern of normal ventricular contraction visualized by caridovascular magnetic resonance. Axial bright blood images in diastole (**A**) and systole (**B**) from a normal volunteer. Note the differences in the contraction patterns of the right ventricle (RV) and the left ventricle (LV). The LV contraction involves significant contribution from both circumferential

and longitudinal shortening. However, the majority of the RV contraction results from longitudinal shortening from the base toward the apex, best seen in the axial images. Thus, the RV maintains its triangular shape with a smaller change in the short axis, but is significantly changed in the long-axis direction. RA—right atrium.

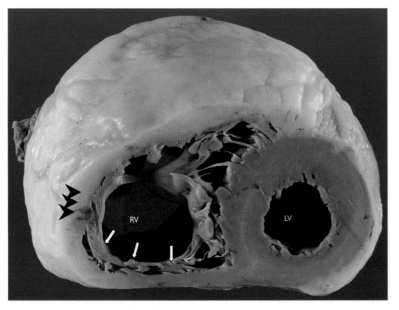

Figure 14-4. Gross anatomy of arrhythmogenic right ventricular cardiomyopathy (ARVC). This image shows an explanted heart from a patient with ARVC. Cardiac chambers shown include the right ventricle (RV) and the left ventricle (LV). The RV is massively enlarged compared with the normal sized LV. The RV wall is entirely replaced by yellow fat (*arrowheads*). Note the increased trabeculation within the RV and the grayish appearance of the fibrotic RV endocardium (*arrows*).

CMR PROTOCOL

CMR Protocol in ARVC

Axial and short-axis T1-weighted ECG gated black blood images, with and without fat suppression

Axial and short-axis ECG gated cine images, with and without fat suppression

Administer 0.15–0.12 mmol/kg gadolinium intravenously

Late gadolinium enhancement, axial and short-axis plane

Additional images:

Long-axis cine image of the RV

Horizontal and vertical long-axis cine image of the LV

Figure 14-5. Cardiovascular magnetic resonance (CMR) protocol for arrhythmogenic right ventricular cardiomyopathy (ARVC). CMR protocol provides information related to the various pathologic manifestations of ARVC; namely, abnormal RV morphology, global and regional dysfunction, fat infiltration, and fibrosis of the right ventricle (RV). Image quality is crucial for interpretation of CMR. CMR technicians who educate patients regarding breath holding techniques, as well as taking measures to ensure proper electrocardiogram (ECG) gating are invaluable for high-quality CMR examinations. In patients with frequent premature ventricular contractions, use of a cardioselective β-blocker such as metoprolol 30 minutes prior to CMR is recommended. Black blood images with and without fat suppression obtained in the axial and short-axis orientation provide tissue characterization (*ie*, depiction of intramyocardial fat). Bright blood images in the axial, four-chamber, two-chamber, and short-axis views are used to visually assess global and regional function. Short-axis views allow for volumetric assessment. Late gadolinium enhancement images in the axial and short-axis views are also used to detect fibrosis in the RV. LV—left ventricle.

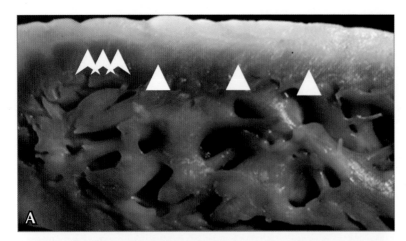

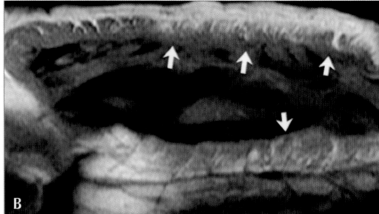

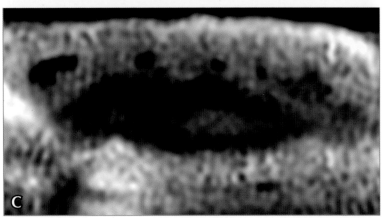

Figure 14-6. Gross pathologic abnormalities in arrhythmogenic right ventricular cardiomyopathy (ARVC) visualized by cardiovascular magnetic resonance (CMR). Intramyocardial fat and fibrosis within the right ventricular (RV) wall is the histopathologic hallmark of ARVC. CMR has the unique advantage over other conventional imaging modalities in its ability to characterize fat in the RV wall. However, fat infiltration in early ARVC tends to be microscopic, and current resolution of CMR is often inadequate in in vivo imaging of fat infiltration, especially in early ARVC. This image reveals a section of the RV from a 28-year-old man who experienced sudden death; a diagnosis of ARVC was confirmed on autopsy. **A,** This image shows the gross anatomy of the RV. Note the line of separation between the myocardium and the epicardial fat (*arrowheads*) that is disrupted toward the middle RV wall by infiltrating epicardial fat. **B,** This image shows high-resolution CMR, revealing strands of epicardial fat (*arrows*) that infiltrate the RV myocardium corresponding to the regions on the gross anatomic specimen. A similar level of detail is difficult to achieve in in vivo imaging because of limitations of breath-hold, motion artifacts, and field of view. **C,** CMR obtained with lower resolution clinical scanning, revealing significant blurring, making the image uninterpretable.

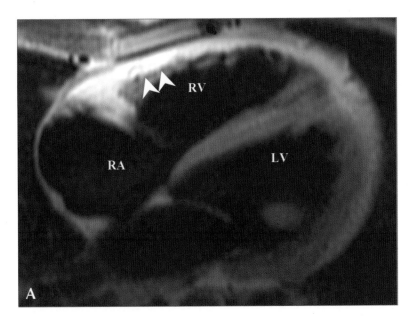

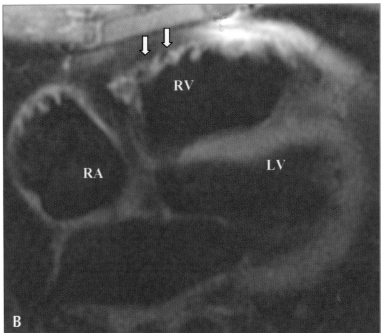

Figure 14-7. Cardiovascular magnetic resonance (CMR) of the normal heart. Differentiation of normal fat distribution from pathologic intramyocardial fat is often difficult as fat is normally distributed around the heart and is most abundant near the atrioventricular groove and the right ventricular (RV) apex. Caution should be exercised when interpreting intramyocardial fat, as pathologic and some degree of intramyocardial fat infiltration is also seen in elderly subjects and with long-term steroid therapy. Thus, intramyocardial fat on CMR lacks specificity for diagnosis of arrhythmogenic right ventricular cardiomyopathy (ARVC). An example of intramyocardial fat infiltration in ARVC is shown in this figure (**B**). **A**, Axial black blood image from a 33-year-old athlete who presented with sustained ventricular tachycardia. Note the epicardial fat infiltrating the RV myocardium (*arrowheads*) and the lack of a clear line of demarcation between the epicardial fat and the RV wall closer to the RV inflow region. **B**, A fat-suppressed image at the same location reveals a signal void in the region of hyperintense signal (*arrows*), confirming the diagnosis of intramyocardial fat. LV—left ventricle; RA—right atrium.

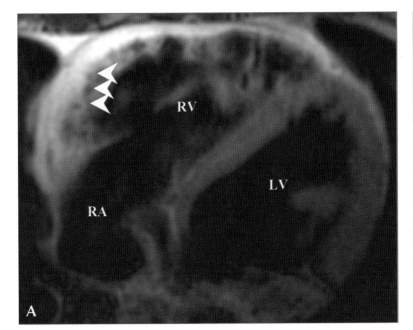

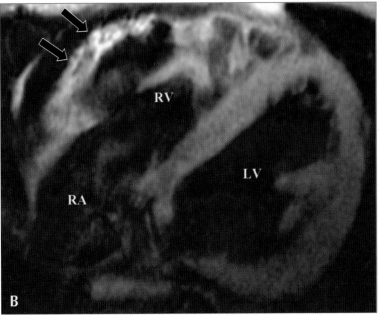

Figure 14-8. Arrhythmogenic right ventricular cardiomyopathy (ARVC) abnormalities of the right ventricle (RV) identified by cardiovascular magnetic resonance. **A**, Axial black blood image from a 40-year-old man who met task force criteria for ARVC (*arrows*). The RV wall appears hypertrophied with a diffuse heterogeneous signal. No clear separation between the epicardial fat and the RV endocardium is seen. Also note the enlarged RV with increased trabeculations within the RV. Morphologic changes such as global and regional dilatation and functional changes such as regional wall motion abnormalities often accompany fat infiltration. The presence of regional contraction abnormalities corresponding to the region of fat infiltration is more suggestive of the diagnosis than fat infiltration alone. **B**, A fat-suppressed image at the same location shows several signal voids (*arrows*) within the RV corresponding to the regions of hyperintense signals in the non–fat-suppressed image. LV—left ventricle; RA—right atrium.

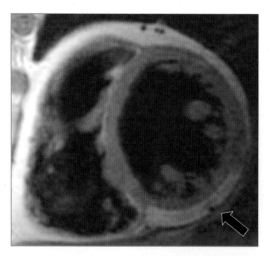

Figure 14-9. Arrhythmogenic right ventricular cardiomyopathy (ARVC) involvement of the left ventricle (LV) indentified by cardiovascular magnetic resonance. Autopsy studies have reported a high prevalence of LV involvement on histology in patients with ARVC. However, LV involvement detected on in vivo imaging is seen in less than 15% of patients. LV involvement appears uncommon during early stages of the disease and is often seen in conjunction with severe right ventricular (RV) involvement. The differential involvement of the RV by the disease process is thought to be related to the relative thickness of the LV wall compared with the thin RV wall, which is more vulnerable to dysfunction because of replacement of myocardial cells by fibrofatty tissue. LV involvement in ARVC characteristically spares the interventricular septum and is often located in the inferolateral wall as shown in this figure. A short-axis black blood image from the base of the heart in a 30-year-old man with ARVC is shown. Fat replacement of the inferior and posterolateral wall of the LV (*arrow*) is seen extending from the epicardial surface. Note the decreased thickness of the LV wall in the region of fat infiltration. Other diagnostic features in this image include the enlarged RV with diffuse fat infiltration of the RV wall.

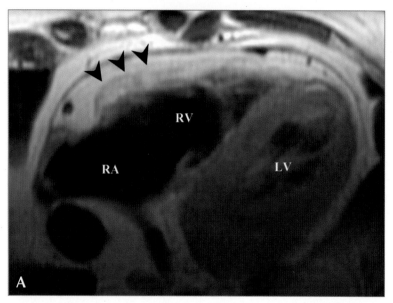

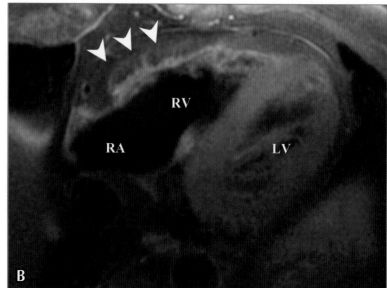

Figure 14-10. Cardiovascular magnetic resonance (CMR) of lipomatous infiltration of the myocardium. Fat replacement of the right ventricular (RV) wall on CMR is not unique to arrhythmogenic right ventricular cardiomyopathy (ARVC) and can also be seen in obese individuals, elderly individuals, and in patients on long-term steroid therapy. Fat may also be interspersed with RV myocardial fibers without fibrosis or signs of inflammation. Minor amounts of fat were reported in up to 85% of elderly patients terminally ill with noncardiac causes. Marked lipomatous infiltration of the RV was also described without global or regional functional abnormalities [13]. Lipomatous infiltration of the RV could be a distinct CMR-defined disorder, apart from ARVC. These patients often lack other electrocardiographic manifestations of ARVC. Overdiagnosis of ARVC can be avoided by adhering to the task force criteria. **A,** An example of "fat dissociation syndrome" is shown in this axial black blood CMR of a 42-year-old woman who was evaluated for presyncope. Note the abundance of epicardial fat that replaces the entire RV myocardium (*arrowheads*). **B,** A fat-suppressed image at the same location reveals the underlying RV myocardial wall (*arrowheads*). LV—left ventricle; RA—right atrium.

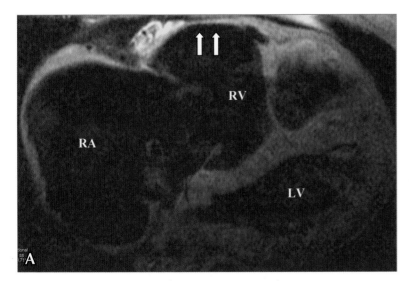

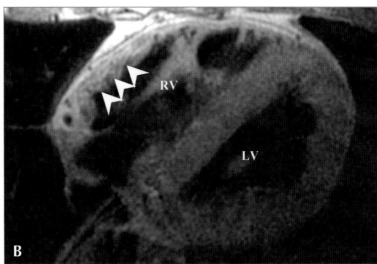

Figure 14-11. Cardiovascular magnetic resonance findings in arrhythmogenic right ventricular cardiomyopathy (ARVC): wall thinning, wall hypertrophy, and trabecular disarray. These findings are less frequent than fat infiltration and were observed in less than a quarter of patients with ARVC in our series. Normal right ventricular (RV) wall thickness is 4 mm to 5 mm. RV wall thinning is defined as a focal abrupt reduction in wall thickness to less than 2 mm, surrounded by regions of normal wall thickness. Wall thinning is thought to result from loss of myocytes because of apoptosis or fat infiltration. Occasionally myocardial infiltration by fibrofatty tissue gives the appearance of increased wall thick-

ness (> 8-mm thickness). Abnormal trabeculation is a consequence of abnormal stress experienced by the surviving myocytes in the endocardial layers of the RV. **A**, An example of focal wall thinning and severe RV dilatation. Note the abrupt decrease in RV wall thickness, best seen on the fat-suppressed images (*arrows*). **B**, An example of wall hypertrophy. The RV wall has a diffuse heterogeneous signal because of infiltration by fibrofatty tissue. Also note the increased trabeculation of the RV (*arrowheads*). These findings are rarely seen in the absence of global functional abnormalities; thus, there is a lack of sensitivity for ARVC diagnosis. LV—left ventricle; RA—right atrium.

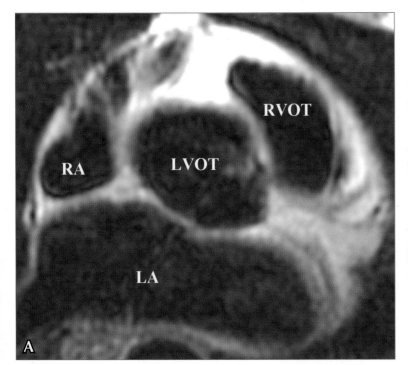

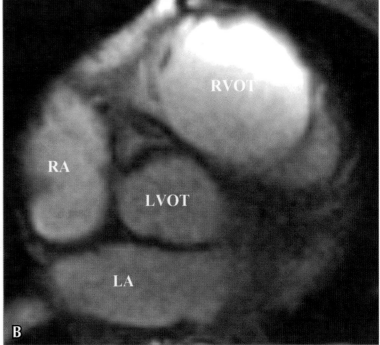

Figure 14-12. Right ventricular outflow tract (RVOT) enlargement by cardiovascular magnetic resonace (CMR) in arrhythmogenic right ventricular cardiomyopathy (ARVC). The RVOT is a common location for localized ARVC. The RVOT is usually smaller than the aortic outflow tract at the level of the aortic valve. An exception to this rule is pediatric patients in whom the RVOT may be larger than the left ventricular outflow tract (LVOT). Presence of an enlarged RVOT beyond adolescence is uncommon. RVOT enlargement in ARVC may be a part of generalized dilation involving the right side of the

heart. More important than a simple enlargement is a dysmorphic appearance of the outflow tract. Abnormal appearance of the RVOT, which is dyskinetic in systole, is highly suggestive of ARVC in the absence of pulmonary hypertension.
A, An axial black blood CMR of a healthyS volunteer at the level of the aortic valve. Note that the RVOT is marginally larger than the LVOT at this level. **B**, Axial black blood CMR from a patient with ARVC. Note the dysmorphic appearance of the RVOT, which is clearly bigger than the LVOT. LA—left atrium; RA—right atrium.

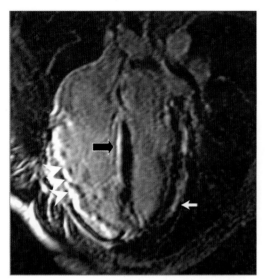

Figure 14-13. Cardiovascular magnetic resonance (CMR) fibrosis in arrhythmogenic right ventricular cardiomyopathy (ARVC). One of the pathologic hallmarks of ARVC is fibrosis of the right ventricle (RV) that accompanies fatty infiltration. Late gadolinium enhancement (LGE) CMR allows for noninvasive detection of fibrosis in the RV that may improve the specificity of ARVC diagnosis. Our group imaged 12 ARVC patients with LGE CMR. Eight (67%) of the 12 patients with ARVC demonstrated increased signal consistent with fibrosis in the RV [12]. The areas of fibrosis on CMR corresponded with regions containing kinetic abnormalities, and the extent of fibrosis showed an inverse correlation with global RV function. An important finding of this study revealed that 18 patients with idiopathic ventricular tachycardia who underwent LGE CMR showed no evidence of fibrosis, highlighting the negative predictive value of LGE CMR in evaluating patients with suspected ARVC. Presence of fibrosis detected on LGE CMR predicted inducibility of sustained ventricular tachycardia during electrophysiologic testing, thus providing information on arrhythmic risk. Shown in this image is an example of LGE CMR in a 19-year-old patient who presented with ventricular tachycardia. Note the diffuse enhancement of the RV wall (*arrowheads*), the enhancement of the interventricular septum (*black arrow*), and the left ventricular lateral wall (*white arrow*) suggestive of biventricular involvement.

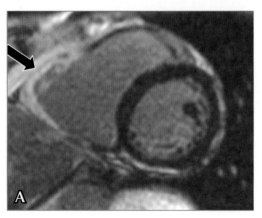
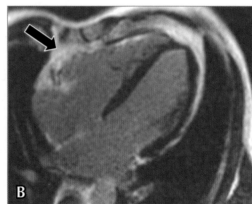

Figure 14-14. **A** and **B**, Delayed enhanced images from a patient with arrhythmogenic right ventricular cardiomyopathy (ARVC) who met the Task Force Criteria. Late gadolinium enhancement (LGE) of the right ventricular myocardium can be seen in the basal anterior wall. LGE in ARVC can be useful in directing the site of biopsy for a definitive diagnosis and for electrophysiologic localization of scar tissue for ablative therapy in patients with ventricular arrhythmias.

REGIONAL AND GLOBAL RIGHT VENTRICULAR DYSFUNCTION

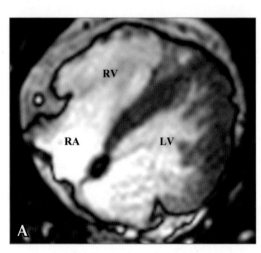
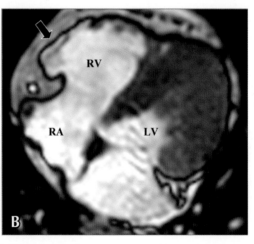

Figure 14-15. Abnormalities of regional and global ventricular dysfunction in arrhythmogenic right ventricular cardiomyopathy (ARVC). Fibrofatty infiltration and loss of myocytes result in wall thinning with focally reduced contraction and aneurysm formation. These findings precede changes in global ventricular function. Thus, accurate identification may improve the sensitivity of the diagnosis. In fact, studies have consistently reported a high incidence of regional dysfunction in ARVC, which appears more sensitive than morphologic findings such as fat infiltra-tion. Regional functional abnormalities of the right ventricle described in ARVC include focal hypokinesis, akinesis, dyskinesis (myocardial segment, which moves outward in systole), and aneurysms (segments with persistent bulging in diastole, and dyskinetic in systole).

A and **B**, Systolic and diastolic four-chamber cine images from a patient with ARVC. Note the discrete aneurysmal out-pouching in the anterior wall close to the diaphragm in systole (B) (*arrow*). LV—left ventricle; RA—right atrium.

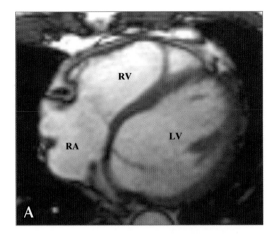 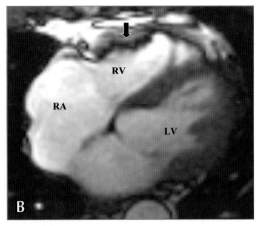

Figure 14-16. Regional dysfunction in arrhythmogenic right ventricular dysplasia/cardiomyopathy (ARVC) involving the triangle of dysplasia (*ie,* the subtricuspid region, the apex, and the right ventricular outflow tract). The importance of careful evaluation of the peritricuspid region cannot be overstated because minor contraction abnormalities limited to this region may be the only early manifestations of ARVC. Shown is a cine axial cardiovascular magnetic resonance of a 32-year-old first degree relative of a patient with ARVC with a plakophillin mutation who was diagnosed with ARVC after meeting the task force criteria. **A,** Note the normal right ventricular morphology in diastole. **B,** Focal wall motion abnormality limited to the peritricuspid region is seen in systole (*arrow*). LV—left ventricle; RA—right atrium.

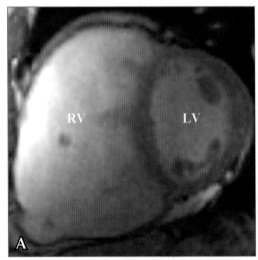 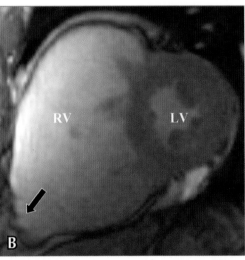

Figure 14-17. Global dysfunction in arrhythmogenic right ventricular cardiomyopathy (ARVC). ARVC is a progressive cardiomyopathy, and eventually most patients develop global right ventricular (RV) dysfunction. Several factors such as genetic factors, environmental factors, exercise, and viral myocarditis superimposed on ARVC have been proposed to affect the rate of progression of RV dysfunction. The severity of RV dilation and dysfunction also correlates with the risk of ventricular arrhythmias and the need for cardiac transplantation. Accurate and reproducible quantification of RV volumes and function by cardiovascular magnetic resonance plays an important role not only in diagnosis but also in assessing the long-term prognosis of patients with ARVC. **A,** Diastolic midcavity short-axis cine image from a patient with ARVC. Note the disproportionate enlargement of the RV compared with the left ventricle (LV). **B,** Systolic frame at the same location shows akinesis of the entire RV wall (*arrow*) with severe global RV dysfunction. The LV, in contrast, shows normal global contraction.

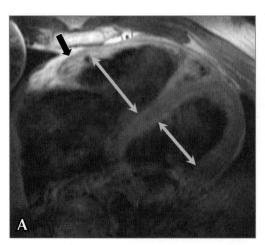 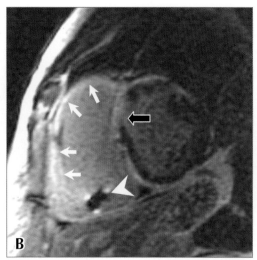 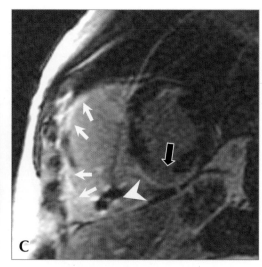

Figure 14-18. Long-term follow-up of patients with arrhythmogenic right ventricular cardiomyopathy (ARVC). The majority of patients with ARVC who meet task force criteria receive implantable defibrillator therapy for prevention of sudden cardiac death. Further evaluation of right ventricular (RV) function can be challenging, because current cardiovascular magnetic resonance (CMR) is contraindicated in patients with implantable devices. In addition, device hardware–related artifacts interfere with image quality. The authors have performed CMR in selected patients on an investigational basis both to diagnose ARVC and for follow-up evaluation of RV function. In our experience, the artifacts are generally confined to the region of the pulse generator and do not interfere significantly with image interpretation. Shown in the figures are CMR obtained from ARVC patients with implantable defibrillators that validate the use of CMR in diagnosis and follow-up of these patients.

A, Black blood image of a 21-year-old man with biopsy-proven ARVC who received implantable defibrillator therapy. Hyperintense signals in the basal RV wall indicative of fat infiltration are clearly seen. Also note the enlarged RV compared with the left ventricle (LV). *B* and *C*, Short-axis late gadolinium enhanced (LGE) images from a patient with ARVC who has an implantable defibrillator. Note the artifact caused by the RV lead that appears as a signal void in the image (*arrowheads*). Diffuse LGE of the RV free wall (*white arrows*) can be seen in the images with focal enhancement of the anterior interventricular septum and the inferior wall (*black arrows*). Also note the enlarged RV compared with the left ventricle.

Thus, despite the presence of an implantable cardiodefibrillator, hardware morphologic and tissue characterization of the RV is possible by cardiovascular magnetic resonance, enabling its use in diagnosis and follow-up of patients with ARVC.

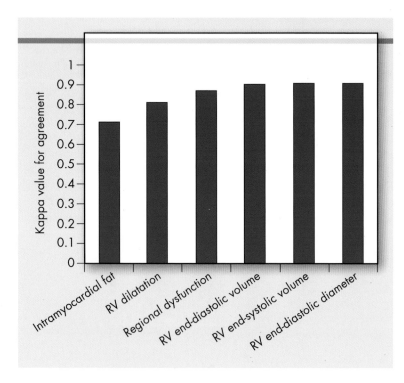

Figure 14-19. Reader agreement of cardiovascular magnetic resonance (CMR) for patients with arrhythmogenic right ventricular cardiomyopathy (ARVC). The diagnostic utility of qualitative CMR findings such as fat infiltration, wall thinning, and regional dysfunction is controversial. Considerable variation exists among observers in the definition of abnormal intramyocardial fat, resulting in significant interobserver variability in the reporting of fat on CMR. Reporting of fat infiltration on CMR performed in patients evaluated for ARVC has resulted in a serious overdiagnosis of ARVC, subsequently resulting in inappropriate therapy with implantable defibrillators. Among experienced CMR readers, reproducibility is excellent. The reproducibility for reporting fat infiltration can be further improved by utilizing chemical shift fat suppression. Quantitative CMR findings such as right ventricular (RV) end-diastolic volumes and RV diameters show a high degree of interobserver reproducibility. This figure shows the interobserver reproducibility for qualitative and quantitative CMR findings in ARVC. Among the qualitative findings, fat infiltration was the least reproducible parameter (κ value of 0.73) compared with RV dilation ($\kappa = 0.86$) and regional dysfunction ($\kappa = 0.85$). All the quantitative parameters showed excellent interobserver reproducibility with κ values greater than 0.90 for all the quantitative variables.

CONCLUSIONS

Cardiovascular magnetic resonance (CMR) offers unique advantages over other conventional imaging modalities in evaluating patients with suspected right ventricular (RV) dysplasia. Good image quality and interpretation made by experienced CMR readers are crucial in the CMR evaluation of arrhythmogenic right ventricular cardiomyopathy (ARVC). Among the qualitative CMR variables, regional RV dysfunc-tion is more sensitive and reproducible compared with fat infiltration. Quantitative RV analyses are highly reproducible and useful in clinical follow-up of patients with ARVC, as well as their first degree relatives. Finally, the diagnosis of ARVC should be made by using the task force criteria and should not be made based on CMR features alone.

REFERENCES

1. Marcus FI, Fontaine GH, Guiraudon G, *et al.*: Right ventricular dysplasia: a report of 24 adult cases. *Circulation* 1982, 65:384–398.

2. Laurent M, Descaves C, Biron Y, *et al.*: Familial form of arrhythmogenic right ventricular dysplasia. *Am Heart J* 1987, 113:827–829.

3. Corrado D, Thiene G, Nava A, *et al.*: Sudden death in young competitive athletes: clinicopathologic correlations in 22 cases. *Am J Med* 1990, 89:588–596.

4. Thiene G, Nava A, Corrado D, *et al.*: Right ventricular cardiomyopathy and sudden death in young people. *N Engl J Med* 1988, 318:129–133.

5. McKenna WJ, Thiene G, Nava A, *et al.*: Diagnosis of arrhythmogenic right ventricular dysplasia/cardiomyopathy. Task Force of the Working Group Myocardial and Pericardial Disease of the European Society of Cardiology and of the Scientific Council on Cardiomyopathies of the International Society and Federation of Cardiology. *Br Heart J* 1994, 71:215–218.

6. Casolo GC, Poggesi L, Boddi M, *et al.*: ECG-gated magnetic resonance imaging in right ventricular dysplasia. *Am Heart J* 1987, 113:1245–1248.

7. Tandri H, Calkins H, Nasir K, *et al.*: MR Imaging findings in patients meeting task force criteria for arrhythmogenic right ventricular dysplasia. *J Cardiovasc Electrophysiol* 2003, 14:476–483.

8. Midiri M, Finazzo M, Brancato M, *et al.*: Arrhythmogenic right ventricular dysplasia: MR features. *Eur Radiol* 1997, 7:307–312.

9. van der Wall EE, Kayser HW, Bootsma MM, *et al.*: Arrhythmogenic right ventricular dysplasia: MR imaging findings. *Herz* 2000, 4:356–364.

10. Blake LM, Scheinman MM, Higgins CB: MR features of arrhythmogenic right ventricular dysplasia. *AJR Am J Roentgenol* 1994, 162:809–812.

11. Molinari G, Sardanelli F, Gaita F, *et al.*: Right ventricular dysplasia as a generalized cardiomyopathy? Findings on magnetic resonance imaging. *Eur Heart J* 1995, 16:1619–1624.

12. Tandri H, Saranathan M, Rodriguez ER, *et al.*: Noninvasive detection of myocardial fibrosis in arrhythmogenic right ventricular cardiomyopathy using delayed-enhancement magnetic resonance imaging. *J Am Coll Cardiol* 2005, 45:98–103.

13. Macedo R, Prakasa K, Tichnell C, *et al.*: Marked lipomatous infiltration of the right ventricle: MRI findings in relation to arrhythmogenic right ventricular dysplasia. *AJR Am J Roentgenol* 2007, 188:W423–W427.

15

Valvular Heart Disease

Kevin J. Duffy Jr and Victor A. Ferrari

Cardiovascular magnetic resonance (CMR) provides an accurate depiction of cardiac morphology and function, and has an emerging new role in the assessment of cardiac valvular disease. CMR provides improved anatomic description of cardiac chambers, particularly in hearts deformed or distorted by disease or previous surgery. Qualitative and quantitative evaluation of stenotic and regurgitant valves is readily performed, as the multiplanar imaging capability of CMR permits an almost infinite number of imaging planes. A recent European Society of Cardiology Task Force Recommendation on CMR suggested that although echocardiography remains the technique of choice for overall valvular assessment, supravalvular pulmonic stenosis and supravalvular aortic stenosis are best assessed with CMR. The report emphasized the important role of CMR in noninvasively quantifying shunts and assessing physiology, especially following repair of congenital heart disease. Presently, cine imaging using a steady-state free-precession technique is the most common pulse sequence for initial valvular evaluation. This pulse sequence provides a movie-like image to assess leaflet excursion and identify turbulent flow in the valvular area.

CMR is particularly useful in cases involving eccentric jets. In many cases, evaluation of eccentric jet severity by echocardiography is very difficult, but the quantitative capabilities of CMR techniques provide a numerical value for the regurgitant volume, regardless of the jet orientation. Thus, interpreters are not limited to the visual depiction of a jet, which can vary significantly based on both echocardiographic and CMR imaging parameters [1]. CMR's larger field of view is especially useful in assessing the mechanism of aortic regurgitation. Aortic segment diameters and dilatation may be quantified, aortic valve morphology can be determined, and the presence or absence of an aortic coarctation may be confirmed.

Flow voids (signal drop outs caused by turbulence) are usually one of the first indications of valvular dysfunction. A series of scout images are performed to select an optimal plane perpendicular to the valve of interest. The imaging plane is placed approximately 1 cm to 1.5 cm from the valve plane, depending on the valve excursion, not to interfere with normal through-plane valve motion. This permits an accurate examination of the valve morphology, as well as centering the area of interest on the stenotic or regurgitant jet. A phase-contrast velocity encoded image is next obtained to determine the directions and magnitudes of blood flow velocities as well as to calculate flow volumes.

Recent work shows that CMR-estimated mitral and aortic regurgitant fractions correlate well with Doppler echocardiographic techniques [1-13]. Using these tools, comparisons between Doppler echocardiography and CMR, respectively, are as follows: mild < 15%, moderate 16% to 25%, moderate-severe 26% to 48%, and severe > 48%. A recent study also validated the use of the continuity equation for CMR assessment of the aortic valve area (stroke volume/aortic velocity time integral) compared with Doppler echocardiography. The results found a very good correlation ($r^2 = 0.83$) between the two.

CMR quantitative flow assessment permits several checks and balances. For example, in the absence of valvular disease, left ventricular (LV) stroke volume should equal the aortic flow volume, the flow volumes in the left and right pulmonary arteries should match the flow volume in the main pulmonary artery, and in the absence of a shunt, the pulmonary artery stroke volume should match the aortic stroke volume.

Also of great importance is CMR's highly accurate assessment of global and regional ventricular function, as well as LV mass. These data provide critical parameters for following patients serially with valvular disease to identify progression of dysfunction.

In summary, CMR provides a unique combination of accurate morphologic and quantitative valvular assessment, as well as serial evaluation of ventricular function. The following cases will highlight several of these points.

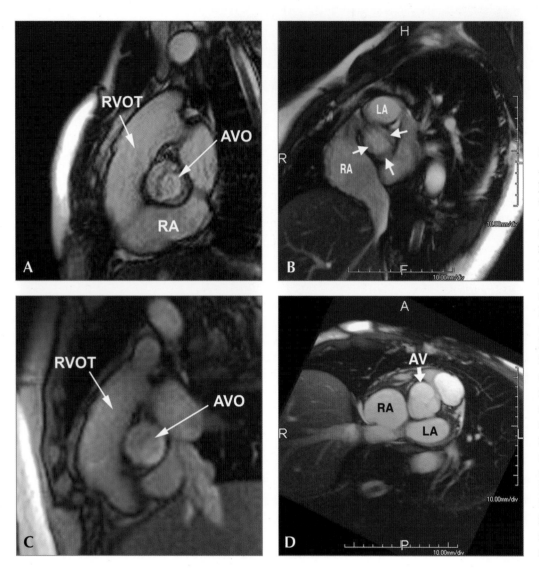

Figure 15-1. Bicuspid aortic valve (BAV). **A**, Short-axis plane steady-state free precession images of a BAV with a vertical commisure in a 40-year-old patient. At peak systole, the two leaflets open in an elliptical or "football-shaped" manner with minimal stenosis (peak gradient 12 mm Hg) and no regurgitation. A small amount of calcium (dark signal) is noted on the leaflet edges, and the right ventricular outflow tract (RVOT) and aortic valve orifice (AVO) are also noted. In **B**, the three leaflets of a normal aortic valve are seen in the typical triangular position (*arrows*) during systole. The left atrium (LA) and right atrium (RA) are also identified. Cardiovascular magnetic resonance (CMR) is an excellent technique for assessing leaflet morphology and the degree of stenosis or regurgitation, as well as in assessing complications following valve replacement [2-7]. CMR also permits evaluation of the thoracic aorta despite dilatation or tortuosity, particularly when examining patients for coarctation or pseudocoarctation associated with BAV disorder [8].

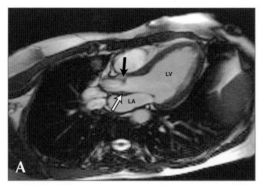
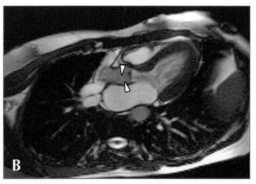

Figure 15-2. Dysmorphic aortic valve with aortic stenosis. Axial plane steady-state free precession (SSFP) images of a patient with an abnormal aortic valve. In **A** (end diastole) and **B** (end systole), a poorly visible aortic valve on transthoracic echocardiography was identified with cardiovascular magnetic resonance (CMR) as a thickened and calcified "functionally bicuspid" valve with three individual leaflets, but with fusion of the right and left cusps. In these images, the thickening and calcification is seen as dark areas on the aortic leaflets (*arrows*), and turbulent flow is visible, distal to the aortic valve (AV) with several jets (*arrowheads*), indicative of some stenosis. Moderate aor-

tic stenosis was identified using phase velocity pulse sequences. There was good correspondence between the peak AV gradients with echocardiography and CMR (36 mm Hg and 30 mm Hg, respectively). The phase velocity profile was measured at a slice location of 1.5 cm distal to the aortic valve at peak systole and perpendicular to the aortic stenosis jet direction (to detect the maximum jet velocity). A maximum encoding velocity limit (V_{ENC}) of 400 to 500 cm/s was used to avoid aliasing. LA—left atrium; LV—left ventricle. There is an excellent correlation between CMR planimetry of SSFP images and Doppler echocardiography determination of the aortic valve area [6,9-10].

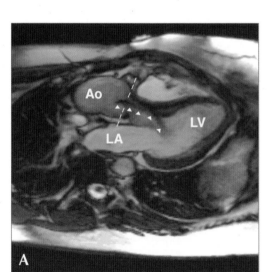
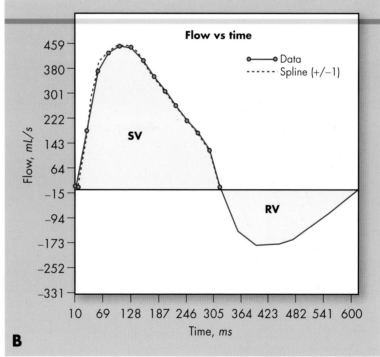

Figure 15-3. Aortic regurgitation. **A,** Axial steady-state free precession images in diastole demonstrate moderate aortic regurgitation (dark jet) in a 40-year-old patient with a bicuspid aortic valve, a dilated aortic root, and chronic aortic regurgitation. The dilated aortic root (Ao), left atrium (LA), and left ventricle (LV) are identified. The eccentric aortic regurgitation jet, which courses along the anterior mitral valve leaflet, is indicated by the *arrowheads*, and is clearly depicted using cardiovascular magnetic resonance (CMR). The *dotted line* identifies the optimal imaging plane (perpendicular to the regurgitant jet) for severity assessment of aortic regurgitation using the phase-contrast or velocity-encoded method. Quantitative assessment of antegrade

systolic or regurgitant flow is performed by integrating the instantaneous velocity over time across the vessel in systole and diastole, respectively, and subsequently multiplying this value by the vessel cross-sectional area. **B,** Antegrade systolic flow per heartbeat (or stroke volume [SV]) and retrograde diastolic regurgitant volume (RV). The regurgitant fraction is calculated as RV/SV. The cardiac output (CO) may be calculated by multiplying the SV by the heart rate (CO = SV × HR). There is excellent correlation between CMR-derived valvular regurgitation and Doppler techniques using echocardiography [13]. A major clinical benefit of CMR is the accurate noninvasive and serial assessment of LV volume and function. (**B,** *adapted from* [14] Scott, *et al* [14].)

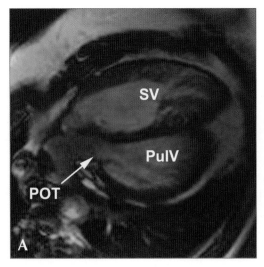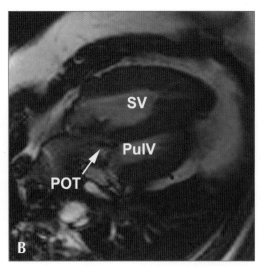

Figure 15-4. Subvalvular pulmonic stenosis in transposition of the great arteries. Steady-state free precession images in the four-chamber view from a patient with transposition of the great arteries (TGA) following Mustard procedure (atrial switch via baffle technique), at end diastole (**A**) and late systole (**B**). In diastole, the pulmonic outflow tract (POT) is shown as widely patent, without pulmonic regurgitation. In systole, there is a signal void (dark signal within the POT just beyond the *arrow*) signifying high velocity flow from functional subvalvular pulmonic stenosis caused by obstruction from the adjacent anterior mitral valve leaflet. In TGA, the morphologic left ventricle (LV) delivers blood to the pulmonic circulation, and the morphologic right ventricle (RV) supplies the systemic circulation. A dilated RV with decreased RV ejection fraction (EF) is frequently seen in this disorder, as the elevated systemic afterload and other factors lead to progressive RV dysfunction. In this patient, the RV end diastolic volume was severely enlarged at 304 mL (113 mL/m2). The RVEF was reduced at 35%, whereas the LVEF was preserved at 60%. PulV—pulmonic ventricle; SV—systemic ventricle.

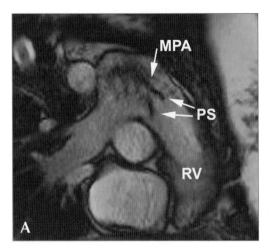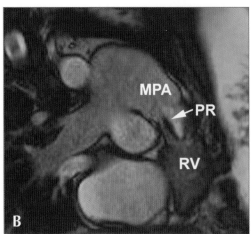

Figure 15-5. Valvular pulmonic stenosis and pulmonic regurgitation with two-dimensional cine imaging. Steady-state free precession images in a parasagittal orientation at the level of the right ventricular outflow tract (RVOT) during early systole (**A**) showing signal void of moderate pulmonic stenosis, and during early diastole (**B**) showing signal void of moderate pulmonic regurgitation. The chest wall is located to the right of the image (plane orientation is from cephalad [*top*] to caudad [*bottom*]). Note the severely dilated main pulmonary artery (5.7 cm at maximum diameter), as well as branch pulmonary artery dilatation. Cardiovascular magnetic resonance allows accurate depiction of the location of pulmonic stenosis (subvalvular, valvular, or supravalvular) and assists clinical decision making for selection of the optimal therapeutic approach. Technical factors such as stenosis location, leaflet morphology, and degree of calcification may influence the decision to proceed with a percutaneous balloon versus surgical treatment. Peak pulmonary artery stenotic gradient = 25 mm Hg, and pulmonary valve regurgitant fraction = 17% (regurgitant volume/stroke volume, using quantitative measures described in the next case). These techniques are especially useful in the assessment of postoperative patients [11]. MPA—main pulmonary artery; PR—pulmonic regurgitation; PS—pulmonic stenosis (*arrows*); RV—right ventricle.

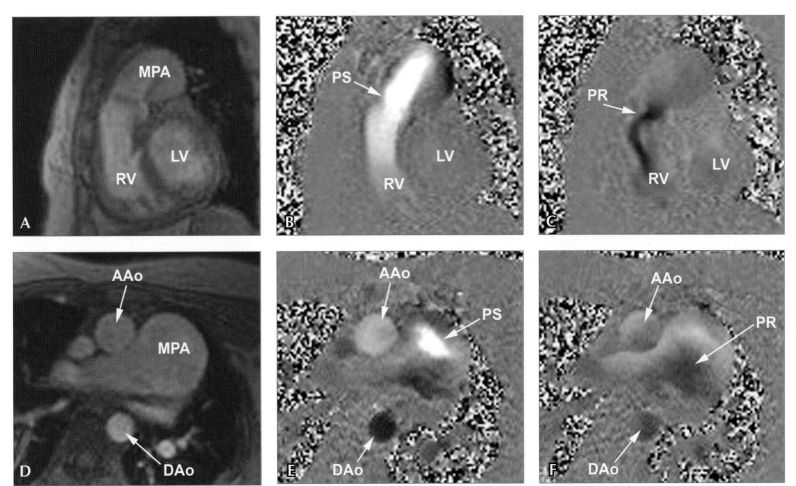

Figure 15-6. Valvular pulmonic stenosis and pulmonic regurgitation: phase contrast velocity maps. Cine phase contrast velocity mapping can further characterize and provide quantitate data regarding the severity of valvular lesions. A parasagittal right ventricular outflow tract view of a two-dimensional magnitude image (**A**) and its corresponding phase-encoded velocity maps during systole (**B**) and diastole (**C**) demonstrating the stenotic (*white*) and regurgitant jets (*black*), respectively. Velocities may be encoded in 1, 2, or 3 directions. In **B** and **C**, velocities are encoded as positive (*white*) in the cephalad direction, and negative (*black*) in the caudad direction. When performed orthogonal to the direction of blood flow (**D**), velocity-encoded images can quantify forward flow (**E**) and the greatest velocity jet (PS, brightest white or most stenotic), as well as abnormal regurgitant flow (**F**), as indicated by the dark area (PR). Note that flow in the ascending thoracic aorta (AAo) is of lower velocity (less white) than that of the main pulmonary artery (MPA), and that flow is white in the AAo (toward the observer), and black in the descending thoracic aorta (away from the observer). With accurate measures of vessel diameters, MPA antegrade and retrograde flow may be determined from velocity-time integral curves. Note the severely dilated MPA relative to the normal-sized AAo (**D**). DAo—descending thoracic aorta; LV—left ventricle; MPA—main pulmonary artery; PR—pulmonic regurgitation; PS—pulmonic stenosis; RV—right ventricle.

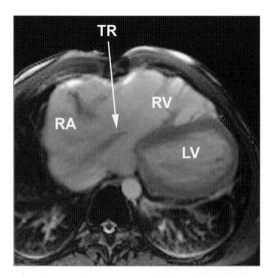

Figure 15-7. Tricuspid regurgitation (TR). Axial steady-state free precession images during systole demonstrating moderate to severe TR (*dark jet*) in a patient with a history of repaired tetralogy of Fallot. Note the very severely dilated right atrium, right ventricle, and tricuspid valve (TV) annulus. Those interpreting cardiovascular magnetic resonance studies must appreciate newer and more rapid acquisition techniques such as steady-state free precession sequences may underestimate the severity of regurgitation because of short echocardiography times, as compared with conventional techniques. When necessary, the echo time and TR may be lengthened to better ascertain the degree of regurgitation. For accurate measurement of the peak velocity of the TR jet to estimate the TV pressure gradient (and subsequently, the pulmonary artery systolic pressure [PASP]), the maximum velocity encoding limit (V_{ENC}) must exceed the peak velocity of the jet. Using the principle of the modified Bernoulli equation, the pressure gradient = $4 \times$ (Peak TR velocity)^2. RV systolic pressure is the sum of the TR pressure gradient and an estimated RA pressure, often determined with echocardiography using the degree of inspiratory collapse of the inferior vena cava. In the absence of pulmonic stenosis, the RV systolic pressure will also represent the PASP. However, technical factors such as reduced temporal resolution compared with echocardiography may result in an underestimate of actual PASP. LV—left ventricle.

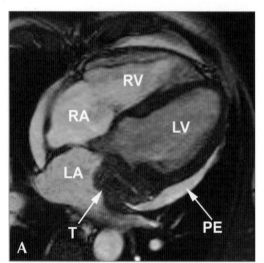
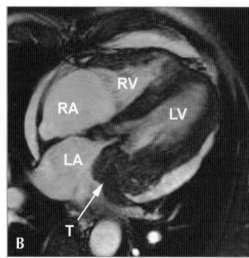
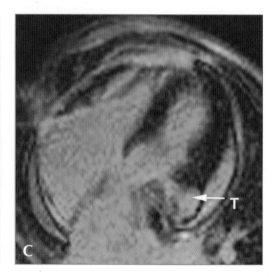

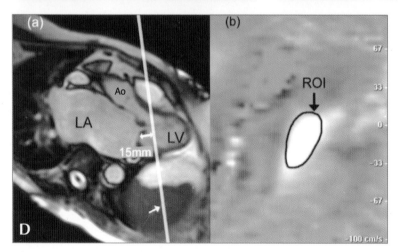

Figure 15-8. Metastatic carcinoid tumor causing functional mitral stenosis. Axial steady-state free precession images at end-diastole (**A**) and late systole (**B**) showing a large carcinoid tumor involving the atrioventricular groove, extending onto the body of the mitral valve (MV), and invading the left atrium (LA). Signal void in the diastolic image at the level of the MV signifies a significant degree of functional mitral stenosis caused by outflow obstruction from posterior leaflet restriction and mass effect by the tumor. A small circumferential pericardial effusion is present (*arrow*). Various cardiovascular magnetic resonance (CMR) sequences can further characterize tumors, including late gadolinium enhanced imaging (**C**), which demonstrates hyper enhancement within the center of the tumor, likely caused by necrosis. To assess the degree of mitral stenosis (caused by valvular disease or other obstruction), the diastolic phase velocity profile is measured approximately 1.5 cm below the MV, and perpendicular to the inflow jet (*see* line in **D**, *left*). A region of interest (ROI) is placed as shown (*right*). The velocity scale represented by the pixel intensities is at the right of the figure in cm/s. The correspondence was very good between Doppler ultrasound and velocity-encoded CMR measures of mitral valve area using the pressure half-time method (r = 0.80), which improved (r= 0.92) when patients with significant aortic regurgitation were excluded [12]. Ao—aortic root; LV—left ventricle; PE—pericardial effusion; RA—right atrium; RV—right ventricle; T—tumor. (**D**, *adapted from* [12], Lin SJ *et al* [12].)

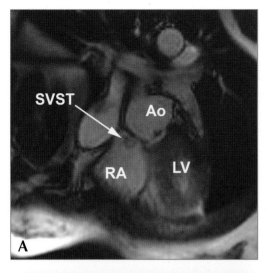

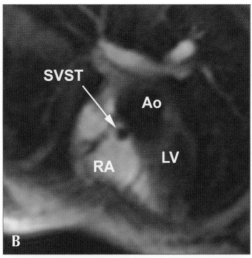

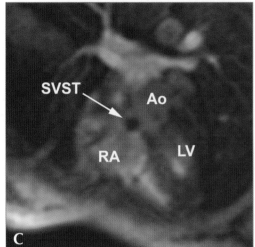

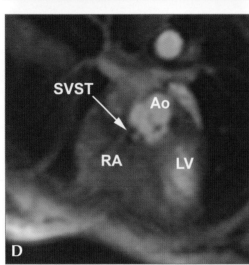

Figure 15-9. Right coronary sinus of Valsalva aneurysm with partially thrombosed fistula to the right atrium.

Steady-state free precession image in an oblique axial view demonstrating the aortic root (Ao) and sinus of Valsalva aneurysm with a 1.1 cm mass above the tricuspid valve. Signal characteristics were similar to blood on the T1-weighted images (**A**), and the mass was initially hypoenhanced on first-pass contrast-enhanced imaging (**B, C**), then hyperenhanced (**D**) following cardiovascular magnetic resonance contrast administration. These findings are consistent with a partially thrombosed fistula (sinus of Valsalva sessile thrombus [SVST]) between the right sinus of Valsalva and the right atrium (RA), and were corroborated at surgery. The surgeon found a windsock-type membrane at the fistula site that restricted flow from the sinus of Valsalva to the RA, explaining the absence of the usual findings of significant right-sided heart volume overload in this disorder. LV—left ventricle.

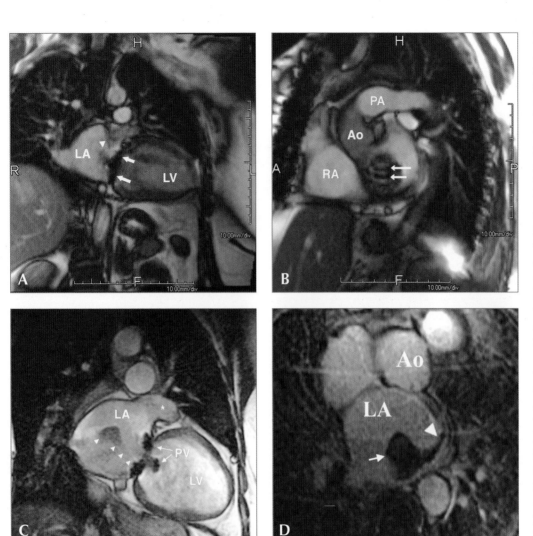

Figure 15-10. Prosthetic valve artifacts. Artifact associated with a St. Jude's bileaflet mechanical mitral valve prosthesis in cine steady-state free precession (SSFP) coronal (**A**, *arrows*) and short-axis (**B**, *arrows*) views. The left (LA) and right atria (RA) atria, left ventricle (LV), and pulmonary artery (PA) are identified. An *arrowhead* shows a flow void in the LA representing a small leaflet closing jet. In **C** and **D**, a stenotic Hancock mitral valve bioprosthesis is visible with an associated large thrombus attached to the sewing ring. In **C**, a two-chamber SSFP image demonstrates the LA, LA appendage (*), LV, and the artifact related to the bioprosthesis (pulmonary valve, *arrows*). The thin stalk and large body of the thrombus are identified by the *arrowheads*. Highly mobile structures such as this "ball on a string"-type thrombus are not as well seen on routine SSFP sequences (**C**), but are more discernible on postcontrast SSFP images (**D**). **D** shows a contrast-enhanced axial image of the stalk (*arrowhead*) and main body of the thrombus (*arrow*), now well delineated. The artifact related to the Hancock valve is smaller compared with the St. Jude's mechanical prosthesis due to the smaller amount of paramagnetic material in the bioprosthesis. The valve-associated artifact obscures only a small region of the perivalvular area, and important clinical information (such as valve leaflet opening, **B** [*arrows*]) may still be derived from cardiovascular magnetic resonance studies in patients following valve replacement or repair. (**C** and **D** adapted from Abdel-Aty H *et al* [15].)

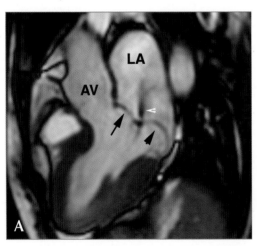

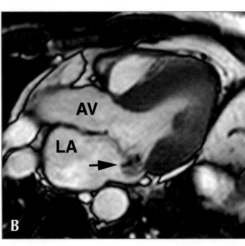

Figure 15-11. Mitral valve prolapse. Steady-state free precession images in the apical (**A**) and parasternal (**B**) long-axis views from patients with mitral valve (MV) prolapse. In **A**, the prolapsing posterior (*black arrowhead*), greater than anterior (*arrow*) MV leaflet is seen. A jet of mitral regurgitation (*white arrowhead*) is also seen during systole. In **B**, a partially flail posterior leaflet is identified (*arrow*) as it prolapses significantly above the valve plane. Cardiovascular magnetic resonance (CMR) can accurately depict the location and degree of prolapse compared with transesophageal echocardiography (TEE) and surgical findings, as well as the severity of MR [13,16]. In one study, TEE and CMR were highly comparable except for detection of small, highly mobile structures such as ruptured chords, where TEE was superior [16]. CMR can accurately quantify the degree of mitral regurgitation, particularly with highly eccentric jets, because of the ease of prescribing imaging planes in three dimensions without the constraints of imaging windows as in TTE. In addition, CMR is highly useful as a clinical tool in assessing the degree and extent of left ventricular (LV) remodeling following surgical MV repair including LV mechanics, which can be performed with two- and three-dimensional methods [17-19].

(*Courtesy of* Yuchi Han, MD, Beth Israel-Deaconess Medical Center, Boston, MA.)

ACKNOWLEDGMENTS

The authors would like to thank Harold Litt, MD, PhD, Sridhar Charagundla, MD, PhD, Saurabh Jha, MD, David Freeman, MD, Sharyn Katz, MD, and Scott Steingall of the Department of Radiology for assistance with image acquisition.

REFERENCES

1. Kon MW, Myerson SG, Moat NE, Pennell DJ: Quantification of regurgitant fraction in mitral regurgitation by cardiovascular magnetic resonance: comparison of techniques. *J Heart Valve Dis* 2004, 13:600–607.

2. Caruthers SD, Lin SJ, Brown P, *et al.*: Practical value of cardiac magnetic resonance imaging for clinical quantification of aortic valve stenosis: comparison with echocardiography. *Circulation* 2003, 108:2236–2243.

3. Arai AE, Epstein FH, Bove KE, Wolff SD: Visualization of aortic valve leaflets using black blood MRI. *J Magn Reson Imaging* 1999, 10:771–777.

4. Yap SC, van Geuns RJ, Meijboom FJ, *et al.*: A simplified continuity equation approach to the quantification of stenotic bicuspid aortic valves using velocity-encoded cardiovascular magnetic resonance. *J Cardiovasc Magn Reson* 2007, 9:899–906.

5. Robles P, Sonlleva A: Aneurysm of the intervalvular mitroaortic fibrosa after aortic valve replacement diagnosed by cardiovascular magnetic resonance imaging. *Intern Med* 2007, 46:1825.

6. Pouleur AC, le Polain de Waroux JB, *et al.*: Planimetric and continuity equation assessment of aortic valve area: Head to head comparison between cardiac magnetic resonance and echocardiography. *J Magn Reson Imaging* 2007, 26:1436–1443.

7. Kozerke S, Schwitter J, Pedersen E, *et al.*: Aortic and mitral regurgitation: Quantification using moving slice velocity mapping. *J Magn Reson Imaging* 2001, 14:106–112.

8. Tung R, Siegel RJ: Aortic pseudocoarctation associated with a stenotic congenitally bicuspid aortic valve. *Am J Cardiol* 2007, 100:157–158.

9. Reant P, Lederlin M, Lafitte S *et al.*: Absolute assessment of aortic valve stenosis by planimetry using cardiovascular magnetic resonance imaging: comparison with transesophageal echocardiography, transthoracic echocardiography, and cardiac catheterization. *Eur J Radiol* 2006, 59:276–283.

10. John AS, Dill T, Brandt R, *et al.*: Magnetic resonance to assess aortic valve area in aortic stenosis: how does it compare to current diagnostic standards? *J Am Coll Cardiol* 2003, 42:519–526.

11. Rebergen SA, Chin JG, Ott enkamp J, *et al.*: Pulmonary regurgitation in the late Postoperative follow-up of tetralogy of Fallot. Volumetric quantitation by nuclear magnetic resonance velocity mapping. *Circulation* 1993, 88:2257–2266.

12. Lin SJ, Brown PA, Watkins MP, *et al.*: Quantification of stenotic mitral valve area with magnetic resonance imaging and comparison with Doppler ultrasound. *J Am Coll Cardiol* 2004, 44:133–137.

13. Gelfand EV, Hughes S, Hauser TH, *et al.*: Severity of mitral and aortic regurgitation as assessed by cardiovascular magnetic resonance: optimizing correlation with Doppler echocardiography. *J Cardiovasc Magn Reson* 2006, 8:503–507.

14. Scott CH, Lorenz C, Ferrari VA: CMR evaluation of cardiac valvular disease. In *MRI of the Cardiovascular System*. Edited by Lardo A, *et al.* London: Martin Dunitz Ltd; 2003:179–200.

15. Abdel-Aty H, Boye P, Bock P, *et al.*: Stenotic mitral valve prosthesis with left atrial thrombus. *J Cardiovasc Magn Reson* 2005, 7:421–423.

16. Stork A, Franzen O, Ruschewski H, *et al.*: Assessment of functional anatomy of the mitral valve in patients with mitral regurgitation with cine magnetic resonance imaging: comparison with transesophageal echocardiography and surgical results. *Eur Radiol* 2007, 17:3189–3198.

17. Guenzinger R, Wildhirt SM, Voegele K, *et al.*: Comparison of magnetic resonance imaging and transthoracic echocardiography for the identification of LV mass and volume regression indices 6 months after mitral valve repair. *J Card Surg* 2008, 23:126–132.

18. Westenberg JJ, van der Geest RJ, Lamb HJ, *et al.*: MRI to evaluate left atrial and ventricular reverse remodeling after restrictive mitral annuloplasty in dilated cardiomyopathy. *Circulation* 2005, 112(Suppl):I437–I442.

19. Mankad R, McCreery CJ, Rogers WJ Jr, *et al.*: Regional myocardial strain before and after mitral valve repair for severe mitral regurgitation. *J Cardiovasc Magn Reson* 2001, 3:257–266.

16
CHAPTER

Pericardium in Health and Disease

Kevin E. Steel, Otavio Rizzi Coelho Filho, *and* Raymond Y. Kwong

The pericardium consists of two distinct layers that surround the heart. The fibrous pericardium composes the outer sac, encircling the heart, and extending up to the proximal portions of the great vessels. The serous pericardium is an exceptionally thin layer of tissue that reflects upon itself to create two layers: the visceral layer, adjacent to the myocardium, and a parietal layer, which is in contact with the inner surface of the fibrous pericardium. Pericardial fat can be found on the surface of the fibrous pericardium, within the pericardial space, or on the epicardial surface between the heart and visceral pericardial layer. As a result of the limited thickness of the pericardial layers, the tissue characteristics of both the fat and the pericardial fluid are typically used to aid in the visualization of these structures. The normal thickness of the fibrous and parietal pericardium upon pathologic inspection is less than 1 mm. Because of the technical limitation of current cardiovascular magnetic resonance (CMR) techniques, including partial volume averaging, cardiac motion, and chemical shift artifact, the normal pericardium measures up to 4 mm by CMR. Currently, no imaging modality can capture an image of the visceral pericardium unless it is thickened by inflammation or malignancy [1].

Because of the superior spatial resolution and unobstructed imaging planes, CMR is a valuable tool in pericardial imaging. Normal pericardium typically appears as a hypointense linear structure on T1-weighted imaging. The pericardium is most prominent adjacent to the right ventricular (RV) free wall and the inferior and apical aspects of the left ventricle (LV). Abnormal pericardium may appear thickened and can be associated with increased pericardial effusions. Primary masses can arise from the pericardium, or it can be invaded by adjacent malignancies. The pericardium can also be congenitally absent and, rarely, it can lead to the strangulation of cardiac chambers. CMR can assess the impact that the diseased pericardium may have on cardiac physiology through the evaluation of structural changes involving the cardiac chambers, the mechanical relationship of both the RV and the LV, and alterations in chamber filling patterns. Various examples of pericardial diseases will be demonstrated in this chapter.

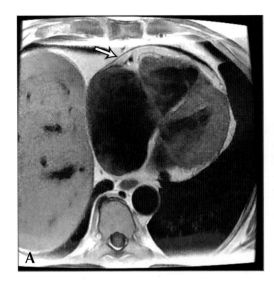
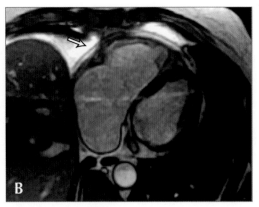

Figure 16-1. Normal pericardium. The parietal pericardium appears as a thin, dark line surrounding the heart (*arrows*), measuring less than four millimeters in thickness. It is best viewed with axial images and often is clearly seen when surrounded by bright fat on T1-weighted spin echo images (**A**) or in the presence of pericardial effusions, using a steady-state free precession sequence (**B**). The visceral pericardium is a very thin-layered tissue adjacent to the myocardium and can only be seen in pathologic states that may increase its thickness.

CMR Pericardial Sequences

SSFP cine

T1- and T2-weighted black blood fast spin echo

Myocardial cine tagging

Contrast-enhanced myocardial perfusion if pericardial mass present

Late gadolinium enhancement

Phase contrast of vena caval flow

Figure 16-2. Recommended pericardial sequences in cardiovascular magnetic resonance. A variety of sequences are used to characterize the qualities of the pericardium, pericardial effusion,

and pericardial space. The sequences may be tailored for a specific study depending on the question that is answered [2]. Steady-state free precession (SSFP)-type cine technique can assess cardiac sizes, function, and structural changes of the ventricles from constrictive physiology. T1-weighted fast spin echo technique can assess the pericardial thickness and compare it with the imaging data of the cine SSFP technique acquired in similar scan planes. When moderate- to large-sized pericardial effusion is present, T1-and T2-weighted fast spin echo techniques can characterize the content of the effusion (transudate versus exudate). Myocardial cine tagging can provide information regarding presence of regional myocardial adhesion, while late gadolinium enhancement imaging can assess for any regional myocardial fibrosis or pericardial inflammation. Finally, other evidence of constriction can be assessed by phase-contrast imaging of vena cavae blood flow.

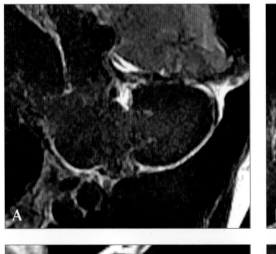
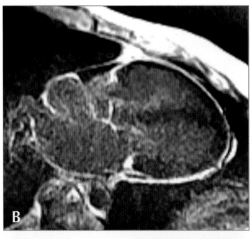
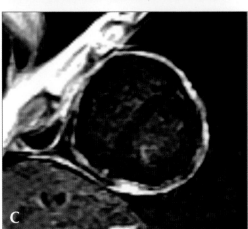
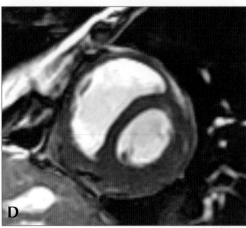

Figure 16-3. Acute pericarditis. The retention of gadolinium diethylenetriamine penta-acetic acid (DTPA) throughout the pericardium on late gadolinium enhancement (LGE) imaging strongly suggests diffuse pericardial inflammation (**A–C**). Because adipose tissue also has high-signal intensity on T1-weighted inversion recovery pulse sequences, comparison with steady-state free precession imaging (**D**) at the same slice location is essential to differentiate adipose from true LGE. Pericarditis can also be accompanied by pericardial effusions and a thickened pericardium [3,4].

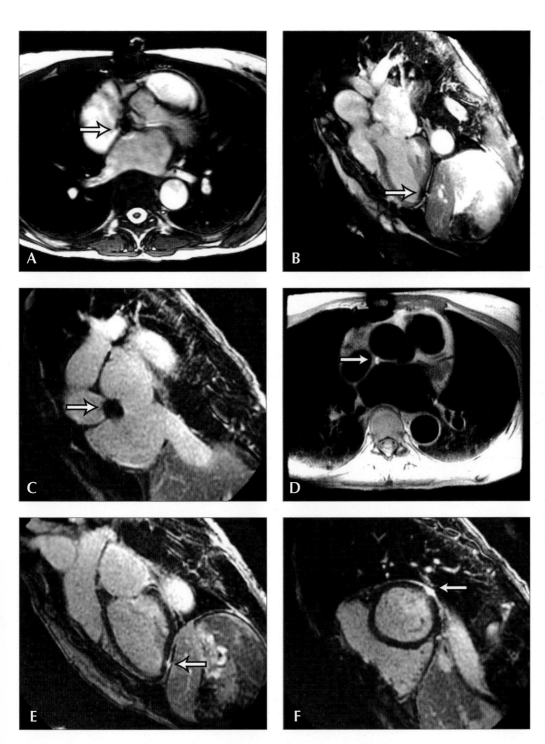

Figure 16-4. Retained epicardial pacing wire. The images were taken from an individual with a history of coronary artery bypass grafting (note the artifact from the anterior sternotomy wires on the axial images). The epicardial pacing wires, routinely used during the surgical procedure, were retained with the distal portion of the wires cut at the level of the skin. While selected reports have indicated safety in cardiovascular magnetic resonance (CMR) in patients with retained epicardial pacing wires, patients need to be monitored closely throughout the study. Further, performance of CMR study should be reserved for important clinical indication without an alternative imaging method (as in this patient's case) [5]. Steady-state free precession gradient echo is more sensitive to metallic artifacts, and it shows a large signal void within the transverse pericardial sinus (A) and inferoapex (B). The spin echo sequence (D) is notable for a focal area of high signal intensity in the same area as in A. Late gadolinium enhancement (LGE) imaging sequences (E,F) also show focal areas of increased signal of both the inferoapical and mid-lateral walls. These findings can be misinterpreted as LGE, but are only related to the presence of the pacing wire running along the cardiac border.

Characteristics of Pericardial Effusions by CMR

Pericardial Effusion	T1-weighted Fast Spin-echo Signal Intensity	T2-weighted Fast Spin-echo Signal Intensity
Transudative	Low	High
Exudative	Medium	High
Proteinaceous	High	Very high
Acute hemorrhagic	Homogeneous, high	Homogeneous, low
Subacute/chronic hemorrhagic	Heterogeneous	Subacute: heterogeneous Chronic: homogenously dark

Figure 16-5. Characteristics of moderate to large sized pericardial effusions by cardiovascular magnetic resonance (CMR). CMR can differentiate tissue characteristics with the use of various sequences. Pericardial effusions can be evaluated by the degree of signal intensity compared with the myocardium (hyper-, iso-, hypointense) and the homogeneity of the signal [6].

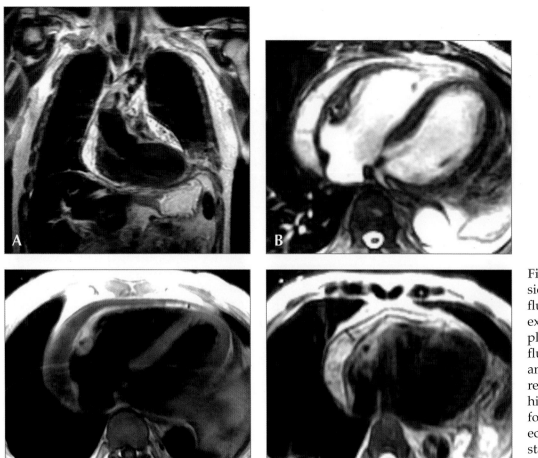

Figure 16-6. Transudative pericardial effusion. Tissue characterization of pericardial fluid can distinguish transudative from exudative pericardial effusions. This example demonstrates differences in pericardial fluid signal intensity through T2-weighted and T1-weighted cardiovascular magnetic resonance sequences. **A**, **B**, and **C** show a high signal within the pericardial space for the sequences of T2-weighted fast spin echo (coronal and axial views) and steady-state free precession, respectively. The low signal intensity of the T1-weighted fast spin echo sequence is seen in **D** [7,8].

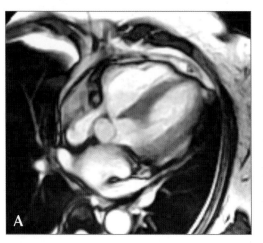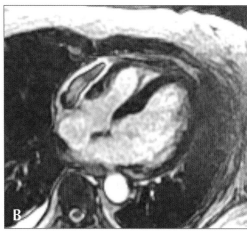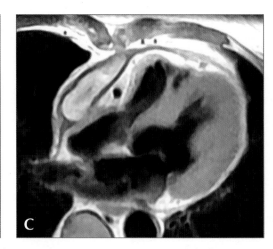

Figure 16-7. Pericardial hematoma. Loculated blood within the pericardial space is usually the result of trauma: postsurgical or postpercutaneous intervention. The patient seen in this figure recently had a complex percutaneous intervention of her right coronary artery. Steady-state free precession imaging (**A**) shows a fluid collection within the pericardial space with heterogeneous signal intensity. T1-weighted spin echo sequences, without (**C**)

Continued on the next page

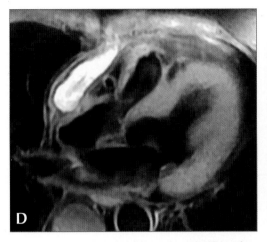
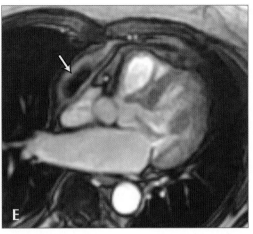

Figure 16-7. *(Continued)* and with (**D**) a fat saturation prepulse, show moderate to bright fluid collection intensity, suggestive of an exudative content. Note the suppression of fat within the adjacent atrioventricular groove, but not within the fluid collection itself (**D**). There is an associated inflammatory reaction of the adjacent pericardium, which is demonstrated late gadolinium enhancement (LGE) (**B**). Using different inversion times in LGE imaging (250 and 400 ms in **B** and **D**, respectively), the presence of a dark mass (*arrow*) can be seen within the pericardial space, which is consistent with a pericardial clot (**E**) [9,10].

CMR Features of Pericardial Constriction

Pericardial thickness > 4 mm
Epicardial and pericardial adhesions
Atrial enlargement
Tubular right ventricle
Dilated inferior vena cava
Septal bounce or "shiver"
Septal inversion with inspiration

Figure 16-8. Cardiovascular magnetic resonance (CMR) features of pericardial constriction. There are a number of CMR findings associated with pericardial constriction. The specificity for significant physiologic constriction increases as more elements are noted, given concurrent clinical signs and symptoms of constrictive physiology [11,12].

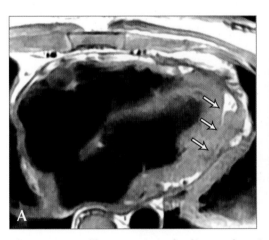
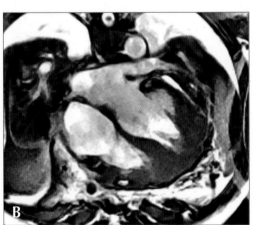
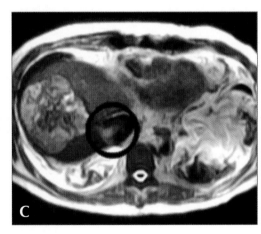

Figure 16-9. Characteristic findings of pericardial constriction. In this case, T1-weighted fast spin echo (**A**) demonstrates a markedly thickened pericardium (*arrows*). While a thickened pericardium is a common feature in patients with pericardial constriction, reports have shown that up to 18% of constriction can occur with normal pericardial thickness [13,14]. Cine steady-state free precession images (**B**) show findings of biatrial enlargement, small ventricles, and a tubular appearing right ventricle. The inferior vena cava is also dilated (*black circle*), using a black blood spin echo technique (**C**). Real time cine cardiovascular magnetic resonance may demonstrate abnormal septal flattening in early diastole during inspiration. This finding differentiates constriction from restrictive cardiomyopathy at high accuracy (*see* 16-7) [15,16].

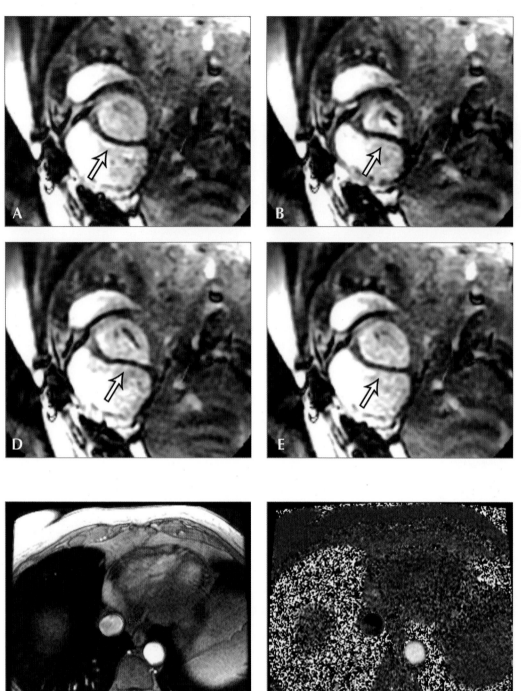

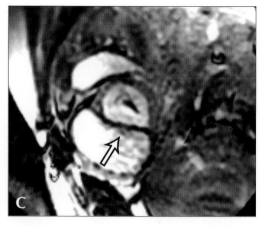

Figure 16-10. Abnormal septal motion in pericardial constriction. A useful finding associated with constrictive pericarditis is the respiratory effects on septal position during early ventricular filling seen with real time cine cardiovascular magnetic resonance. Leftward motion of the intraventricular septum, giving a sigmoid-shaped appearance, is absent in restrictive cardiomyopathy and has a sensitivity of 81%, and specificity of 100%, to diagnose pericardial constriction [17,18]. The example illustrates abnormal septal motion through time (**A–E**) and evidence of a septal "bounce." (*Courtesy of* Dr. Andrew E. Arai, Bethesda, MD.)

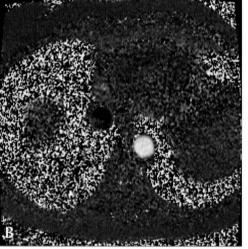

Figure 16-11. Inferior vena cava velocity profile in constriction. Velocity flow mapping can demonstrate alterations in diastolic velocities and flow during end-inspiration and end-expiration. The cross sectional area of the inferior vena cava should also be enlarged. This example was obtained at end-inspiration and depicts phase-contrast cardiovascular magnetic resonance of the inferior vena cava (*circled*) with the associated velocity profile (**A** and **B**).

Continued on the next page

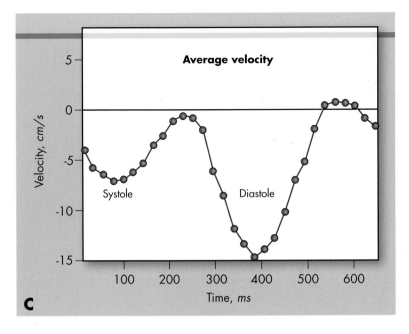

C

Figure 16-11. *(Continued)* Note the pronounced diastolic component of flow during end-inspiration in this patient, with constrictive pericarditis (**C**) [19].

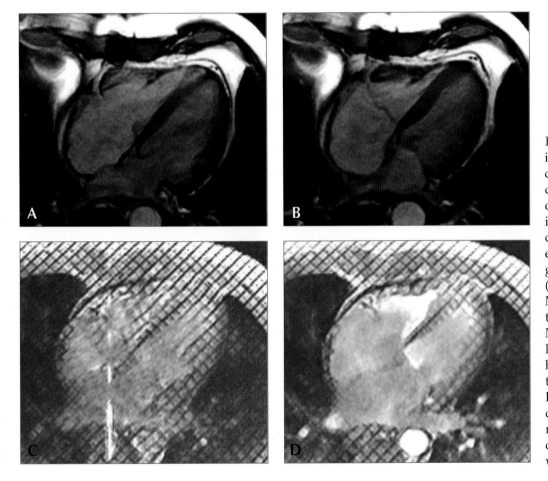

Figure 16-12. Adherent right ventricle in pericardial constriction. Long-axis cine steady-state free precession images demonstrate the functional consequence of an adherent pericardium on surrounding tissues. Limited RV systolic function can be seen when comparing the differences of right and left atrioventricular groove descent from diastole (**A**) to systole (**B**) cardiovascular magnetic resonance. Myocardial tagging is another tool used to demonstrate an adherent pericardium. Note the lack of deformation of the tagging lines that pass along the RV free wall as the heart contracts from diastole (**C**) to systole (**D**). Assessing the tagged lines of the RV myocardium in the adjacent anterior chest wall and the pericardium, as well as regional concordance during the cardiac cycle can also be seen, which is consistent with adhesion of the RV free wall [20].

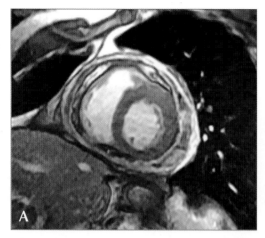 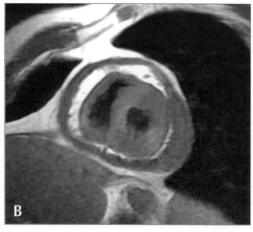

Figure 16-13. Diffuse pericardial thickening and circumferential effusion associated with effusive-constrictive pericarditis. The pericardial fluid demonstrates a moderate signal intensity on steady-state free precession (**A**) and bright signal intensity on the

T1-weighted spin echo (**B**) and are features of exudative pericardial effusions. Effusive-constrictive pericarditis is a progressive condition that has varying degrees of hemodynamic consequences initially because of the collection of pericardial fluid and ultimately because of pericardial constriction. It is typically suspected in cases where pericardiocentesis fails to normalize intracardiac pressures. In the example, pericardial fluid analysis resulted in a rSterile exudate of leukocytes and erythrocytes [11].

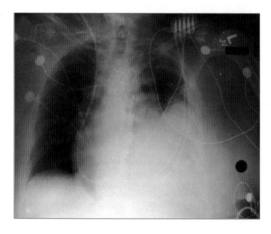

Figure 16-14. Cardiac tamponade secondary to a very large left pleural effusion. A 15-year-old boy with a history of malignancy presented with tachycardia before and after chemotherapy. Chest radiograph revealed a large, left sided pleural effusion. Cardiovascular magnetic resonance was performed to evaluate for metastatic disease, and revealed regional diastolic compression of the LV adjacent to the pleural effusion. The left ventricle (LV) is more resistant to external compression from the pleural fluid than the right ventricle because of higher LV chamber pressure and the thicker myocardial wall. Clinical signs such as hypotension and pulsus paradoxus are insensitive in this situation [21-23].

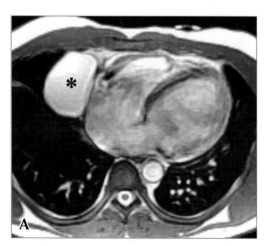 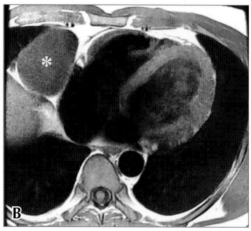 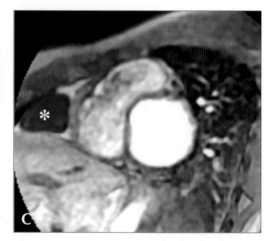

Figure 16-15. Pericardial cyst. The high signal intensity on cine (**A**) and T2-weighted spin echo images and low intensity on T1-weighted spin echo images (**B**) are characteristics of transudative contents of pericardial cysts (*see asterisks*). Perfusion imaging demonstrates the absence of gadolinium within the structure consistent with its avascular qualities (**C**). Pericardial cysts are also frequently compressed by the heart during diastole, whereas tumors are typically not compliant to compression [24].

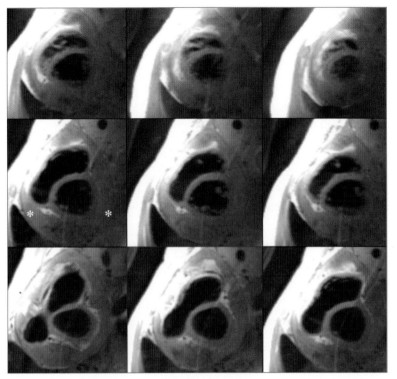

Figure 16-16. Angiosarcoma involving the pericardium. These short axis T1-weighted fast spin echo images were acquired on a young man who presented with increasing dyspnea. The pericardium is abnormal with focal areas of significant thickening. As opposed to the hyperintense signal of exudative effusions and the hypointense signal of transudate effusions, the signal within the focal areas (*asterisk*) is isointense, making the differentiation of the mass more difficult to determine. This patient underwent pericardial resection, and the mass was later diagnosed as primary angiosarcoma [25,26].

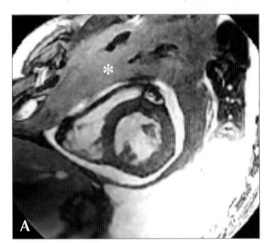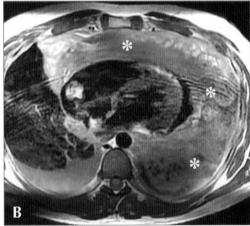

Figure 16-17. Mediastinal mass without pericardial involvement. Determination of pericardial invasion is an important aspect in the assessment of mediastinal masses. Elements such as pericardial thickness and late enhancement may provide insight for the aggressiveness of the tumor. These images were taken from a 30-year-old man with a history of acute lymphocytic leukemia and a prior bone marrow transplant. Cine steady-state free precession cardiovascular magnetic resonance (**A**) and T1-weighted spin echo images (**B**) show a large mass (*asterisk*) encasing the heart and great vessels, although no pericardial thickening is seen. The interface of the pericardium and mass is well demarcated. Biopsy later revealed a thymoma [27].

REFERENCES

1. Kumar V, Fausto N, Abbas A: *Robbins and Cotran Pathologic Basis of Disease,* edn 7. Philadelphia: WB Saunders; 2005.

2. J Barkhausen, S Flamm, R Kim, *et al.*: CMR Image Acquisition Protocols — Pericardial disease. Accessible at: www.scmr.org/documents/scmr_protocols_2007.pdf. Accessed February 27, 2008.

3. Kovanlikaya A, Burke LP, Nelson MD, Wood J: Characterizing chronic pericarditis using steady-state free-precession cine MR imaging. *AJR Am J Roentgenol* 2002, 179: 475–476.

4. Taylor AM, Dymarkowski S, Verbeken EK, Bogaert J: Detection of pericardial inflammation with late-enhancement cardiac magnetic resonance imaging: initial results. *Eur Radiol* 2006, 16:569–574.

5. Hartnell GG, Spence L, Hughes LA, *et al.*: Safety of MR imaging in patients who have retained metallic materials after cardiac surgery. *AJR Am J Roentgenol* 1997, 168:1157–1159.

6. Kwong RY: Cardiovascular magnetic resonance self-assessment program (CMRSAP). 2004; 1.

7. Axel L: Assessment of pericardial disease by magnetic resonance and computed tomography. *J Magn Reson Imaging* 2004, 19:816–826.

8. Frank H, Globits S: Magnetic resonance imaging evaluation of myocardial and pericardial disease. *J Magn Reson Imaging* 1999, 10:617–626.

9. Arata MA, Reddy GP, Higgins CB: Organized pericardial hematomas: magnetic resonance imaging. J *Cardiovasc Magn Reson* 2000, 2:1–6.

10. Takami Y, Ina H, Tanaka Y, Terasawa A: Constrictive pericarditis caused by calcification and organized hematoma 30 years after cardiac surgery. *Circ J*, 2002, 66:610–612.

11. LeWinter MM, Kabbani S: Pericardial diseases. Zipes DP, Libby P, Bonow RO, Braunwald E, eds., edn 7. Philadelphia: WB Saunders, 2005: 1757.

12. Masui T, Finck S, Higgins CB: Constrictive pericarditis and restrictive cardiomyopathy: evaluation with MR imaging. *Radiology* 1992, 182:369–373.

13. Talreja DR, Edwards WD, Danielson GK, *et al.*: Constrictive pericarditis in 26 patients with histologically normal pericardial thickness. *Circulation* 2003, 108:1852–1857.

14. Steel K, Duming SJ, DeMott C, Haigney M: Symptomatic pericardial constriction without active pericarditis. *Mil Med* 2005, 170:668–671.

15. Francone M, Dymarkowski S, Kalantzi M, *et al.*: Assessment of ventricular coupling with real-time cine MRI and its value to differentiate constrictive pericarditis from restrictive cardiomyopathy. *Eur Radiol* 2006, 16:944–951.

16. Hartnell GG, Hughes LA, Ko JP, Cohen MC: Magnetic resonance imaging of pericardial constriction: comparison of cine MR angiography and spin-echo techniques. *Clin Radiol* 1996, 51:268–272.

17. Giorgi B, Mollet NR, Dymarkowski S, *et al.*: Clinically suspected constrictive pericarditis: MR imaging assessment of ventricular septal motion and configuration in patients and healthy subjects. *Radiology* 2003, 228:417–424.

18. Francone M, Dymarkowski S, Kalantzi M, Bogaert J: Real-time cine MRI of ventricular septal motion: a novel approach to assess ventricular coupling. *J Magn Reson Imaging* 2005, 21:305-309.

19. Nishimura RA: Constrictive pericarditis in the modern era: a diagnostic dilemma. *Heart* 2001, 86:619–623.

20. Chiles C, Woodard PK, Gutierrez FR, Link KM. Metastatic involvement of the heart and pericardium: CT and MR imaging. *Radiographics* 2001, 21:439–449.

21. Alam HB, Levitt A, Molyneaux R, *et al.*: Can pleural effusions cause cardiac tamponade? *Chest* 1999, 116:1820–1822.

22. Schwartz SL, Pandian NG, Cao QL, *et al.*: Left ventricular diastolic collapse in regional left heart cardiac tamponade. An experimental echocardiographic and hemodynamic study. *J Am Coll Cardiol* 1993, 22:907–913.

23. Vaska K, Wann LS, Sagar K, *et al.*: Pleural effusion as a cause of right ventricular diastolic collapse. *Circulation* 1992, 86:609–617.

24. Gilkeson RC, Chiles C: MR evaluation of cardiac and pericardial malignancy. Magn Reson Imaging *Clin North Am* 2003, 11:173–186, viii.

25. Hoffmann U, Globits S, Schima W, *et al.*: Usefulness of magnetic resonance imaging of cardiac and paracardiac masses. *Am J Cardiol* 2003, 92:890–895.

26. Kurian KC, Weisshaar D, Parekh H, *et al.*: Primary cardiac angiosarcoma: case report and review of the literature. *Cardiovasc Pathol* 2006, 15:110–112.

27. Kaminaga T, Takeshita T, Kimura I: Role of magnetic resonance imaging for evaluation of tumors in the cardiac region. *Eur Radiol* 2003, 13 (Suppl 6): L1–L10.

17

CHAPTER

Pediatric Congenital Heart Disease

Tal Geva

Congenital heart disease is among the most common forms of congenital anomalies, affecting approximately eight of every 1000 live births [1]. Of those births, approximately 50% of patients require some form of surgical or transcatheter intervention [2]. Recent developments in hardware design, computer sciences, and imaging sequences mark an expansion of the clinical utility of cardiovascular magnetic resonance (CMR) in patients with congenital and acquired pediatric heart disease [3]. Along with these improved capabilities, the speed and efficiency of imaging have also increased, thereby allowing a comprehensive examination obtained within an acceptable time frame. However, CMR is rarely used as the first or the sole diagnostic imaging test. It complements echocardiography, provides a noninvasive alternative to radiograph angiography, avoids the risk of cancer from exposure to ionizing radiation associated with CT, and overcomes many of the limitations of these modalities [4]. For example, compared with echocardiography, acoustic windows and body size do not limit CMR. In addition, unlike cardiac catheterization, CMR is not invasive, and it clearly depicts soft tissues such as heart and vessel walls [5]. In current clinical practice, CMR is increasingly used in concert with other imaging modalities (most commonly echocardiography) for assessment of cardiac anatomy and function, measurements of blood flow, tissue characterization and, more recently, for the evaluation of myocardial perfusion and viability. This chapter illustrates the clinical use of CMR in a variety of congenital and pediatric heart diseases through a series of illustrations.

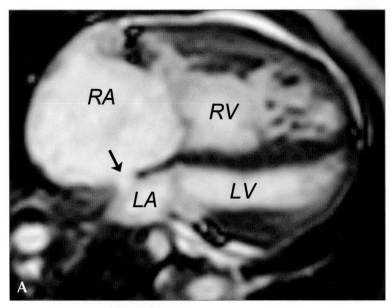

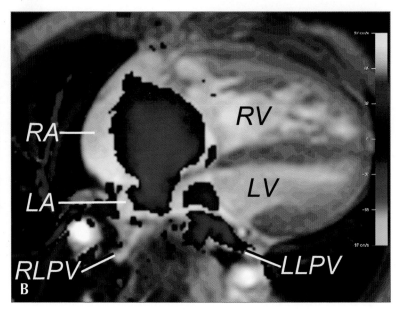

Figure 17-1. Secundum atrial septal defect (ASD). **A,** Electrocardiogram (ECG) gated steady-state free precession cine cardiovascular magnetic resonance (CMR) in the ventricular four-chamber plane showing a secundum ASD (*arrow*). Note the dilated right atrium (RA) and right ventricle (RV). **B,** ECG-gated phase velocity cine CMR in the same location as figure **A** with velocity encoding in the anterior-posterior direction. Flow from posterior-to-anterior is encoded in *blue*, and flow from anterior-to-posterior is encoded in *red*. Note the prominent flow jet from the left atrium (LA) to the RA through the secundum ASD. LLPV—left lower pulmonary vein; RLPV—right lower pulmonary vein.

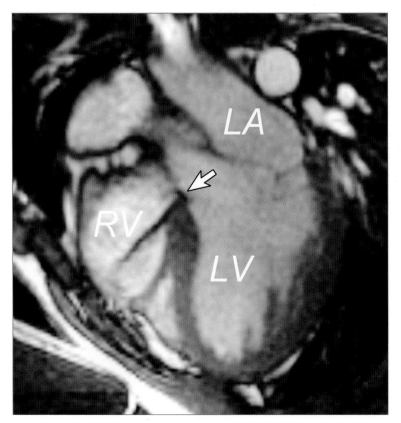

Figure 17-2. Ventricular septal defect: electrocardiogram triggered, breath hold, steady-state free precession cine cardiovascular magnetic resonance of a small membranous ventricular septal defect (*arrow*). Note the systolic signal void through the defect, resulting from a high velocity turbulent flow jet from the left ventricle (LV) to the right ventricle (RV). LA—left atrium.

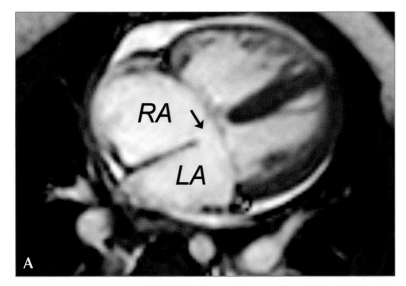

A

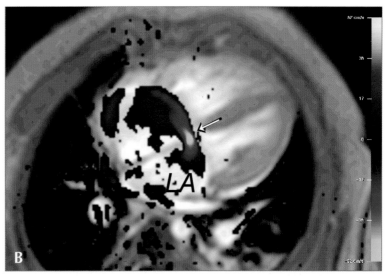

B

Figure 17-3. Partial atrioventricular canal defect comprised of a primum atrial septal defect (ASD) with left-to-right flow. **A,** Electrocardiogram (ECG)-gated steady-state free precession cine cardiovascular magnetic resonance (CMR) in the four-chamber plane showing a primum ASD (*arrow*). In contrast to secundum ASD (Fig. 17-1), primum ASD is bordered inferiorly by the atrio-ventricular valves. **B,** ECG-gated phase velocity cine CMR in the same location as **A** with velocity encoding in the anterior-posterior direction. Flow from posterior-to-anterior is encoded in *blue*, and flow from anterior-to-posterior is encoded in *red*. Note the prominent flow jet from the left atrium (LA) to the right atrium (RA) through the primum ASD.

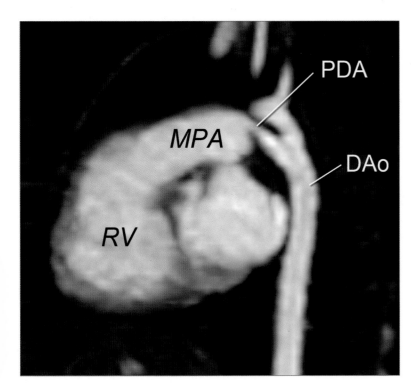

Figure 17-4. Maximal intensity projection gadolinium-enhanced three-dimensional cardiovascular magnetic resonance angiogram showing patent ductus arteriosus (PDA). DAo—descending aorta; MPA—main pulmonary artery; RV—right ventricle.

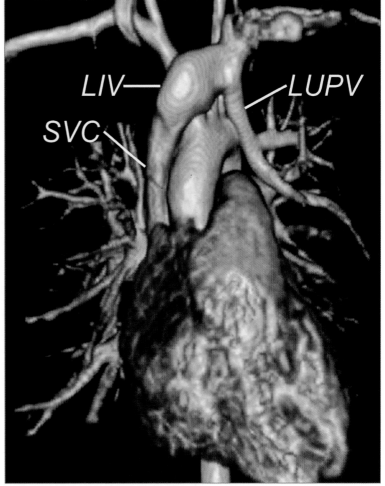

Figure 17-5. Partially anomalous pulmonary venous connection. Volume-rendered reconstruction from gadolinium-enhanced three-dimensional CMR angiogram showing partially anomalous pulmonary venous connection of the left upper pulmonary vein (LUPV) to the left innominate vein (LIV) with subsequent drainage to the superior vena cava (SVC). This is the most common type of partially anomalous pulmonary venous connection [6,7].

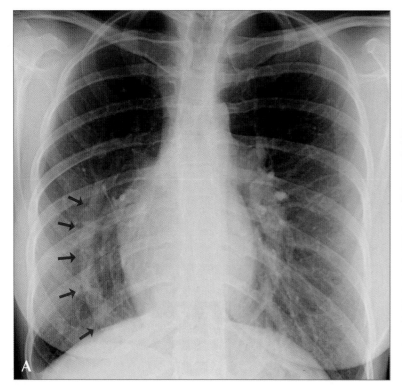

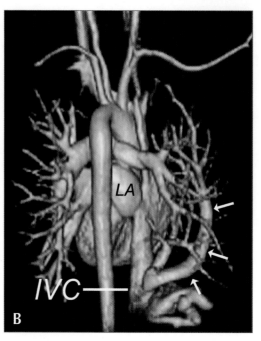

Figure 17-6. Scimitar vein: **A**, Chest radiograph showing meso-cardia and a scimitar sign (*red arrows*). **B**, Posterior view of a volume-rendered reconstruction from gadolinium-enhanced three-dimensional CMR angiogram showing a partially anoma-lous pulmonary venous connection of the right pulmonary vein (*arrows*) to the inferior vena cava (IVC). Note that the left atrium (LA) does not receive a right pulmonary vein, but the left pulmo-nary veins drain normally.

CYANOTIC CONGENITAL HEART DISEASE

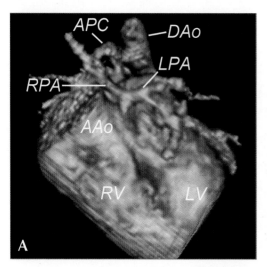

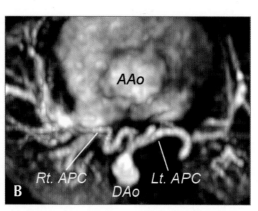

Figure 17-7. Tetralogy of Fallot with pulmonary atresia in a neonate presenting with cyanosis. **A**, Volume-rendered reconstruction from gadolinium-enhanced three-dimensional CMR angiogram showing a blind-ending main pulmonary artery to the left of the ascending aorta (AAo). The left and right pulmonary arteries (LPA and RPA, respectively) are markedly hypoplastic. Note a large aortopulmo-nary collateral vessel (APC) originates from the descending aorta (DAo), communicating with the diminutive right pulmonary artery at the hilum of the right lung. **B**, Maximal intensity projection gado-linium-enhanced three-dimensional CMR angiogram showing large collateral vessels (APC) from the DAo supplying the left (Lt) and right (Rt) lungs. LV—left ventricle; RV—right ventricle.

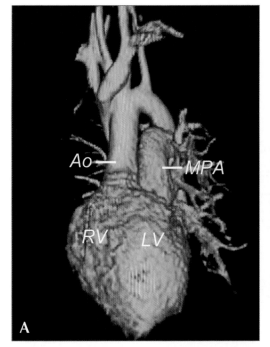

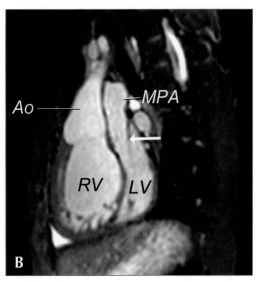

Figure 17-8. D-loop transposition of the great arteries. **A,** Volume-rendered reconstruction from gadolinium-enhanced three-dimensional cardiovascular magnetic resonance (CMR) angiogram showing origin of the main pulmonary artery (MPA) from the left ventricle (LV) and origin of the aorta (Ao) from the right ventricle (RV). The segmental anatomy comprises atrial situs solitus (*not shown*), ventricular D-loop, and D-transposition of the great arteries, or {S,D,D} transposition of the great arteries. **B,** Electrocardiogram-gated steady-state free precession cine CMR in the ventricular short-axis plane showing origin of the MPA from the LV without an intervening infundibulum (note the contiguity between the anterior leaflet of the mitral valve and the pulmonary valve (*arrow*). The Ao originates from the RV and is supported by a large subaortic infundibulum. These anatomic features are common in {S,D,D} transposition of the great arteries. Other anatomic variations include transposition of the great arteries with bilateral infundibulum, transposition of the great arteries with subpulmonary infundibulum, and others [8].

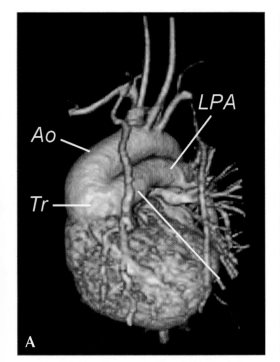

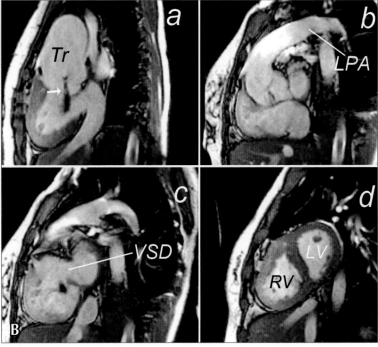

Figure 17-9. Truncus arteriosus. **A,** Volume-rendered reconstruction from gadolinium-enhanced three-dimensional cardiovascular magnetic resonance (CMR) angiogram showing origin of the main pulmonary artery (MPA) and aorta (Ao) from a common trunk (Tr). **B,** Electrocardiogram-gated steady-state free precession cine CMR in the ventricular short-axis plane at four locations: (a) a large truncal root (Tr) is seen with truncal valve regurgitation (*arrow*); (b) the left pulmonary artery (LPA) is seen as a continuation of the MPA off the truncus arteriosus; (c) large ventricular septal defect (VSD) of the conoventricular type; (d) a more apical slice showing the left ventricle (LV) and right ventricle (RV).

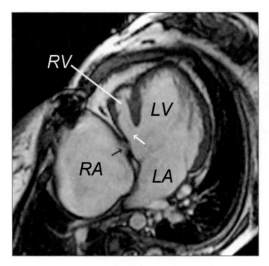

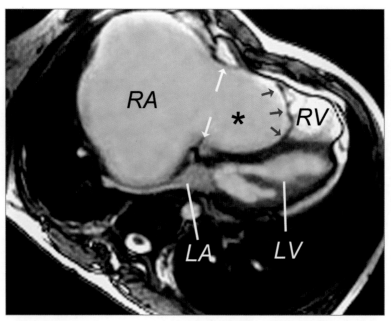

Figure 17-10. Tricuspid atresia. Electrocardiogram-gated steady-state free precession cine cardiovascular magnetic resonance in the ventricular four-chamber view showing a tissue plate between the right atrium (RA) and the hypoplastic right ventricle (RV) with a small central area of membranous atresia (*red arrow*). The left atrium (LA) opens in to an enlarged left ventricle (LV) via the mitral valve. A ventricular septal defect (*white arrow*) is seen.

Figure 17-11. Ebstein anomaly. Electrocardiogram-gated steady-state free precession cine cardiovascular magnetic resonance in the ventricular four-chamber plane showing severe Ebstein anomaly of the tricuspid valve and right ventricular (RV) sinus. The plane of the tricuspid valve annuls is marked by the *white arrows*. The tricuspid valve is displaced toward the RV apex (*red arrows*), leaving a large portion of the RV sinus (*asterisk*) to communicate freely with the right atrium (RA). This "atrialized" segment of the RV does not contribute to RV function. The functional RV comprises the apical segment of the sinus and the infundibulum (not shown). The left atrium (LA) and left ventricle (LV) are compressed by the markedly dilated right-sided chambers.

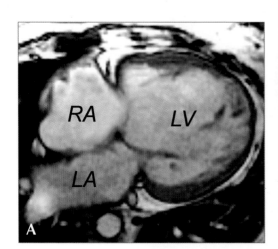

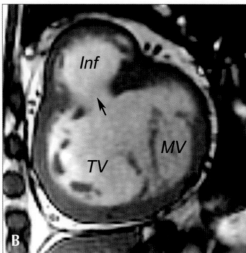

Figure 17-12. Single, double-inlet LV. **A**, Electrocardiogram (ECG)-gated steady-state free precession cine cardiovascular magnetic resonance (CMR) in the ventricular horizontal long-axis view showing the right atrium (RA) connecting to the single left ventricle (LV) through a tricuspid valve (TV) and the left atrium (LA) connecting to the LV through a mitral valve (MV). **B**, ECG-gated steady-state free precession cine CMR in the ventricular short-axis view showing the MV and TVs entering the LV. An infundibular outlet chamber (Inf) is located above the LV, giving rise to the aorta (not shown). The communication between the LV and the infundibular chamber (*arrow*) is termed *bulboventricular foramen.*

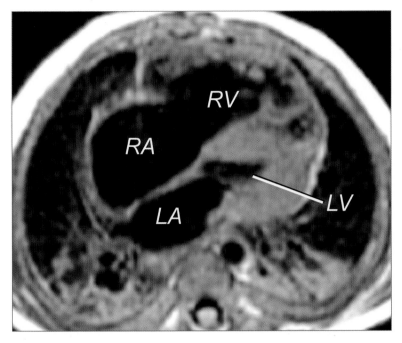

Figure 17-13. Hypoplastic left heart syndrome. Electrocardiogram-gated turbo (fast) spin echo cardiovascular magnetic resonance in the ventricular four-chamber view in a neonate with severe mitral and aortic valve stenosis and hypoplasia, and a diminutive left ventricle (LV). LA—left atrium; RA—right atrium; RV—right ventricle.

ANOMALIES OF THE AORTA

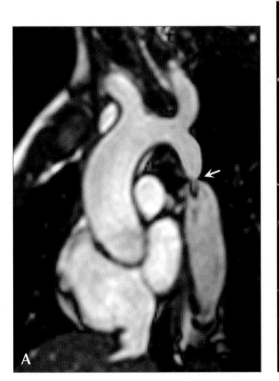
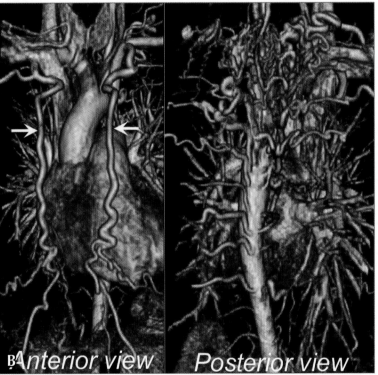

Figure 17-14. Coarctation of the aorta. **A**, Electrocardiogram-gated steady-state free precession cine cardiovascular magnetic resonance (CMR) parallel to the long-axis of the thoracic aorta showing severe coarctation of the aortic isthmus (*arrow*). **B**, Volume-rendered reconstruction from gadolinium-enhanced three-dimensional CMR angiogram showing multiple large collateral vessels that eventually supply blood to the descending aorta. *Anterior view*: markedly dilated left and right internal mammary arteries (*arrows*). *Posterior* *view*: multiple tortuous collateral arteries, including dilated intercostal arteries connecting to the descending aorta. Measurements of blood flow through the collateral vessels correlate with the severity of the coarctation [9]. Another approach for the assessment of coarctation severity is based on measurement of the cross-sectional area of the narrowest aortic segment (from a gadolinium-enhanced three-dimensional CMR angiogram) and determination of the deceleration rate of the flow profile in the descending aorta [10].

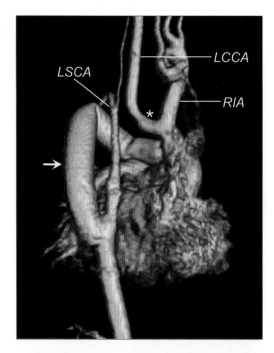

Figure 17-15. Type B interrupted aortic arch. Volume-rendered reconstruction from gadolinium-enhanced three-dimensional CMR angiogram showing the right innominate artery (RIA) as the first branch off the aortic arch, followed by the left common carotid artery (LCCA). The proximal transverse arch is marked (*asterisk*). The distal aortic arch is absent, and the left subclavian artery (LSCA) arises from the descending aorta. Note the large ascending-to-descending aorta conduit, which was used to bypass the interrupted aortic arch segment in this patient. According to the classification proposed by Celoria and Patton in 1959, type A interruption is distal to the left subclavian artery, type B interruption is between the left common carotid and left subclavian arteries, and type C interruption is between the right and left common carotid arteries [11].

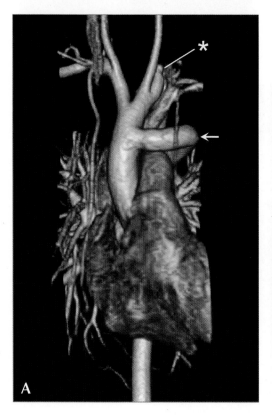

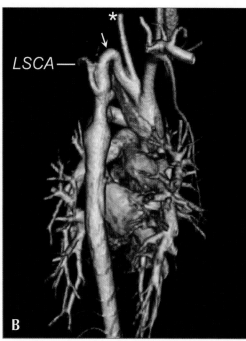

Figure 17-16. Cervical left aortic arch. **A,** Anterior view of a volume-rendered reconstruction from gadolinium-enhanced three-dimensional CMR angiogram showing an elongated distal transverse arch with superior orientation (*asterisk*). Note the ascending-to-descending aorta conduit (*arrow*). **B,** Posterior view of the same dataset showing the elongated, hypoplastic, and tortuous distal transverse arch (*arrow*) with an acute inferior turn before giving rise to the left subclavian artery (LSCA). The left common carotid artery is marked (*asterisk*). Note the hypoplastic aortic isthmus distal to the left subclavian artery.

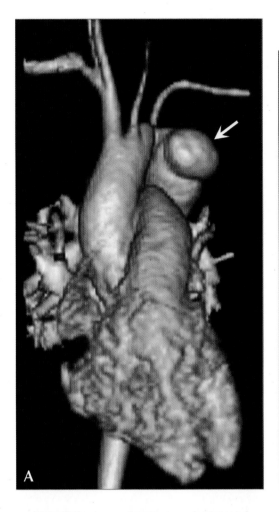

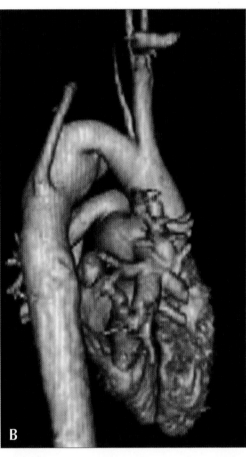

Figure 17-17. Congenital aneurysm of the distal transverse aortic arch in a patients with PHACE syndrome (*ie*, **P**osterior fossa malformations, cervicofacial **H**emangioma, **A**rterial anomalies of the head and neck vessels, **C**oarctation of the aorta and cardiac defects, and **E**ye anomalies). **A,** Anterior view of a volume-rendered reconstruction from gadolinium-enhanced three-dimensional CMR angiogram showing a moderately large aneurysm (*arrow*) of the distal transverse aortic arch between the origins of the left common carotid and left subclavian arteries. **B,** Right lateral view showing the distal transverse arch and the origin of the left subclavian artery.

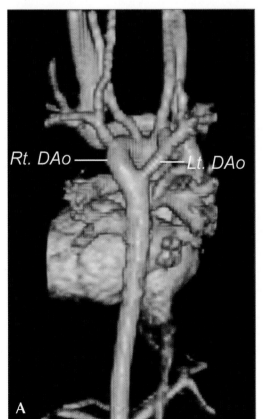

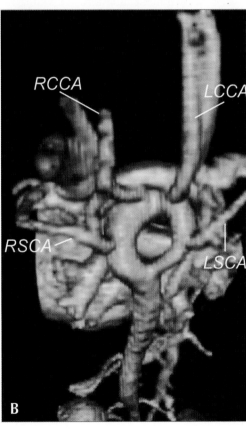

Figure 17-18. Vascular ring comprised of double aortic arch. **A,** Posterior view of a volume-rendered reconstruction from gadolinium-enhanced three-dimensional CMR angiogram showing a large right aortic arch and a smaller left aortic arch. The left and right dorsal aortas (Lt. and Rt. DAo) join the descending aorta. **B,** Superior view of the same dataset showing the right and left aortic arches and the brachiocephalic arteries. LCCA—left common carotid artery; LSCA—left subclavian artery; RCCA—right common carotid artery; RSCA—right subclavian artery.

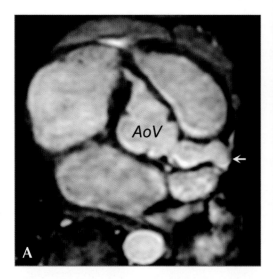

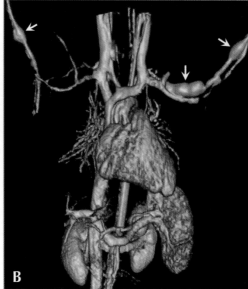

Figure 17-19. Kawasaki disease. **A,** Electrocardiogram- and respiratory navigator-gated, free breathing coronary cardiovascular magnetic resonance showing a giant aneurysm of the left main and left anterior descending coronary arteries (*arrow*) measuring 10 mm in maximal diameter. **B,** Anterior view of a volume-rendered reconstruction from gadolinium-enhanced three-dimensional CMR angiogram showing multiple aneurysms (*arrows*) of the subclavian, axillary, and brachial arteries. AoV—aortic valve.

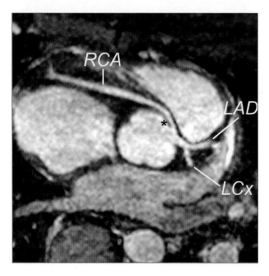

Figure 17-20. Electrocardiogram- and respiratory navigator-gated, free breathing coronary cardiovascular magnetic resonance showing an anomalous origin of the right coronary artery (RCA) from the left aortic sinus of the Valsalva. The RCA originates from the left aortic sinus of the Valsalva, to the left of the intercoronary commissure (*asterisk*), in close proximity to the origin of the left main coronary artery. The RCA takeoff is tangential to the aortic wall and is narrow. The vessel then courses between the aorta and main pulmonary artery (interarterial course) before reaching the right atrioventricular groove. The left anterior descending (LAD) and circumflex (LCx) coronary arteries are seen. This anomaly is associated with an increased risk of sudden death; however, the risk is lower than that associated with anomalous origin of the left main coronary artery from the right aortic sinus of the valsalva with an interarterial course [12].

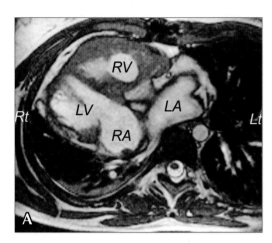

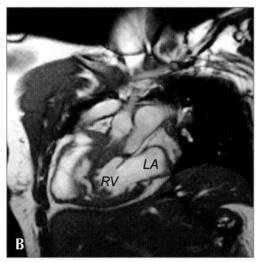

Figure 17-21. Dextrocardia in a 15-year-old patient with physiologically corrected transposition of the great arteries (TGA) with {S,L,L} TGA (atrial situs solitus, L-ventricular loop, and L-transposition of the great arteries); ventricular septal defect (VSD); and pulmonary stenosis. The patient underwent patch closure of the VSD and placement of a left ventricular (LV)-to-pulmonary artery conduit. **A,** Electrocardiogram (ECG)-gated steady-state free precession cine cardiovascular magnetic resonance (CMR) in the axial plane showing dextrocardia. Note the majority of the cardiac mass is located in the right hemithorax, and the apex points to the right. **B,** ECG-gated steady-state free precession cine CMR in the coronal plane showing the dextrocardia. LA—left atrium; Lt—left; RA—right atrium; Rt—right; RV—right ventricle.

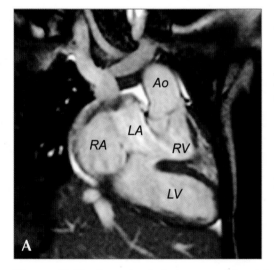

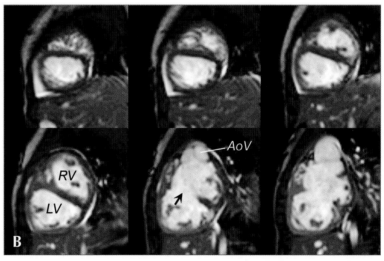

Figure 17-22. Superior-inferior ventricles (also known as upstairs-downstairs ventricles). **A,** Electrocardiogram (ECG)-gated steady-state free precession cine cardiovascular magnetic resonance (CMR) in the coronal plane showing that the right-sided right atrium (RA) is aligned with the left venticle (LV), and the left-sided left atrium (LA) is aligned with the right ventricle (RV), which is superior to the LV and is hypoplastic. The aorta (Ao) arises from the RV. **B,** ECG-gated steady-state free precession cine CMR in the ventricular short-axis plane showing the superior-inferior relationship between the ventricles and the nearly horizontal septum. Note that atrial situs is solitus, and there is atrioventricular alignment discordance (RA-to-LV and LA-to-RV) (*arrow*). However, instead of the expected L-ventricular loop, the ventricular topology is right-handed (D-loop). In other words, there is atrioventricular situs concordance (atrial situs solitus and ventricular D-loop) but atrioventricular alignment discordance. This rare anatomic arrangement is referred to as atri*oventricular situs-alignment disharmony* [13]. AoV—aortic valve.

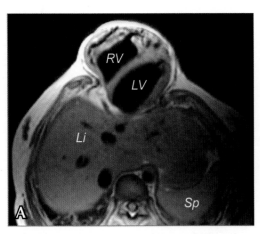 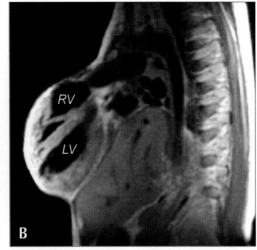 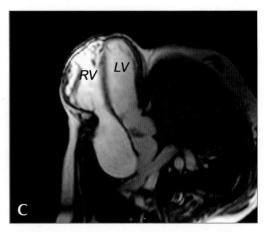

Figure 17-23. Ectopia cordis. **A,** Electrocardiogram (ECG)-gated turbo (fast) spin echo image in the axial plane showing a midline defect in the anterior chest wall through which part of the ventricles herniates. **B,** Same imaging sequence as **A,** in the sagittal plane, showing exteriorization of the ventricles through the chest wall defect. **C,** ECG-gated steady-state free precession cine cardiovascular magnetic resonance in the ventricular four-chamber plane showing the left venticle (LV) and right ventricle (RV) partially outside the thorax. Li—liver; Sp—spleen.

REFERENCES

1. Hoffman JI, Kaplan S: The incidence of congenital heart disease. *J Am Coll Cardiol* 2002, 39:1890–1900.

2. Hoffman JI, Kaplan S, Liberthson RR: Prevalence of congenital heart disease. *Am J Heart* 2004, 147:425–439.

3. Geva T: Magnetic resonance imaging: historical perspective. *J Cardiovasc Magn Reson* 2006, 8:573–580.

4. Brenner D, Elliston C, Hall E, Berdon W: Estimated risks of radiation-induced fatal cancer from pediatric CT. *AJR Am J Roentgenol* 2001, 176:289–296.

5. Geva T, Kreutzer, J: Diagnostic pathways for evaluation of congenital heart disease. In *Cardiology.* Edited by Crawford M, DiMarco, JP. London: Mosby International; 2001:4.1–4.22.

6. Greil GF, Powell AJ, Gildein HP, Geva T: Gadolinium-enhanced three-dimensional magnetic resonance angiography of pulmonary and systemic venous anomalies. *J Am Coll Cardiol* 2002, 39:335–341.

7. Geva T, Van Praagh S: Anomalies of the pulmonary veins. In *Moss & Adams' Heart Disease in Infants, Children, and Adolescents, 6th ed.* Edited by Allen HD, Gutgessel HP, Clark EB, Driscoll DJ. Philadelphia: Lippincott Williams & Wilkins; 2001:736–772.

8. Pasquini L, Sanders SP, Parness IA, *et al.*: Conal anatomy in 119 patients with d-loop transposition of the great arteries and ventricular septal defect: an echocardiographic and pathologic study. *J Am Coll Cardiol* 1993, 21:1712–1721.

9. Steffens JC, Bourne MW, Sakuma H, *et al.*: Quantification of collateral blood flow in coarctation of the aorta by velocity encoded cine magnetic resonance imaging. *Circulation* 1994, 90:937–943.

10. Nielsen JC, Powell AJ, Gauvreau K, *et al.*: Magnetic resonance imaging predictors of coarctation severity. *Circulation* 2005, 111:622–628.

11. Celoria GC, Patton RB: Congenital absence of the aortic arch. *Am J Heart* 1959, 58:407–413.

12. Angelini P: Coronary artery anomalies: an entity in search of an identity. *Circulation* 2007, 115:1296-305.

13. Geva T, Sanders SP, Ayres NA, *et al.*: Two-dimensional echocardiographic anatomy of atrioventricular alignment discordance with situs concordance. *Am J Heart* 1993, 125:459–464.

18

Congenital Heart Disease in Adults

Richard Eldridge Slaughter

Adult congenital heart disease is a fast growing and challenging area of cardiology. No longer are adults with congenital heart disease a rarity. Some patients develop congenital heart disease symptoms only during adult life. Many others have presented with heart disease in infancy and have undergone surgical repairs prior to adulthood. This group poses new challenges in disease management that have not been previously encountered.

Nowhere in cardiology does cardiovascular magnetic resonance (CMR) offer more than in this area. CMR provides a global perspective on complex cardiac problems, which is appealing to both the cardiologist and the surgeon. High-resolution images of cardiac morphology can now be obtained. CMR has an advantage over echocardiography because it can better capture images of the structures outside the heart, such as the aorta, the pulmonary arteries, and the pulmonary and systemic veins. Knowledge of these structures is often essential to properly manage the disease. Many studies can be conducted without using intravenous injection, but the superb contrast resolution afforded by gadolinium-enhanced CMR angiography allows the demonstration of obstructed or narrowed vessels, which may not be shown by other techniques. CMR techniques for the measurement of ventricular volume and function are now the gold standard. Measurement of right ventricular (RV) volumes and function is important in congenital heart dis-

ease. However, CMR techniques also apply to complex and single ventricles. The measurement of flow in individual vessels such as the right and left pulmonary arteries, shunts, and other smaller vessels is essential in understanding the physiology in many of these patients. Velocity-encoded phase contrast (PC) imaging is also of value in quantitating valve regurgitation. PC imaging is particularly helpful with the pulmonary and tricuspid valves.

The large chambers, as well as a lack of acoustic windows, present challenges for echocardiography in many adult patients with congenital heart disease. Catheterization also has limitations in displaying morphology in many of these patients. Sternal wires, valve replacements, and most stents do not pose significant limitations on CMR techniques. This chapter addresses specific examples of congenital defects presenting during adult life, as well as patients who have had surgery for previous congenital abnormalities and who require regular follow-up. In areas such as postoperative tetralogy of Fallot, transposition of the great arteries, Fontan connections, and cavopulmonary shunts, CMR is quickly becoming the imaging technique of choice for ongoing clinical management. No longer should CMR be reserved for those cases in which other imaging techniques have been unsuccessful. CMR has now been accepted as the primary imaging modality in many circumstances.

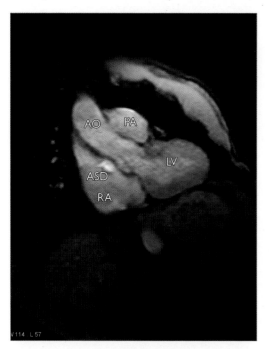

Figure 18-1. A single frame from an electrocardiogram (ECG) gated fast gradient echo cine of the heart with the imaging plane parallel to the interatrial septum and on the right atrial side. A secundum-type atrial septal defect (ASD) is present. Blood flowing through the defect has produced an area of high signal that corresponds to the ASD. Measurements of the size and position of the defect from such images have shown good correlation with surgical observation and balloon sizing at device closure [1].

Ostium secundum defects are the most common type of ASD. They are caused by a deficiency in septum primum and often present in adult life. Ostium secundum defects are usually oval in shape and may have several fenestrations. Large defects can extend beyond the confines of the fossa ovalis. Ostium secundum defects are usually seen as deficiencies in the atrial septum on axial or four-chamber steady-state free precession images. Small defects, however, may be difficult to detect and may be evident only as a small jet of signal loss best seen on fast gradient echo images. The degree of left to right shunting can be measured using phase contrast imaging through the ascending aorta and pulmonary artery. Measurements of ventricular volumes can also be used for this purpose in the absence of other shunts. CMR measured parameters in conjunction with patient symptoms are important determinants of the need for defect closure. AO—aorta; LV—left ventricle; PA—pulmonary artery; RA—right atrium.

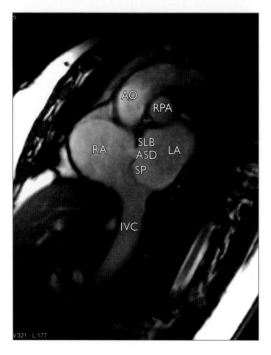

Figure 18-2. A frame from an electrocardiogram gated steady-state free precession cine cardiovascular magnetic resonance (CMR) taken through an ostium secundum defect in the atrial septum and passing through the inferior vena cava (IVC). Septum primum (SP) is shown, ballooning into the right atrium. The margins of the defect that comprise the superior lip of SP and the superior limbic band can clearly be seen in this plane. The distance between the inferior margin of the atrial septal defect (ASD) and the IVC can be measured. Similar projections through the ASD and other adjacent structures such as the superior vena cava, the right upper lobe pulmonary vein, and the ascending aorta can be used to measure the septal rim around the ASD accurately and can aid in planning for device closure. CMR may provide an alternative to transesophageal echo in accurately sizing and locating ASDs.

Patent foramen ovale is more difficult to detect as there may be no blood flow across the abnormality at rest. Real-time imaging through the atrial septum following an intravenous bolus of a gadolinium-based contrast agent while the patient performs the Valsalva maneuver has demonstrated this abnormality by contrast detection prematurely in the left atrium. AO—aorta; PA—pulmonary artery; RPA—right pulmonary artery; SLB—superior limbic band.

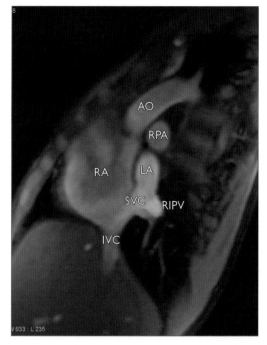

Figure 18-3. A single frame from an electrocardiogram (ECG) gated fast gradient echo cine CMR taken in a sagittal oblique plane through the atrial septum. This image shows a defect in the inferior sinus septum. The defect is closely related to the inferior vena cava and the right inferior pulmonary vein (RIPV). The inferior sinus venosus defect allows communication between the RIPV, left atrium (LA), and right atrium.

Sinus venosus defects are less common than ostium secundum defects. They occur most commonly in the superior sinus septum adjacent to the superior vena cava right atrial junction and are best seen in axial ECG gated images directly beneath this region. Sinus venosus defects are commonly associated with anomalous pulmonary venous drainage from the right upper lobe to the superior vena cava. Demonstration of the pulmonary venous return is important for defects of this type. Three-dimensional contrast-enhanced CMR angiography may be necessary to accurately define all the draining veins. Identification of four veins draining into the LA is inadequate to exclude anomalous drainage to the superior vena cava, as extra veins may exist. AO—aorta; IVC—inferior vena cava; RPA—right pulmonary artery; SVD—sinus venosus defect.

UNROOFED CORONARY SINUS

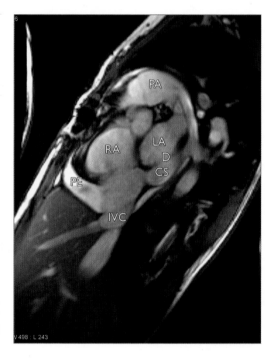

Figure 18-4. A single frame from an electrocardiogram (ECG) gated steady-state free precession (SSFP) cardiovascular magnetic resonance in a parasagittal oblique projection through the atrial septum. The coronary sinus (CS) can be seen entering the right atrium (RA). A deficiency is present in the roof of the CS and there is communication between the CS and the left atrium (LA) via this defect. This allows shunting of blood between the LA, the CS, and the RA. The orifice of the CS is usually enlarged under these circumstances. Occasionally a left superior vena cava is present, draining directly into the CS. These defects are rare but are well demonstrated in SSFP images in the plane of the CS. CMR has the ability to demonstrate complex anatomy in this region if carefully orientated views are taken through the abnormalities. A pericardial effusion is also present in this case.

Ostium primum atrial septal defect is a partial atrioventricular canal defect. The atrioventricular valve leaflets are tethered to the septal crest, resulting in a communication between the two atria. No ventricular septal defect is present. The absence of the atrioventricular septum and abnormal attachment of the atrioventricular valve leaflets causes a characteristic deformity of the LV outflow tract (LVOT). This deformity can be well demonstrated with ECG gated SSFP imaging through the LVOT. D—deficiency; IVC—inferior vena cava; PA—pulmonary artery; PE—pericardial effusion.

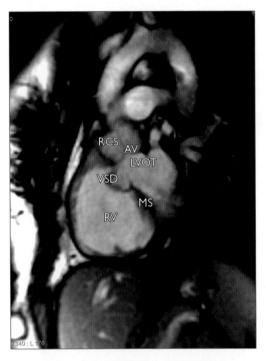

Figure 18-5. An electrocardiogram (ECG) gated steady-state free precession (SSFP) LV short-axis cine cardiovascular magnetic resonance, through the membranous septum in an adult. Proliferation of membranous tissue around the margins of the ventricular septal defect (VSD) has resulted in effective closure with a windsock protruding into the right ventricle (RV) in ventricular systole. Membranous VSDs are the most common type of VSD; they occur in the membranous septum beneath the right coronary sinus at the junction of the conal septum and muscular septum and often close spontaneously, as in this example.

VSDs may occur in several locations in the interventricular septum [2]. Conoventricular VSDs also involve the membranous septum but are often larger and commonly involve some malalignment of the conal and muscular septa. In tetralogy of Fallot, there is anterior displacement of the conal septum narrowing the RV outflow tract and creating a conoventricular VSD directly beneath the noncoronary and right coronary attachments of the aortic valve. Such relationships are well demonstrated with SSFP imaging prescribed through these regions. AV—aortic valve; LA—left atrium; LVOT—left ventricular outflow tract; MS—muscular septum; RV—right ventricle; RCS—right coronary sinus.

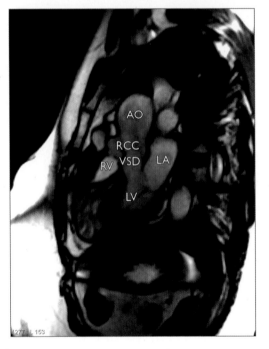

Figure 18-6. A frame from an electrocardiogram gated steady-state free precession cine cardiovascular magnetic resonance (CMR) through the left ventricular outflow tract. A ventricular septal defect (VSD) is present involving the membranous septum and conal septum. It lies directly below the right coronary cusp of the aortic valve. The cusp is prolapsing into the VSD, partially closing it. A central jet of aortic regurgitation was evident during ventricular diastole and this can be quantified by phase contrast imaging through the ascending aorta. Flow through the VSD was evident during ventricular systole. Defects involving the conal septal or supra crystal defects are often better seen with CMR than with other imaging modalities [3]. The size and location of VSDs in various locations in the interventricular septum can be readily appreciated because of the excellent morphological image characteristics of CMR. AO—aorta; RCC—right coronary cusp.

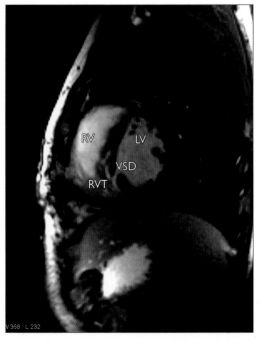

Figure 18-7. An electrocardiogram (ECG) gated steady-state free precession (SSFP) LV short-axis cine cardiovascular magnetic resonance through the ventricles of a patient with a muscular ventricular septal defect (VSD). Muscular VSDs can occur in any area of the muscular interventricular septum, most commonly in the mid muscular septum. They may occur anterior to the septal band or at the apex. Muscular VSDs often have a single orifice on the LV side, but enter the RV among the trabeculae as in this case. At the apex, they can open into a heavily trabeculated area. Muscular VSDs are often multiple and are usually well demonstrated on a series of LV short-axis SSFP images. However, other views may be necessary for more precise localization. VSDs may occur in the atrioventricular canal tissue beneath the septal leaflet of the tricuspid valve, or large membranous VSDs may extend into the adjacent muscular septum. They may be isolated defects and may present in adult life. However, they often occur as part of more complex cardiac abnormalities. RVT—right ventricular trabeculae.

AORTIC ROOT

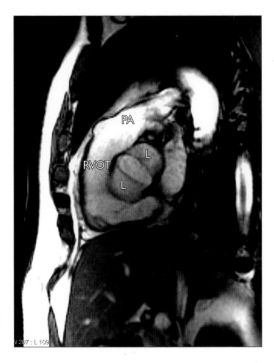

Figure 18-8. A steady-state free precession (SSFP) cine cardiovascular magnetic resonance (CMR) through the aortic valve orthogonal to the long axis of the aortic root. The aortic valve is bicuspid with two leaflets of approximately equal size (L). There is no significant fusion at the commissures in this case. The aortic annulus is not reduced in size, but the free margins of the leaflets are shorter than usual. One of the cusps is often larger than the other and there is often a raphe dividing the larger cusp. Bicuspid aortic valve occurs in 1% of the population. Abnormal stresses on the valve leaflets may predispose to their degeneration and calcification, and resultant aortic valve stenosis commonly presents in adult life. Bicuspid aortic valve is often associated with abnormalities of tissue in the aortic root and eventual dilation; possible dissection of the ascending aorta and aortic coarctation. CMR is an ideal technique for the demonstration of both the aortic valve and the associated aortic root dilation and coarctation. Subvalvar aortic stenosis and supravalvar aortic stenosis such as occurs in William's syndrome or following arterial switch operation, are also well displayed with SSFP imaging or three-dimensional contrast-enhanced CMR angiography. L—leaflets; PA—pulmonary artery; RVOT—right ventricular outflow tract.

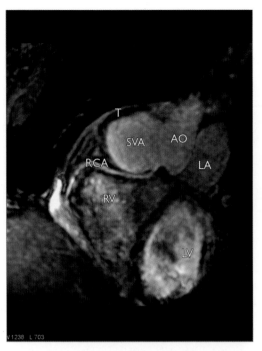

Figure 18-9. A maximum intensity projection image from a three-dimensional steady-state free precession cardiovascular magnetic resonance (CMR) of the aortic root in an adult with a congenital sinus of Valsalva aneurysm arising from the right coronary sinus. The relationship of the lesion to the orifice and course of the right coronary artery can be demonstrated by this technique without the need for catheterization. A small amount of thrombus (T) is present in the superior aspect of the aneurysm. Sinus of Valsalva aneurysms usually arise as a dilation of the right sinus and occasionally the noncoronary sinus between the aortic annulus and the sinotubular junction. Sinus of Valsalva aneurysms may be congenital or acquired. These aneurysms may extend into the right venticular outflow tract (RVOT) and cause RVOT obstruction. Rupture is the major complication. CMR is also of value in assessing other areas around the aortic root in patients with conditions such as paravalvar abscess and paravalvar aortic regurgitation occurring following aortic valve replacement. Most mechanical valves are able to be imaged at 1.5 T, and CMR has some advantages over echocardiography in evaluating paravalvar abnormalities. The hemodynamic effects of aortic valvar and paravalvar lesions and aortic root abnormalities can be assessed with phase contrast imaging to measure peak velocities and quantitate regurgitation. Planimetry of the aortic valve area from an orthogonal view through the tips of the leaflets and measurement of LV size and function can also be performed. AO—aorta; RCA—right coronary artery; RV—right ventricle; SVA—sinus of Valsalva aneurysm; T—thrombus.

Thoracic Aorta

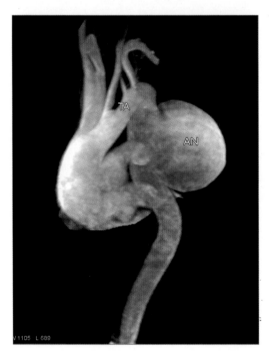

Figure 18-10. A maximum intensity projection image from a three-dimensional contrast-enhanced cardiovascular magnetic resonance (CMR) angiography of the thoracic aorta in a 40-year-old woman who had an aortic coarctation repair with a Dacron patch in childhood. A large aneurysm has developed at the repair site. Postoperative aneurysm formation is a recognized complication of repaired coarctation particularly following patch repair [4]. Recurrent stenosis at the repair site can also occur. This image also demonstrates a narrow transverse arch. Failure of the transverse arch to grow following coarctation repair is a complication seen in adults who may have persisting hypertension. Treatment of mild hypoplasia of the transverse arch and recurrent stenosis remains controversial. Aortic coarctation is a common abnormality often associated with other congenital heart lesions such as obstructive lesions in the left side of the heart including supravalvar mitral membrane, parachute mitral valve, and subaortic stenosis. Bicuspid aortic valve occurs in approximately 50% of cases. CMR is the technique of choice for imaging many aortic abnormalities including native and postoperative aortic coarctation and Marfan's syndrome. Imaging of obstructive lesions and aortic dilation can be carried out with functional assessment including measurements of collateral aortic flow at a single CMR examination. AN—aneurysm; TA—transverse arch.

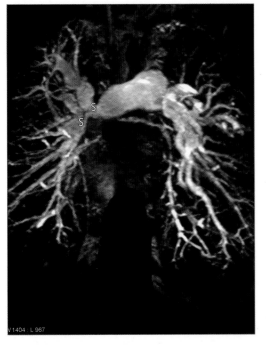

Figure 18-11. A maximum intensity projection (MIP) image from a three-dimensional contrast-enhanced cardiovascular magnetic resonance angiography (CE-MRA) of the pulmonary arteries in a young adult following previous repair of pulmonary atresia with ventricular septal defect (VSD). Arterial focalization with complete repair has been performed previously. The pulmonary arteries are adequate in size with good arborization. There are multiple focal stenoses resulting in proximal pulmonary hypertension. The anatomy of complex pulmonary arteries may be better demonstrated with a three-dimensional CE-MRA acquisition rather than a two-dimensional catheter angiographic image due to overlap of segments. Pulmonary artery morphology varies considerably in patients with pulmonary atresia VSD) which is often regarded as the extreme end of the tetralogy spectrum. The pulmonary artery supply to the lungs may be from native pulmonary arteries and from aortopulmonary collaterals. Staged surgical treatment is aimed at establishing a functional pulmonary arterial tree using native pulmonary arteries or focalized aortopulmonary collaterals. Often residual stenoses, areas of poor perfusion, or systemic collaterals remain. CMR has an important role in demonstrating the variations and is helpful in planning endovascular treatment. Following stent placement, CMR may still be of value in assessing residual stent patency and stenoses. S—stenoses.

PULMONARY VEINS

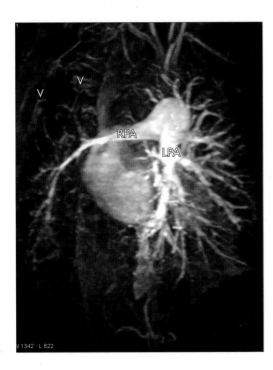

Figure 18-12. A maximum intensity projection image from a three-dimensional contrast-enhanced cardiovascular magnetic resonance angiography (CE-MRA) of a patient with previous repaired Scimitar syndrome with rerooting of the anomalous draining vein from the right lung to the left atrium. Obstruction to the repair has resulted in decreased flow to the right lung and a further reduction in size of the right pulmonary artery. No right pulmonary veins have been demonstrated, and the right lung vessels are decompressed by small systemic veins and lymphatics. In the presence of normal pulmonary vascular resistance in the left lung, the lung can readily accommodate the increased flow without elevation of pulmonary artery pressures; such venous obstruction may have minimal symptoms. The superb contrast resolution of CE-MRA enables the demonstration of the small vessels decompressing the right lung pulmonary arteries. Phase contrast imaging allows measurement of flow in both pulmonary arteries.

Anomalous pulmonary venous drainage may also present in adults. Multiple variations occur, the most common being from the right upper lobe to the superior vena cava. Abnormal drainage to the inferior vena cava/right atrial junction (IVC/RA) junction from an abnormal right lung as in the above case, and to the innominate vein from the left lung, is also a common presentation. Anomalies of venous drainage, abnormal systemic artery supply, and postsurgical complications are well demonstrated with three-dimensional CE-MRA even if venous obstruction is present. LPA—left pulmonary artery; RPA—right pulmonary artery; V—veins.

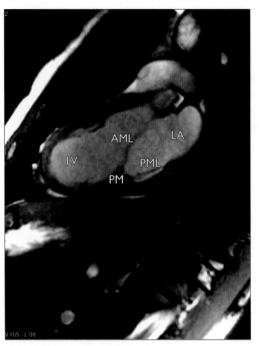

Figure 18-13. A diastolic frame from a steady-state free precession (SSFP) cine cardio-vascular magnetic resonance (CMR) in the left ventricle (LV) in a patient presenting for assessment following aortic coarctation repair. A single complex papillary muscle is present with a parachute deformity of the mitral valve. Ballooning of the anterior mitral leaflet and posterior mitral leaflet is present. Parachute mitral valve occurs when all the chordae insert into a single or complex papillary muscle restricting leaflet opening. The chordae are often thickened and the commissures not well developed. Parachute mitral valve occurs often in association with other obstructive lesions of the left side of the heart [5].

Most cases of congenital mitral stenosis are diagnosed in childhood, but forms with less severe obstruction may present in adult life. Two papillary muscles may be present. They often appear to insert directly into the mitral valve leaflets. SSFP cine CMR in two-chamber long-axis, LV outflow tract, and LV short-axis planes are used to demonstrate the anatomy. Short-axis views enable accurate delineation of the papillary muscles. Assessment of the severity of stenosis may be difficult but planimetry at the valve tips in the LV short axis may be useful.

Primary mitral valve prolapse is classified by some as a congenital abnormality. CMR has a role in evaluating this condition. Images through the scallops of the valve leaflets can define the prolapsing segment. Regurgitant volumes can be measured indirectly by comparison of LV stroke volumes with measurements of aortic flow volumes. AML—anterior mitral leaflet; PM—papillary muscle; PML—posterior mitral leaflet.

COR TRIATRIATUM

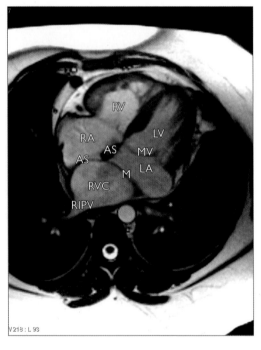

Figure 18-14. An electrocardiogram gated steady-state free precession (SSFP) cardio-vascular magnetic resonance of an adult presenting with obstruction to left atrial inflow due to cor triatriatum. The abnormality is because of inadequate incorporation of the common pulmonary vein with the primitive left atrium (LA). A membrane across the LA separates the atrium into a trabeculated chamber giving rise to the LA appendage and communicating with the mitral valve, and a posterior pulmonary venous confluence receiving the pulmonary veins. The right inferior pulmonary vein is evident. The size of the defect in the obstructing membrane determines the severity of the obstruction and the age of presentation. SSFP images in axial, four-chamber or two-chamber long axis, combined with phase contrast flow images, can usually demonstrate the anatomic variants. In this patient, there was a small atrial septal defect not demonstrated in this view between the right atrium (RA) and low pressure LA chamber. Defects in the atrial septum commonly occur in conjunction with cor triatriatum and have been reported between the RA and both left-sided chambers. Demonstration of all four pulmonary veins is also important. AS—atrial septum; M—membrane; MV—mitral valve; PVC—pulmonary venous confluence; RIPV—right inferior pulmonary vein.

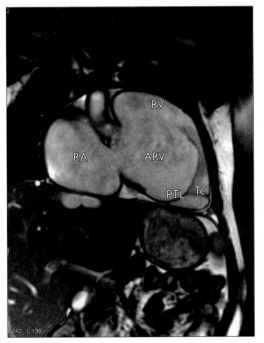

Figure 18-15. A steady-state free precession (SSFP) long-axis view of the right ventricle (RV) in an adult with Ebstein's anomaly of the tricuspid valve. The spectrum of abnormalities in this condition is large with patients presenting at any time from infancy to old age [6]. Older patients may present with arrhythmias, tricuspid regurgitation, and right-sided heart failure. The tricuspid valve annulus is usually large. In this patient, the posterior leaflet and septal leaflet attachments are displaced toward the apex. The anterior leaflet arises normally and is mobile. The anterior and posterior leaflets are tethered to the RV free wall (Te). The trabecular RV chamber is small, and the wall is thinned with reduced systolic function. The dilated atrial portion of the RV is thin walled. Severe tricuspid regurgitation is present, resulting in marked right-sided heart enlargement. Ebstein's anomaly can occur as an isolated abnormality or in conjunction with other congenital heart abnormalities such as congenitally corrected transposition. An atrial septal defect may be present, and right to left shunting may occur. The condition arises from failure of the tricuspid valve leaflet tissue to differentiate from the developing RV muscle.

SSFP cine cardiovascular magnetic resonance in axial, RV long axis, and RV short axis may be necessary to evaluate the complex tricuspid valve anatomy. Imaging series with increased temporal resolution may be helpful. Measurement of RV volumes of both portions of the RV and the RA may be performed from a series of images through the ventricle and may aid understanding of this condition. ARV—atrial right ventricle; PTL—posterior leaflet; Te—teathering trabeculae

TETRALOGY OF FALLOT

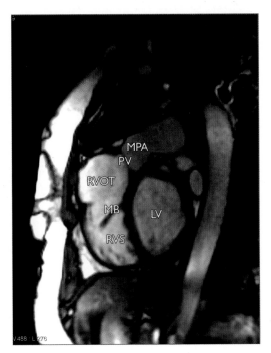

Figure 18-16. An electrocardiogram (ECG) gated steady-state free precession (SSFP) cine cardiovascular magnetic resonance (CMR) in a parasagittal plane through the right ventricular outflow tract (RVOT), pulmonary valve and main pulmonary artery in a patient with previously repaired tetralogy of Fallot. An extensive repair of the RVOT involving a transannular patch to relieve the sub pulmonary and pulmonary stenosis has resulted in scarring and RV outflow tract dilation and dyskinesia. Late gadolinium enhancement can be used to delineate scarring in such areas. Dyskinesia of the RVOT adversely affects the RV ejection fraction. It is possible using CMR to calculate the ejection fraction for the sinus of the RV below the moderator band while excluding the RVOT in patients in whom repair of pulmonary valve regurgitation is contemplated. Surgery in infancy to relieve RVOT and pulmonary valve obstruction often results in free pulmonary regurgitation, RV dilation and decreased RV function with tricuspid regurgitation. The long term natural history of pulmonary regurgitation in this group of patients is still not fully understood. The timing of pulmonary valve replacement is also controversial. However, CMR using a series of SSFP images and phase contrast imaging flow measurements allows accurate measurement of RV size and systolic function as well as the quantitation of pulmonary regurgitation and tricuspid regurgitation and the demonstration of RVOT and pulmonary artery morphology.[7] MB—moderator band; MPA—main pulmonary artery; PV—pulmonary valve; RVS—sinus of the right ventricle.

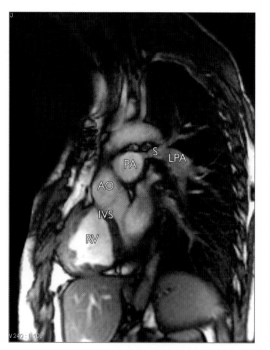

Figure 18-17. An electrocardiogram (ECG) gated steady-state free precession cine cardio-vascular magnetic resonance (CMR) in an oblique plane through the left pulmonary artery of a patient with previous repair of Tetralogy of Fallot. There is a proximal left pulmonary artery stenosis. The main pulmonary artery and distal LPA are of good size. In most cases of tetralogy of Fallot, pulmonary artery stenoses lie centrally and can be seen using ECG gated SSFP imaging without the need for three-dimensional contrast enhanced CMR angiography. The ventricular septal defect (VSD) has been repaired and the interventricular septum is intact. Phase contrast imaging through the main pulmonary artery can be used to quantitate the volumes of forward and reverse flow in patients with pulmonary regurgitation following repair of tetralogy of Fallot. The pulmonary regurgitant fraction has very different implications from the measurements of regurgitant fraction with left-side heart valvular leaks. It is dependant on RV compliance. It has been recently shown that RV volumes and ejection fraction are better predictors of outcomes following pulmonary valve replacement in tetralogy of Fallot than the pulmonary regurgitant fraction.[8] Flow through individual pulmonary arteries, however, is an important measure of the effects of right or left pulmonary artery stenoses, because measurements of pressure gradients are unreliable in a low pressure system with considerable flow reserve. In cases with severe RV impairment, filling of the left ventricle may be reduced. CMR has fast become the technique of choice for follow up of patients with postoperative tetralogy of Fallot. AO—aorta; IVS—interventricular septum; LPA— left pulmonary artery; PA—pulmonary artery; S—stenosis.

DOUBLE-CHAMBERED RV

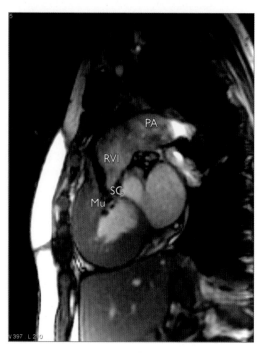

Figure 18-18. An electrocardiogram (ECG) gated steady-state free precession cine cardiovascular magnetic resonance in the sagittal oblique plane of an adult patient presenting with muscular RV outflow tract (RVOT) obstruction. It demonstrates a markedly hypertrophied high pressure RV chamber and a low pressure infundibular RV chamber. The RV obstruction is caused by anomalous muscle bundles usually arising from the septal band of the crista and passing to the RV free wall [9]. The muscle bundles are usually distinct from the moderator band and are thought to represent hypertrophied septoparietal trabeculations. A ventricular septal defect (VSD) is commonly present and may communicate with either RV chamber. However, the VSD is usually membranous in nature and communicates with the high pressure chamber. It is thought that in those patients presenting in adult life without evidence of a VSD, a previous VSD may have closed due to muscular hypertrophy of the septal band or membranous proliferation. The condition differs from tetralogy of Fallot where the VSD and RVOT obstruction are due to malalignment of the conal septum. It was suggested that the presence of a high moderator band may be the causative factor. Double-chambered RV may present in adult life with variable symptoms including those similar to pulmonary hypertension. Mu—muscle bundles; PA—pulmonary artery; RVI—right ventricular infundibular chamber; SC—septal band of the crista.

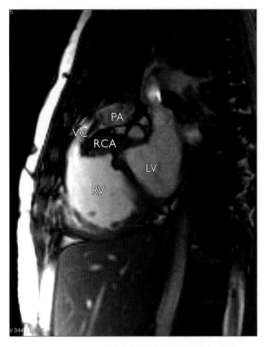

Figure 18-19. An electrocardiogram (ECG) gated steady-state free precession (SSFP) sagittal cine cardiovascular magnetic resonance (CMR) of a patient following Rastelli repair for transposition of the great arteries with pulmonary stenosis and ventricular septal defect. A valved conduit was placed between the right ventricle (RV) and the pulmonary artery. The conduit lies directly behind the sternum. In this position, it may be difficult to assess with transthoracic echocardiography. Despite the presence of sternal wires, satisfactory assessment of this region is usually possible with CMR. In this case, the conduit is narrowed and the tissue valve leaflets are thickened. Peak velocities of greater than 4.5 metres per second were obtained distal to the valve using phase contrast imaging. The RV is hypertrophied, and flattening of the interventricular septum is present in systole indicating elevation of RV systolic pressures due to conduit obstruction. The right coronary artery can also be seen running behind the conduit in a position where it might be vulnerable during surgical upgrade of the conduit. Conduit regurgitation can be assessed in a similar fashion to pulmonary valve regurgitation in postoperative tetralogy of Fallot. As part of the Rastelli repair, the aorta is baffled to the left ventricle (LV) by an existing or enlarged ventricular septal defect. SSFP imaging through the LV outflow tract may demonstrate sub aortic narrowing or residual ventricular septal defects following this type of repair. PA—pulmonary artery; RCA—right coronary artery; VC—valved conduit.

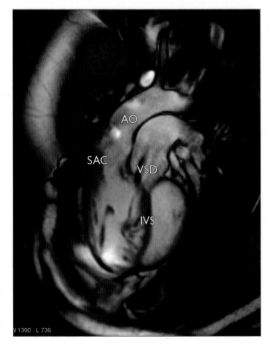

Figure 18-20. An electrocardiogram (ECG) gated steady-state free precession (SSFP) cardiovascular magnetic resonance (CMR) in an oblique plane through the aorta and main pulmonary artery in a patient with transposition of the great arteries who had a previous atrial baffle repair in childhood. The aorta arises high up from the right ventricle (RV), above a sub aortic conus. The ventricular septal defect (VSD) has been repaired but a small residual VSD beneath the pulmonary valve is evident by the turbulent jet passing between the high-pressure systemic RV and the lower pressure LV. The interventricular septum can be seen bulging toward the left side. Following atrial baffle repair for transposition of the great arteries, the morphologic RV remains the systemic ventricle and is subject to systemic pressure. Remodelling of the RV occurs with dilation and rounding of the tricuspid valve annulus with resultant tricuspid regurgitation. RV hypertrophy and impairment of RV function are of ongoing concern in this group of patients in adult life. Late gadolinium enhanced imaging may demonstrate scarring in the impaired systemic RV. Because of the ability of CMR to accurately measure RV volumes and function and to quantitate valve regurgitation, CMR is an ideal technique for follow up of patients when a morphologic RV or a common ventricle is the systemic pumping chamber [10]. AO—aorta; IVS—interventricular septum; SAC—sub aortic conus; VSD—ventricular septal defect.

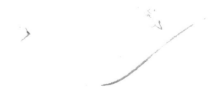

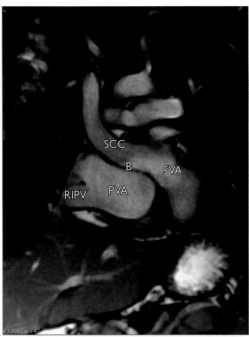

Figure 18-21. An electrocardiogram (ECG) gated steady-state free precession cine cardiovascular magnetic resonance (CMR) taken in an oblique plane through the superior caval channel of a patient following Mustard atrial baffle repair for transposition of the great arteries. A section of the baffle repair and the superior caval channel communicating with the systemic venous atrium are demonstrated. Stenoses may occur in the superior caval channel and are amenable to endovascular dilation and stenting. A section of the pulmonary venous atrium (PVA) receiving a right inferior pulmonary vein is also shown. The PVA however, is better shown in a series of axial or sagittal images. Although obstruction to the PVA can occur, it is uncommon. Two different techniques for atrial switch operation are regularly performed. The Mustard repair uses autologous pericardium, whereas the Senning repair uses atrial tissue to create the baffle. Although these have slightly different appearances on the CMR examination, the overall imaging features are similar. B—baffle repair; PVA—pulmonary venous atrium; RIPV—right inferior pulmonary vein; SCC—superior caval channel; SVA—systemic venous atrium.

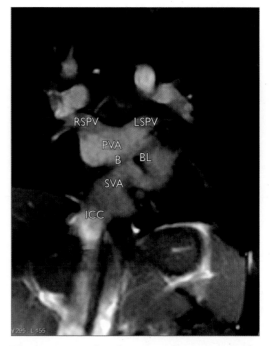

Figure 18-22. An electrocardiogram gated steady-state free precession oblique cine cardiovascular magnetic resonance which was prescribed from an axial view in a patient following Mustard repair. The inferior caval channel baffles the inferior vena caval blood through the systemic venous atrium and subsequently to the morphologic left ventricle. A small baffle leak is present. Such leaks are usually not of hemodynamic significance. The right superior pulmonary vein and the left superior pulmonary vein can be seen draining into the pulmonary venous atrium which is separated by the baffle from the systemic venous atrium. B—baffle; BL—baffle leak; ICC—inferior caval channel; IVC—inferior vena cava; LSPV—left superior pulmonary vein; PVA—pulmonary venous atrium; RSPV—right superior pulmonary vein; SVA—systemic venous atrium.

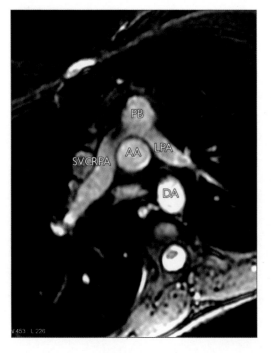

Figure 18-23. A maximum intensity projection image from a three-dimensional fat suppressed steady-state free precession (SSFP) cine cardiovascular magnetic resonance of the pulmonary arteries in a patient who has had an arterial switch operation in infancy for transposition of the great arteries. In this procedure, both the ascending aorta and the main pulmonary artery are divided. A Le Compte maneuver is used to bring the pulmonary bifurcation anterior to the ascending aorta. The descending aorta lies posteriorly. The coronary arteries are reimplanted using coronary buttons. The right and left pulmonary arteries curve around the ascending aorta, and are sometimes difficult to demonstrate with two-dimensional imaging. These vessels can also be imaged in cross section and are usually oval in shape. Stenoses may occur at the anastomosis site and occasionally in either the right or the left pulmonary arteries. SSFP images through the left ventricular and right ventricular outflow tracts, proximal aorta, and pulmonary artery are useful in demonstrating postoperative changes in these vessels. Some deformity is often present in the aorta, and dilation may occur. Neoaortic regurgitation is usually mild. Phase contrast imaging through these vessels may be used to quantitate the severity of regurgitation or obstruction. AA—ascending aorta; DA—descending aorta; LPA—left pulmonary artery; PB—pulmonary bifurcation; RPA—right pulmonary artery; SVC—superior vena cava.

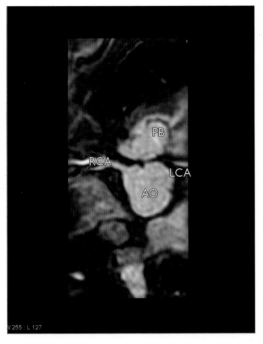

Figure 18-24. A maximum intensity projection image from a three-dimensional fat suppressed steady-state free precession cardiovascular magnetic resonance (CMR) through the coronary arteries following arterial switch procedure for transposition of the great arteries. The left coronary artery is severely stenosed at its origin. The right coronary artery is large and shows no narrowing. Coronary artery stenosis following the switch procedure is a recognized complication and has been reported in up to 18% of patients [11]. It is important to include imaging of the coronary artery origins in all patients examined with CMR for follow-up of previous arterial switch procedures. Occasionally, a coronary artery is evident passing between the neoaorta and the right or left pulmonary artery. The significance of these findings is uncertain. In this patient the pulmonary bifurcation is present anterior to the ascending aorta (AO) and the pulmonary arteries are running superior to the coronary arteries. AO—aorta; LCA—left coronary artery; PB—pulmonary bifurcation; RCA—right coronary artery.

SINGLE VENTRICULAR REPAIR

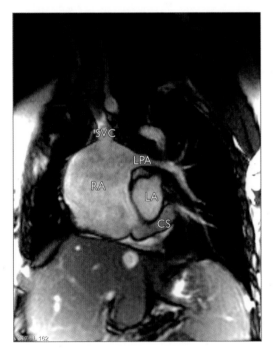

Figure 18-25. An electrocardiogram gated steady-state free precession (SSFP) cine cardiovascular magnetic resonance (CMR) of an adult patient with a single ventricle who had atriopulmonary Fontan connection in infancy. The left pulmonary artery is anastomosed directly to the right atrium (RA) and the atrial septal defect has been closed. The RA is markedly dilated. Dilation of the RA and coronary sinus commonly occur with such procedures with subsequent risk of atrial arrhythmia and possibly reduced coronary perfusion.

The Fontan operation and its modifications, as well as cavopulmonary connections were introduced to provide passive lung perfusion and to preserve the single ventricle or ventricles as the systemic pumping chamber. Various modifications of these procedures have been carried out to minimize complications and to produce an energy-efficient pathway. The venous anatomy can be complex in adult patients. CMR using SSFP cine imaging and three-dimensional contrast enhanced CMR angiography or black blood CMR in different planes usually accurately depicts the previous surgical procedures and demonstrates many of the problems that may occur in the adult patient. Direct atriopulmonary connections as seen in this patient are rarely performed today. CS—coronary sinus; LPA—left pulmonary artery; SVC— superior vena cava.

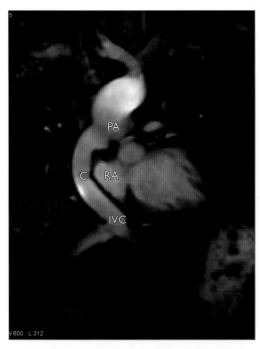

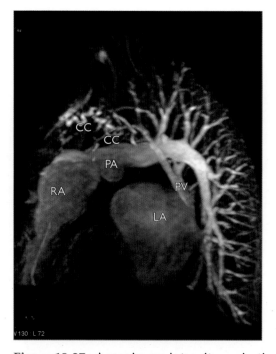

Figure 18-26. An electrocardiogram gated steady-state free precession (SSFP) coronal cardiovascular magnetic resonance of a patient who had a Fontan operation in infancy using an extra cardiac conduit to connect the inferior vena cava to the pulmonary artery. The conduit lies outside the right atrium (RA). This technique, the more commonly used lateral tunnel, and intra right atrial conduits attempt to reduce right atrial enlargement, minimize right atrial suturing, and provide a more energy-efficient pathway for inferior vena caval blood to enter the pulmonary artery circuit. The extra cardiac Fontan conduit may be difficult to evaluate with echocardiography. On occasions, turbulence in venous channels causes signal loss in SSFP imaging and three-dimensional contrast enhanced CMR angiography or black blood CMR may be necessary to fully demonstrate the morphology. C—cardiac conduit; IVC—inferior vena cava; PA—pulmonary artery.

Figure 18-27. A maximum intensity projection (MIP) image from a three-dimensional contrast enhanced cardiovascular magnetic resonance (CMR) angiography of a patient with a long-standing Fontan operation with collateral channels which have developed from the systemic venous circulation to the pulmonary veins. These may cause systemic desaturation [12]. Large channels are amenable to embolization. Arteriovenous malformations may also develop in the smaller vessels in the lungs, again causing systemic desaturation. These anastomoses are small and are difficult to demonstrate with CMR techniques. They are reported as more prevalent when hepatic venous blood is excluded from the pulmonary artery circulation. Desaturation may also occur via shunting through a surgically created atrial fenestration. Such fenestrations can usually be demonstrated on electrocardiogram gated steady-state free precession. Thrombosis can develop in areas of slow flow and in a dilated right atrium. In some patients where a small right ventricle is present, a one and a half ventricular repair is possible using the hypoplastic RV to perfuse the lungs via the main pulmonary artery and left pulmonary artery and a cavopulmonary connection to perfuse the lungs via the right pulmonary artery. Patients with single ventricular repair are an important group where CMR can shed light on complications and lead to better understanding of the morphology and outcomes by monitoring ventricular performance and pulmonary artery and venous connections. CC—collateral channels; PA—pulmonary artery; PV—pulmonary veins.

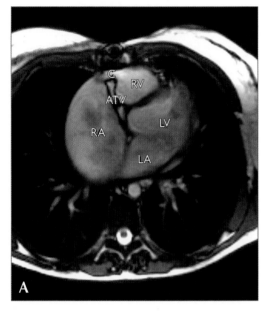

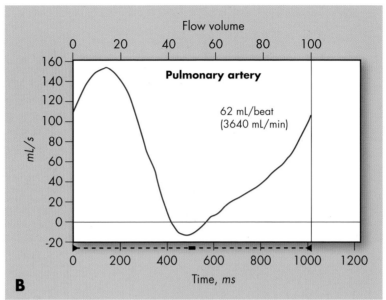

Figure 18-28. A patient with tricuspid atresia. Figure **A** is an electrocardiogram (ECG) gated steady-state free precession (SSFP) axial cine cardiovascular magnetic resonance (CMR). Fibro fatty tissue has replaced the tricuspid valve. A valved conduit has been placed between the right atrium and the right ventricle (RV). The left ventricle (LV) and left atrium are normal. CMR measurements of the RV demonstrated a RV volume at the lower limit of normal with an ejection fraction also at the lower limit of normal for an adult patient. Marked right atrium (RA) enlargement with enlargement of the inferior vena cava and hepatic dysfunction were present. **B,** A flow volume curve generated from a phase contrast imaging series through the main pulmonary artery. There is forward flow through the pulmonary artery in ventricular systole with mild reverse flow in early diastole followed by further forward flow through the pulmonary artery throughout much of diastole. A similar phase contrast flow curve through the conduit showed mild conduit regurgitation during ventricular systole without significant conduit obstruction. The pulmonary artery flow curve demonstrates significant diastolic dysfunction of the hypoplastic RV with failure of relaxation. Flow measurements such as this may be helpful in understanding compliance issues with hypoplastic or single ventricles. ATV—atretic tricuspid valve; C—(valved) conduit.

COMPLEX UNOPERATED DISEASE

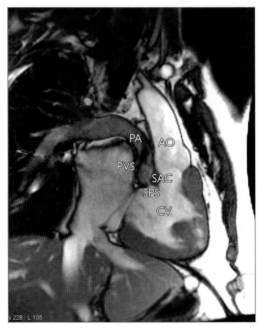

Figure 18-29. An electrocardiogram (ECG) gated steady-state free precession cine CMR in a right ventricular (RV) long-axis view of a 40-year-old patient with a common ventricle. The aorta is arising anteriorly above a muscular sub aortic conus. The pulmonary artery is smaller and is arising posteriorly. Sub pulmonary stenosis and pulmonary valve stenosis are present restricting flow in the pulmonary arteries. In this patient, the pulmonary arteries were protected from pulmonary artery hypertension from the pulmonary stenosis and good mixing of blood occurring in the common ventricle. Ventricular function was well maintained. In spite of some desaturation, the patient was able to lead a functionally useful life. Cases such as pulmonary atresia, truncus, and other complex conditions may survive into adult life in the absence of surgical intervention if appropriate restriction of pulmonary flow, good ventricular function, and venous and arterial mixing of blood can occur. CMR is an ideal technique to evaluate the morphology and functional abnormalities in such patients if surgical or endovascular repair is contemplated. AO—aorta; CV—common ventricle; PA—pulmonary artery; PVS—pulmonary valve stenosis; SAC—sub aortic conus; SPS—sub pulmonary stenosis.

REFERENCES

1. Beerbaum P, Körperich H, Esdorn H, *et al.*: Atrial septal defects in pediatric patients: noninvasive sizing with cardiovascular MR imaging. *Radiology* 2003, 228:361–369. Epub 2003 Jun 11.

2. Van Praagh R, Geva T, Kreutzer J: Ventricular septal defects: how shall we describe, name and classify them? *J Am Coll Cardiol* 1989, 14:1298–1299.

3. Bremerich J, Reddy GP, Higgins CB: MRI of supracristal ventricular septal defects. *J Comput Assist Tomogr* 1999, 23:13–15.

4. von Kodolitsch Y, Aydin MA, Koschyk DH, *et al.*: Predictors of aneurysmal formation after surgical correction of aortic coarctation. *J Am Coll Cardiol* 2002, 4:617–624.

5. Shone JD, Sellers RD, Anderson RC, *et al.*: The developmental complex of "parachute mitral valve," supravalvular ring of left atrium, subaortic stenosis, and coarctation of aorta. *Am J Cardiol* 1963, 11:714–725.

6. Carpentier A, Chauvaud S, Macé L, *et al.*: A new reconstructive operation for Ebstein's anomaly of the tricuspid valve. *J Thorac Cardiovasc Surg* 1988, 96:92–101.

7. Helbing WA, de Roos A.: Clinical applications of cardiac magnetic resonance imaging after repair of tetralogy of Fallot. *Pediatr Cardiol* 2000, 21:70–79.

8. Henkens IR, van Straten A, Schalij MJ, *et al.*: Predicting outcome of pulmonary valve replacement in adult tetralogy of Fallot patients. *Ann Thorac Surg* 2007, 83:907–911.

9. Alva C, Ho SY, Lincoln CR, *et al.*: The nature of the obstructive muscular bundles in double-chambered right ventricle. *J Thorac Cardiovasc Surg* 1999, 117:1180–1189.

10. Strugnell WE, Slaughter RE, Riley RA, *et al.*: Modified Short Axis Series-A new method for cardiac MRI measurement of right ventricular volumes. *J Cardiovasc Magn Reson* 2005, 7:769–774.

11. Bonhoeffer P, Bonnet D, Piéchaud JF, *et al.*: Coronary artery obstruction after the arterial switch operation for transposition of the great arteries in newborns. *J Am Coll Cardiol* 1997, 29:202–206.

12. Magee AG, McCrindle BW, Mawson J, *et al.*: Systemic venous collateral development after the bidirectional cavopulmonary anastomosis. Prevalence and predictors. *J Am Coll Cardiol* 1998, 32:502–508.

19

CMR Venography

Ivan Pedrosa

Cardiovascular magnetic resonance (CMR) represents an excellent alternative to conventional venography, grayscale and Doppler ultrasound, and contrast-enhanced CT for evaluation of the venous system. Noncontrast and contrast-enhanced CMR provides excellent detail of the venous system anatomy, as well as an accurate demonstration of pathology.

CMR offers noninvasive assessments of the venous system with excellent soft tissue contrast, which allows for clear differentiation between the veins and adjacent structures, characterization of thrombus, and delineation of masses affecting the veins. In addition, CMR allows for evaluation of large areas of anatomy, including the central veins of the body.

This chapter will discuss the different CMR techniques available for evaluation of the venous system as well as the imaging findings in common clinical applications, including detection of central venous thrombosis, thrombus characterization, and neoplastic involvement of the venous system.

CARDIOVASCULAR MAGNETIC RESONANCE TECHNIQUES

CMR strategies for evaluation of the venous system include noncontrast and contrast-enhanced techniques. Noncontrast techniques can be classified as dark blood and bright blood sequences depending on the signal intensity of blood on the particular CMR sequence used.

Bright blood sequences may provide intravascular signal from the presence of flow (flow dependent sequences) or based on the T1 and T2 characteristics of blood or thrombus (flow independent sequences). The use of electrocardiographic triggering may reduce pulsatile artifacts and thus improve the homogeneity of the signal within vessels on these acquisitions.

Contrast-enhanced CMRs are usually obtained after administration of a gadolinium-based contrast agent in an antecubital vein during the equilibrium phase, typically 90 to 120 seconds after administration of contrast (indirect CMR venography). Alternatively, a direct contrast-enhanced CMR venography examination can be obtained after administration of diluted gadolinium contrast agents in a peripheral vein of the extremity that is being evaluated. A double dose of gadolinium (0.2 mmol/kg of body weight) administered through an intravenous access in an antecubital vein provides excellent venous enhancement for indirect CMR venography.

CMR Sequences for the Venous System

Noncontrast Methods	Contrast enchanced Methods
Dark blood sequences	Direct MR Venography
Spin echo	3D FS T1-weighted SPGR
Double inversion spin echo	Indirect MR Venography
Bright blood sequences	
Flow dependent	3D FS T1-weighted SPGR
Time of flight (TOF)	
Gradient echo (GRE)*	
Flow independent	
Balanced steady-state precession* (true FISP, FIESTA, balance FFE)	

Figure 19-1. Commonly used cardiovascular magnetic resonance sequences for evaluation of the venous system. Sequences marked with an asterisk can be acquired with electrocardiographic gating and displayed in cine mode. FIESTA—fast imaging employing steady-state acquisition; FISP—fast imaging with steady-state precession; FFE—fast field echo; FS—fat-saturation; SPGR—spoiled gradient echo.

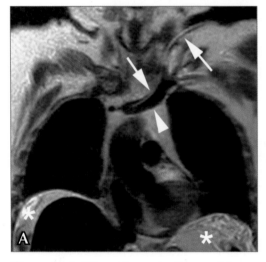
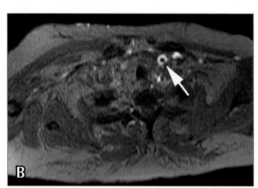
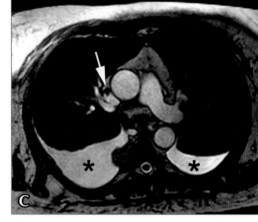

Figure 19-2. Normal venous flow and intravenous catheter on dark blood and bright blood cardiovascular magnetic resonance. **A**, Coronal dark blood single-shot fast spin echo sequence shows a normal flow void in the left brachiocephalic vein (*arrowhead*). In the presence of normal blood flow, the excited protons move out of the imaging slice ("exit phenomenon") causing this characteristic lack of signal on spin echo images [1]. Note a left subclavian catheter (*arrows*) in place. Large amounts of ascites (*see asterisk*) are noted as high-signal intensity fluid in this T2-weighted image. **B**, Axial bright blood time-of-flight image at the level of the upper chest in the same patient as in **A** shows a bright signal in the left brachiocephalic vein, which confirms blood flow. The central filling defect (*arrow*) corresponds to the same catheter in **A**. **C**, Axial bright blood cardiac-gated fast imaging employing steady-state precession (SSFP) of the chest shows the characteristic homogeneous signal intensity of blood vessels on these acquisitions [2]. Thrombus and catheters (*arrow*) are usually of low signal intensity. However, because the intravascular signal on balance SSFP is caused by the T2/T1 contrast of blood and is nearly independent of blood flow [3], detection of blood clots may be challenging when they are isointense to blood [4]. This situation is more common during the subacute stage, between 1 and 2 weeks after the onset of symptoms. Turbulent flow and pulsatility artifacts also cause intravenous filling defects that can be misinterpreted as clots [4].

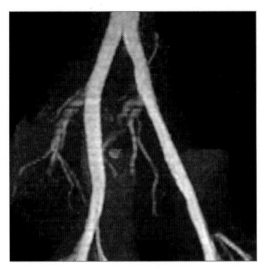

Figure 19-3. Time-of-flight (TOF) cardiovascular magnetic resonance. Maximum intensity projection (MIP) reconstruction from a multislice axial TOF acquisition of the pelvis shows the normal lower inferior vena cava and both internal and external iliac veins, bilaterally. A repetition time shorter than the longitudinal relaxation time of stationary spins in the imaging slice, and a relatively large flip angle cause partial saturation of their magnetization, which leads to decreased signal intensity [5]. Unsaturated moving spins in the flowing blood move into the imaging slice with intact magnetization providing much stronger signal than the partially saturated stationary spins in the imaging slice [5]. The contrast between the decreased signal from partially saturated stationary spins in the imaging slice and the strong signal from unsaturated blood spins entering the imaging slice provides the TOF effect [5]. Thrombus appears as low signal intensity filling defects on TOF imaging. A saturation pulse can be used to selectively eliminate the signal from the flowing spins entering the slice from a chosen direction [6]. In this example, a saturation pulse was applied above the imaging slice to selectively saturate the signal from arterial flow. These images can then be reconstructed using a MIP algorithm to generate conventional venogram-like images.

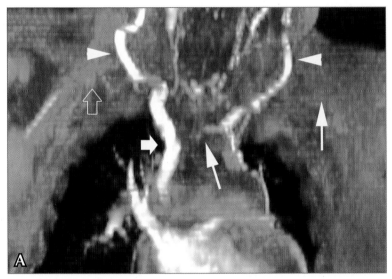

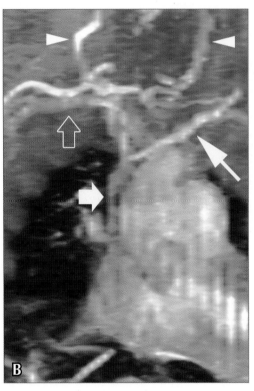

Figure 19-4. Optimization of time-of-flight (TOF) cardiovascular magnetic resonance. The imaging slice should be oriented perpendicular to the vessel of interest to achieve maximum inflow enhancement. Blood spins moving parallel to the imaging slice acquire the excitation history of the stationary spins in the imaging slice, which leads to partial saturation and decreased vessel-to-background contrast. Similarly, the thicker the imaging slice, the longer the blood spins travel within the slice increasing the potential to receive multiple excitation pulses and becoming partially saturated. This effect is more significant with slower flow. **A,** Maximum intensity projection (MIP) from a multislice axial TOF acquisition of the chest shows excellent flow in the right and left internal jugular veins (*arrowheads*) and superior vena cava (SVC) (*short arrow*) because of their vertical orientation perpendicular to the imaging slice. The horizontally oriented right (*open arrow*) and left (*long arrows*) subclavian/brachiocephalic veins are not visualized because of inplane saturation of the blood spins moving parallel to the imaging slice. **B,** MIP reconstruction from a multislice sagittal TOF acquisition in the same patient as in **A** confirms the presence of normal flow in the right subclavian/brachiocephalic vein (*open arrow*) and left brachiocephalic vein (*long arrow*). The sagittal acquisition is now perpendicular to these vessels, which improves the detection of blood flow by minimizing the amount of time the blood spins travel within the imaging slice. However, the vertically oriented right and left internal jugular veins (*arrowheads*) and SVC (*short arrow*) are now partially saturated because of their orientation parallel to the imaging slice.

Certain cardiovascular magnetic resonance features may indicate the chronicity of the venous thrombosis. Acute venous thrombosis fills and typically expands the lumen of the vein [7]. Frequently, acute/subacute venous thrombus demonstrates increased signal intensity on T2-weighted images. Edema (with high signal intensity) in the wall of the thrombosed vein and surrounding tissues is also commonly seen on these images [7]. Chronic thrombus is frequently of low signal intensity on T1- and T2-weighted sequences. Chronically occluded veins decrease in caliber, and not uncommonly are undetectable on cross-sectional imaging studies as they become a thin fibrotic remnant [8]. Collateral vessels are a secondary sign also indicative of subacute to chronic occlusion.

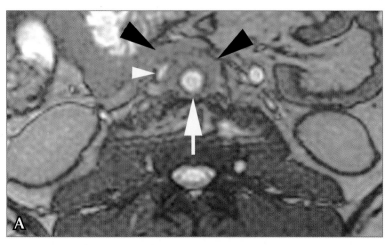

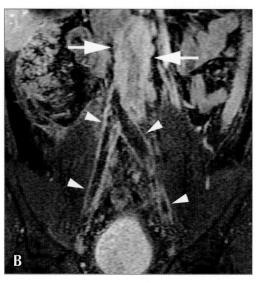

Figure 19-5. Acute thrombosis of the inferior vena cava (IVC)/iliac veins from retroperitoneal fibrosis. **A,** Axial fast imaging employing steady-state free precession of the abdomen shows a soft tissue mass (*black arrowheads*) encasing the distal abdominal aorta (*white arrow*). The IVC (*white arrowhead*) is also encased and attenuated by this mass. **B,** Coronal three-dimensional fat-saturated T1-weighted spoiled gradient echo image during the delayed venous phase after administration of gadolinium confirms the presence of a homogenously enhancing soft tissue mass (*arrows*) encasing the aorta consistent with retroperitoneal fibrosis. The mass also encases the IVC, which is not well identified. The lower IVC, just above the bifurcation, and iliac veins (*arrowheads*) are distended and filled with nonenhancing thrombus. A surgical biopsy confirmed the diagnosis of retroperitoneal fibrosis.

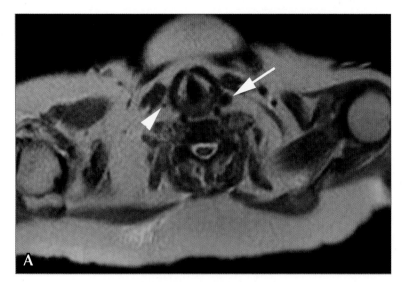

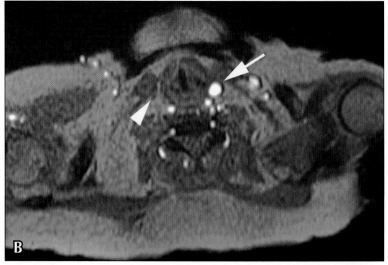

Figure 19-6. Chronic thrombosis of the right internal jugular vein in a patient with prior history of indwelling catheters. **A,** Axial T2-weighted single shot fast spin echo cardiovascular magnetic resonance through the upper chest shows a normal flow void in the left internal jugular vein (*arrow*). A right internal jugular vein (*arrowhead*) is not clearly seen, although a tiny remnant may be present. **B,** Axial two-dimensional time-of-flight image at the same level as **A** confirms the presence of flow in the left internal jugular vein (*arrow*) and lack of flow in the right internal jugular vein (*arrowhead*), which is consistent with chronic occlusion.

Bland thrombus is typically recognized as nonenhancing intravenous filling defects. Tumor thrombus is by definition vascularized, and hence may demonstrate flow on Doppler ultrasound [9], and enhancement on contrast-enhanced CT and cardiovascular magnetic resonance [10].

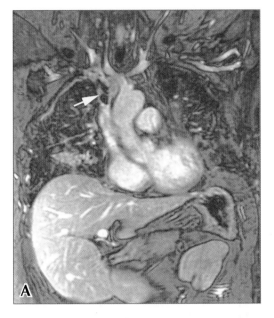

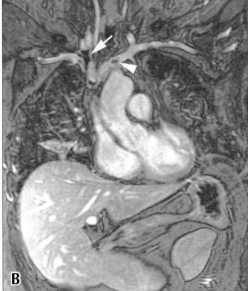

Figure 19-7. Bland thrombus in a patient with prior history of multiple indwelling catheters. **A,** Coronal three-dimensional fat-saturated T1-weighted spoiled gradient echo acquisition of the chest during the venous phase after administration of gadolinium shows a nonenhancing filling defect (*arrow*) in the upper aspect of the superior vena cava. **B,** Coronal image from the same acquisition as shown in **A** at a slightly more posterior location demonstrates additional nonenhancing filling defects in the right internal jugular (*arrow*) and left brachiocephalic (*arrowhead*) veins.

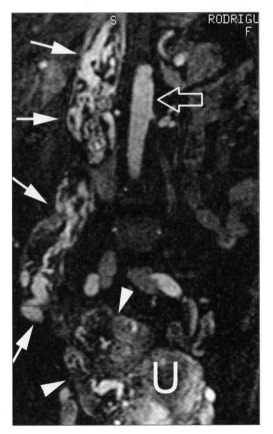

Figure 19-8. Tumor thrombus in the inferior vena cava (IVC) in a patient with intravenous leiomyomatosis. Coronal subtracted (postcontrast minus precontrast) three-dimensional fat-saturated T1-weighted spoiled gradient echo image during delayed venous phase shows a heterogeneous mass (*arrowheads*) during the delayed venous phase arising from the uterus (U) and extending superiorly along the right gonadal vein into the IVC (*arrows*). Note heterogeneous intense enhancement in the mass and tumor thrombus with large abnormal blood vessels. Detection of enhancement in a filling defect within a vein is consistent with the presence of vascularization in tumor thrombus. (*open arrow indicates aorta*).

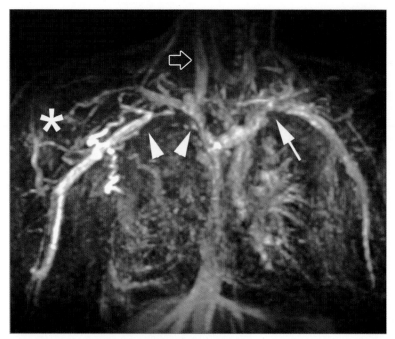

Figure 19-9. Venous roadmap for central catheter placement in a patient with multiple unsuccessful attempts to catheterize the right subclavian vein. Coronal subtracted (postcontrast during venous phase minus postcontrast during the arterial phase) three-dimensional fat-saturated T1-weighted spoiled gradient echo image demonstrates the central veins in the chest. There is occlusion of the distal right subclavian and brachiocephalic vein (*arrowheads*) with increased venous collaterals (*asterisk*). The right internal jugular vein (*open arrow*) is patent while the left internal jugular vein is not visualized. A short segment stenosis (*arrow*) is also present in the left subclavian vein. Cardiovascular magnetic resonance venography provides a roadmap of the venous system that can be used to select the best target vessel for catheterization and/or to plan a venous recanalization [11].

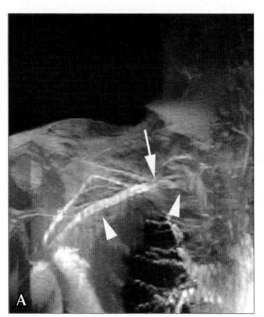

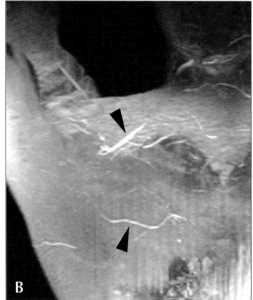

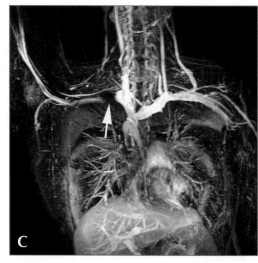

Figure 19-10. Thoracic outlet syndrome in a patient with prior right upper extremity thrombosis. **A,** Maximum intensity projection (MIP) reconstruction from a time-of-flight (TOF) acquisition with the right arm in neutral position shows a patent right brachiocephalic/subclavian vein (*arrowheads*). Note the narrowing (*arrow*) at the level of the thoracic outlet causing heterogeneous signal because of turbulent flow. **B,** MIP reconstruction from a TOF acquisition in the same patient with the right arm in an abducted position demonstrates lack of flow in the brachiocephalic/subcla- vian vein and collateral veins (*arrowheads*). **C,** Coronal subtracted (postcontrast during venous phase minus postcontrast during arterial phase) three-dimensional fat-saturated T1-weighted spoiled gradient echo image obtained with the right arm in the abducted position confirms the presence of a short segment occlusion (*arrow*) of the right brachiocephalic/subclavian vein at the level of the thoracic outlet. These findings are consistent with reversal venous occlusion during abduction maneuvers of the right upper extremity [12].

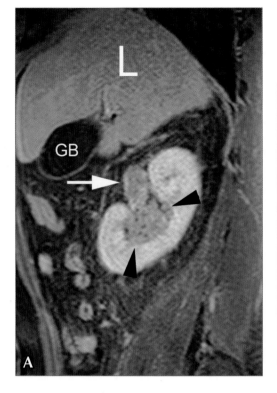

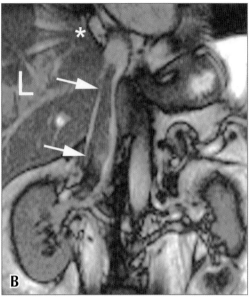

Figure 19-11. Inferior vena cava (IVC) thrombosis in renal cell carcinoma (RCC). Thrombosis of the renal veins and IVC is common in patients with advanced RCC. Cardiovascular magnetic resonance is superior to CT in the detection and characterization of the renal vein and the IVC thrombus in these patients [13]. **A,** Sagittal contrast-enhanced three-dimensional fat-saturated T1-weighted spoiled gradient echo image during the delayed venous phase shows a centrally located infiltrating renal mass (*arrowheads*). The mass extends into the renal hilum and along the proximal right renal vein (*arrow*). **B,** Coronal fast imaging employing steady-state free precession better demonstrates the extension of the tumor thrombus (*arrows*) along the IVC to the level just inferior to the confluence with the hepatic veins (*asterisk*). GB—gallbladder; L—liver.

REFERENCES

1. Miller SW, Holmvang G: Differentiation of slow flow from thrombus in thoracic magnetic resonance imaging, emphasizing phase images. *J Thorac Imaging* 1993, 8:98–107.

2. Carr JC, Simonetti O, Bundy J, *et al.*: Cine MR angiography of the heart with segmented true fast imaging with steady-state precession. *Radiology* 2001, 219:828–834.

3. Plein S, Bloomer TN, Ridgway JP, *et al.*: Steady-state free precession magnetic resonance imaging of the heart: comparison with segmented k-space gradient-echo imaging. *J Magn Reson Imaging* 2001, 14:230–236.

4. Pedrosa I, Morrin M, Oleaga L, *et al.*: Is true FISP imaging reliable in the evaluation of venous thrombosis? *AJR Am J Roentgenol* 2005, 185:1632–1640.

5. Laub GA. Time-of-flight method of MR angiography. *Magn Reson Imaging Clin North Am* 1995, 3:391–398.

6. Felmlee JP, Ehman RL. Spatial presaturation: a method for suppressing flow artifacts and improving depiction of vascular anatomy in MR imaging. *Radiology* 1987, 164:559–564.

7. Froehlich JB, Prince MR, Greenfield LJ, *et al.*: "Bull's-eye" sign on gadolinium-enhanced magnetic resonance venography determines thrombus presence and age: a preliminary study. *J Vasc Surg* 1997, 26:809–816.

8. Polak JF, Fox LA: MR assessment of the extremity veins. *Semin Ultrasound CT MR* 1999, 20:36–46.

9. Dodd GD, 3rd, Memel DS, Baron RL, *et al.*: Portal vein thrombosis in patients with cirrhosis: does sonographic detection of intrathrombus flow allow differentiation of benign and malignant thrombus? *AJR Am J Roentgenol* 1995, 165:573–577.

10. Tublin ME, Dodd GD, 3rd, Baron RL: Benign and malignant portal vein thrombosis: differentiation by CT characteristics. *AJR Am J Roentgenol* 1997, 168:719–723.

11. Shinde TS, Lee VS, Rofsky NM, *et al.*: Three-dimensional gadolinium-enhanced MR venographic evaluation of patency of central veins in the thorax: initial experience. *Radiology* 1999, 213:555–560.

12. Demondion X, Bacqueville E, Paul C, *et al.*: Thoracic outlet: assessment with MR imaging in asymptomatic and symptomatic populations. *Radiology* 2003, 227:461–468.

13. Semelka RC, Shoenut JP, Magro CM, *et al.*: Renal cancer staging: comparison of contrast-enhanced CT and gadolinium-enhanced fat-suppressed spin-echo and gradient-echo MR imaging. *J Magn Reson Imaging* 1993, 3:597–602.

20

CHAPTER

Left Atrium and Pulmonary Veins

Thomas H. Hauser

With the advent of radiofrequency ablation for the treatment of atrial fibrillation, an increased interest developed in the accurate determination of left atrial and pulmonary vein anatomy to help plan the procedure and to monitor for postablation stenosis. Cardiovascular magnetic resonance (CMR) readily demonstrates the left atrium (LA) and pulmonary veins, and is the method of choice for serial imaging studies.

Atrial fibrillation is the most common sustained cardiac arrhythmia, affecting more than 2 million people in the United States, and is a major cause of morbidity and mortality, accounting for more than 400,000 hospitalizations each year, increasing the morbidity rate by 50% [1-3]. Atrial fibrillation quintuples the risk of stroke and is the attributed cause for 15% of all strokes, totaling more than 100,000 per year [2,4]. The hospital costs alone associated with the treatment of atrial fibrillation are estimated at over $1 billion [2]. Although several antiarrhythmic drugs are available for the treatment of atrial fibrillation, all are associated with significant side effects or adverse events, and maintenance of sinus rhythm is frequently suboptimal [5-8].

Although the role of the LA in the development of atrial fibrillation was recognized for some time, recent evidence has shown that the pulmonary veins also play a critical role in the pathophysiology of atrial fibrillation. The pulmonary veins and LA are both derived from the primitive common pulmonary vein and therefore possess many anatomic similarities [9]. Both are smooth-walled structures that have electrically active myocardium. Approximately 90% of pulmonary veins contain atrial myocardium [10].

Although atrial myocardium is uniform, myocardium in the pulmonary veins is frequently discontinuous and fibrotic. Patients with a history of atrial fibrillation uniformly have myocardium in the pulmonary veins and an increased rate of structural abnormalities. These structural abnormalities result in abnormal electrical activation with slow and anisotropic conduction. Proarrhythmic reentrant beats and sustained focal activity can easily be induced [11].

A landmark study demonstrated that the proarrhythmic electrical activity in the pulmonary veins is directly responsible for the generation of atrial fibrillation in many patients [12]. Among those with paroxysmal atrial fibrillation, 94% had ectopic foci in the pulmonary veins that were responsible for the induction of atrial fibrillation. Radiofrequency ablation of these foci resulted in complete suppression of atrial fibrillation in a majority of patients. After the findings were reported, several related procedures were developed for the treatment of atrial fibrillation [12-15]. Each of these procedures uses radiofrequency ablation to electrically isolate the pulmonary veins from the LA, with or without additional ablation in the LA. Short-term success rates range from 65% to 85% in patients with paroxysmal atrial fibrillation, with a reduction in morbidity and improved quality of life [16].

CMR imaging of the LA and pulmonary veins is usually performed before atrial fibrillation ablation to determine the LA and pulmonary vein anatomy, and again after the procedure to screen for pulmonary vein stenosis. In this chapter, normal and variant anatomy of the LA and pulmonary veins will be reviewed, as well as pathology related to atrial fibrillation ablation and congenital disease.

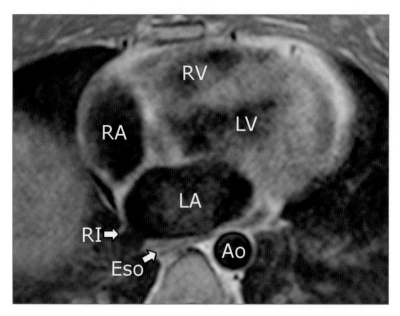

Figure 20-1. Axial spin echo image of the left atrium (LA) and pulmonary veins. The LA and pulmonary veins can easily be identified on standard T1-weighted spin echo cardiovascular magnetic resonance [17]. Shown is an axial image of the LA and right inferior pulmonary vein (RI) in relation to the left ventricle (LV), right ventricle (RV), right atrium (RA), and the descending aorta (Ao). The image was acquired during ventricular systole. The size of the LA is often determined by measuring the maximal anterior-posterior dimension during ventricular systole, a method analogous to echocardiography [18]. Visualization of the pulmonary veins is generally limited to their proximal segments.

The esophagus (Eso) and its relationship to the LA can be readily identified in this image. The formation of an atrial-esophageal fistula is a rare but catastrophic complication of radiofrequency ablation procedures for the treatment of atrial fibrillation that is caused by excessive heating of the LA wall and the adjacent esophagus [19,20]. The esophagus almost always directly abuts the LA and is usually closer to the left-sided pulmonary veins, but the location is highly variable [21,22]. The esophagus is frequently within 5 mm of the pulmonary veins at a location that most likely increases the risk for the formation of an atrial-esophageal fistula [23,24]. The risk of causing an atrial-esophageal fistula may be reduced by avoiding ablation in the region of the LA closest to the esophagus, but this may be difficult as the esophagus is mobile and may move during the course of the procedure [25].

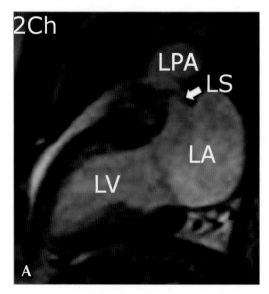
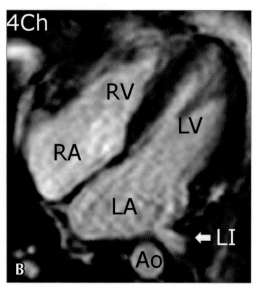

Figure 20-2. Steady-state free precession (SSFP) images of the left atrium (LA) and pulmonary veins. The LA and pulmonary veins can also be visualized using standard SSFP cardiovascular magnetic resonance. These images are usually obtained with electrocardiogram-gating to assess changes in anatomy throughout the cardiac cycle. Although these images can be obtained in any plane, the LA is typically imaged in the two-chamber (2Ch) and four-chamber (4Ch) views. The figure shows still images obtained during ventricular systole. **A,** The two-chamber image shows the relationship of the LA to the left ventricle (LV) and the left pulmonary artery (LPA). **B,** Four-chamber image showing the relationship of the LA to the LV, right ventricle (RV), right atrium (RA), and the descending aorta (Ao). The proximal segments of the left superior (LS) and left inferior (LI) pulmonary veins is visible.

Left atrial cavity size is related to several cardiovascular risk factors and the occurrence of adverse cardiovascular events, especially the occurrence of atrial fibrillation and adverse outcomes associated with atrial fibrillation [26-32]. While the maximal anterior-posterior dimension of the LA obtained from spin echo images is the most commonly used measure of LA size, LA volume may be a better determinant of adverse outcomes [33-35]. Atrial volume is usually determined at ventricular systole, when the LA is at its maximal size. The LA volume can be determined directly by obtaining a stack of images throughout the entire LA using disk summation or estimated from the two-chamber and four-chamber images using the biplane disk method [33,36].

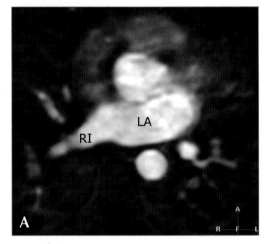
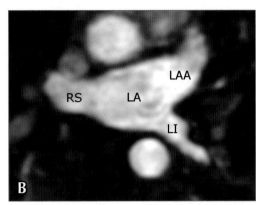
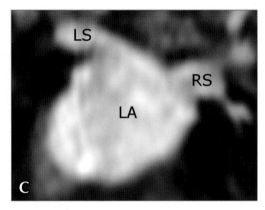

Figure 20-3. Cardiovascular magnetic resonance (CMR) angiography of the pulmonary veins. The pulmonary veins are usually imaged using contrast enhanced CMR angiography. A three-dimensional spoiled gradient echo sequence is acquired during the first-pass of gadolinium contrast [37]. The technique uses short repetition times (3-6 ms), high flip angles (30°-60°), and fractional echoes to provide T1-weighting and minimal flow artifacts. Spatial resolution is typically 2 × 2 mm in-plane with 4-mm slices, before interpolation. A single three-dimensional volume requires a 10- to 20-second breath-hold to suppress ventilatory motion. Electrocardiogram triggering is not employed, although the position and shape of the pulmonary veins changes throughout the cardiac cycle [38,39]. Images obtained with this method appear to reflect the pulmonary veins at their maximal size [40]. Timing of the acquisition to the first pass of contrast through the pulmonary veins is critical, and is achieved using either a bolus timing scan or with fluoroscopic triggering [41,42].

There are usually four pulmonary veins that enter the left atrium (LA): right superior (RS), right inferior (RI), left superior (LS) and left inferior (LI). Each of the veins is directed laterally, with the inferior veins directed posteriorly and the superior veins directed anteriorly. The LS pulmonary vein frequently has a cranial angulation and may appear to arise from the superior portion of the LA. The figures show axial (**A, B**) and coronal (**C**) slices from a three-dimensional cardiovascular magnetic resonance angiography dataset demonstrating the relationship of the pulmonary veins to the LA and the LA appendage (LAA).

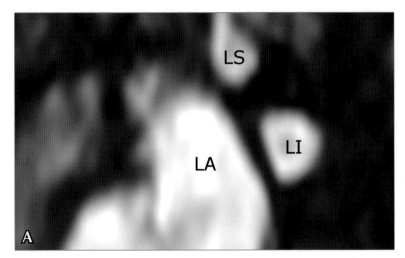
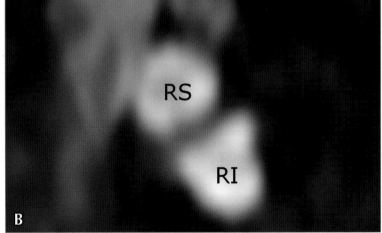

Figure 20-4. Quantification of pulmonary vein size. The accurate measurement of pulmonary vein size is essential for serial assessment of pulmonary vein stenosis. Most investigators have measured pulmonary vein diameters in a specified plane, usually at the ostia [43-45]. These measurements typically have poor reproducibility. A simple method for determining pulmonary vein size in the sagittal plane is highly reproducible. The maximal diameter, perimeter, and cross-sectional area can be measured at the location in the sagittal plane at which the pulmonary veins separate from the left atrium (LA) and from each other. Shown is this location for the left superior (LS) and left inferior (LI) (**A**), and right superior (RS) and right inferior (RI) (**B**) pulmonary veins. The LA extends underneath the left-sided pulmonary veins. Because the measurements are made in a standard plane and location, reproducibility is greatly improved compared with standard diameter measurements [46]. This allows for more accurate determination of inter-study differences in pulmonary vein size and increased statistical power in research studies. Even in the absence of severe stenosis, this method can identify small changes in pulmonary vein size after atrial fibrillation ablation that may be caused by hemodynamic changes related to the restoration of sinus rhythm [47]. The determination of the perimeter and cross-sectional area is also advantageous. Patients with a larger summed total pulmonary vein cross-sectional area are more likely to have recurrent atrial fibrillation after ablation independent of the atrial fibrillation type or LA size [48]. Diameter measurements do not have predictive value [16].

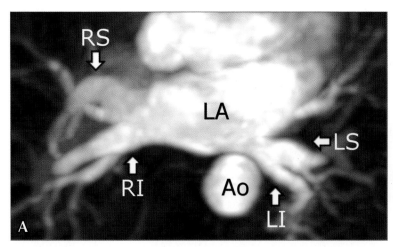

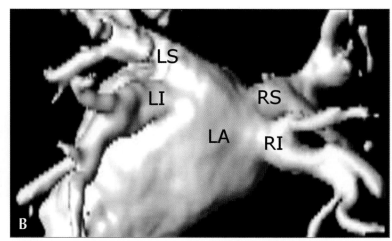

Figure 20-5. Summary images of the left atrium (LA) and pulmonary veins. Shown are maximal intensity projection (**A**) and volume rendered (**B**) images of the LA and the left superior (LS), left inferior (LI), right superior (RS), and right inferior (RI) pulmonary veins. These images take full advantage of the three-dimensional dataset and provide excellent summary images. The volume rendered image is most useful when the displayed volume is limited to the LA and pulmonary veins, with exclusion of the aorta (Ao) from the displayed volume.

The accurate determination of pulmonary vein anatomy is critical for the planning and execution of atrial fibrillation ablation. To achieve success, the operator must place a series of radiofrequency lesions that encircle the pulmonary veins and electrically isolate

them from the LA [49]. This requires that pulmonary vein anatomy be determined prior to the procedure. In the initial development of the procedure, the pulmonary veins are identified using invasive contrast venography [44]. Although this can be done successfully, it greatly increases the procedure time and only provides projection images of the pulmonary veins. Most centers now use cardiovascular magnetic resonance angiography or CT angiography to determine the pulmonary vein anatomy prior to the procedure. Either technique provides high-resolution three-dimensional and tomographic images of the pulmonary veins and other mediastinal structures. These images can also be imported into electrophysiological mapping systems that are an integral part of the procedure to combine anatomic and functional information [50].

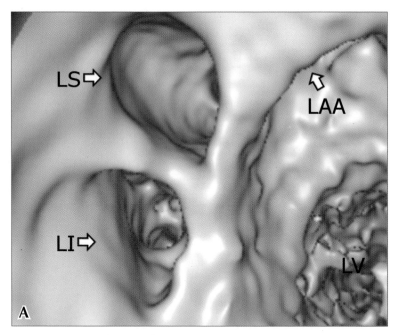

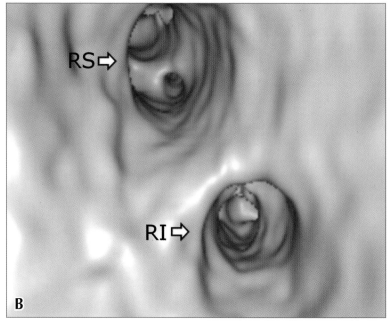

Figure 20-6. Endovascular view of the pulmonary veins. Three-dimensional images can be reformatted so that the pulmonary veins can be viewed from a perspective inside the left atrium (LA). **A**, Left superior (LS) and left inferior (LI) pulmonary veins are adjacent to the LA appendage (LAA) and across from the left ventricle. **B**, Right superior (RS) and right inferior (RI) pulmonary veins are also shown. The embryology of the LA and pulmonary veins is intricately linked. The endovascular view of the pulmonary veins highlights this intimate relationship, as there is no clear anatomic border between them. The pulmonary veins and LA are derived from the primitive common pulmonary vein. The primitive pulmonary venous system initially has no connection with the heart and drains into the cardinal veins

and the umbilicovitelline system. At approximately the fourth week of gestation, the pulmonary venous drainage coalesces into a single vessel [51]. Simultaneously, an outgrowth of the primitive LA extends toward the pulmonary venous system to meet this vessel and to form the primitive common pulmonary vein. The common pulmonary vein then expands to form the smooth-walled body of the LA while the primitive LA forms the trabeculated LA appendage [9]. The branches of the primitive common pulmonary vein form the adult pulmonary veins. The development of the LA and pulmonary veins is asymmetrical, with the two right-sided pulmonary veins developing first, while the left-sided pulmonary venous drainage enters the LA through a single trunk that eventually bifurcates [52].

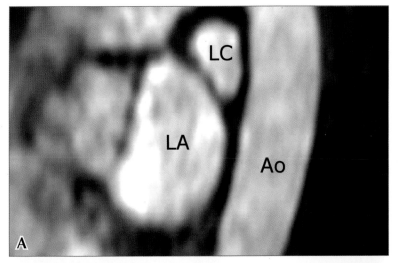

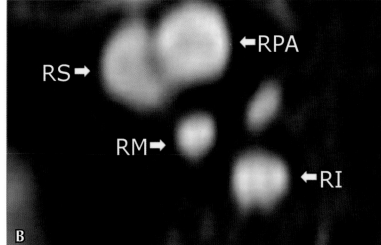

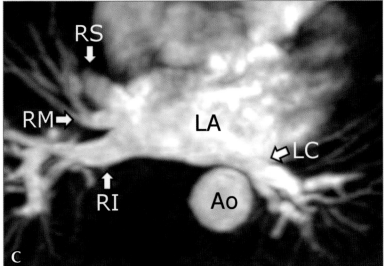

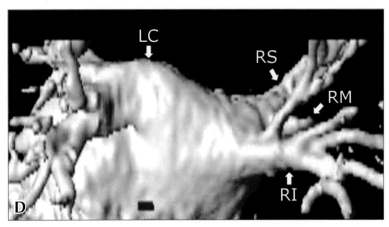

Figure 20-7. Variant pulmonary vein anatomy. Variant, non-pathologic pulmonary vein anatomy is common, present in approximately 40% of patients [45,53]. Although numerous variations have been described, the most common variations are the presence of a single left common pulmonary vein or an additional right middle pulmonary vein [46]. These variations mainly occur from the incorporation of the primitive common pulmonary vein into the left atrium (LA). Less incorporation leads to apparent fusion of pulmonary veins prior to entering the LA, whereas more incorporation results in additional pulmonary veins [54]. Because the right-sided pulmonary veins form first and have more developmental time to incorporate into the LA, it is more common to have additional veins on the right. Converse-

ly, the left-sided pulmonary veins form later and are more likely to have a common trunk.

These images were obtained from a patient with right middle and left common pulmonary veins. **A,** The common left pulmonary vein (LC) is easily identified in the sagittal plane, adjacent to the LA and descending aorta (Ao). **B,** The right middle pulmonary vein (RM) is also identified in the sagittal plane adjacent to the right superior (RS) and right inferior (RI) pulmonary veins and the right pulmonary artery (RPA). All of the pulmonary veins are shown in the axial maximal intensity projection (**C**) and posterior-anterior volume-rendered (**D**) images. The right middle pulmonary vein is obscured somewhat by the right inferior pulmonary vein. It is frequently necessary to manipulate the point of view to see all of the pulmonary veins.

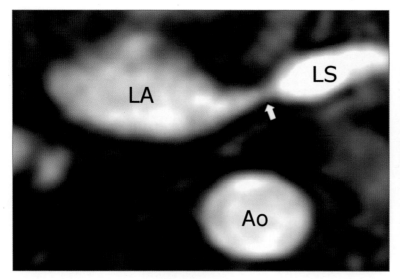

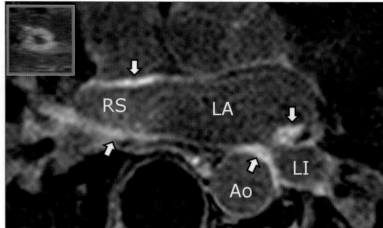

Figure 20-8. Pulmonary vein stenosis. Shown here is the severe stenosis of a left superior pulmonary vein (LS) at its ostium with the left atrium (LA), indicated by the *arrow*, and with prestenotic dilation of the pulmonary vein.

Pulmonary vein stenosis is an uncommon but severe complication of radiofrequency ablation for the treatment of atrial fibrillation [43-45, 53, 55-60]. The application of radiofrequency energy to the pulmonary veins causes intimal proliferation and myocardial necrosis that can result in stenosis or occlusion [61]. Severe stenosis occurs in up to 5% of patients after the procedure, and results in pulmonary hypertension and decreased perfusion of the affected lung segments [62,63]. Patients frequently present with cough or dyspnea, but a significant proportion are asymptomatic [57]. Stenosis is most likely to occur in smaller pulmonary veins in which the ablation lesions were placed further into the pulmonary vein trunk, and with greater extent of ablation [43,60]. If stenosis does occur, pulmonary vein balloon angioplasty is usually successful in restoring normal flow and alleviating symptoms [64]. Newer techniques that have emphasized placing ablation lesions closer to the LA under intracardiac echocardiographic guidance have reduced the rate of pulmonary vein stenosis, but screening is still recommended for all patients [56]. Ao—aorta.

Figure 20-9. Left atrial (LA) and pulmonary vein scar imaging. Radiofrequency ablation for the treatment of atrial fibrillation results in scarring of the pulmonary vein and LA [61]. Scar cardiovascular magnetic resonance (CMR) imaging has the potential to noninvasively assess the completeness of ablation by providing a precise anatomic map of the ablation lines. This could be useful either after the procedure to assess the adequacy of ablation or as a real-time tool to guide ablation during the ablation procedure. Scar can be detected using the late gadolinium enhancement (LGE) technique, in which a strongly T1-weighted CMR is acquired late after the injection of gadolinium contrast [65, 66]. Gadolinium contrast remains concentrated in the regions of scar, compared with muscle or blood, because of reduced clearance and the large contrast volume of distribution in fibrotic regions [67]. To detect scar in the LA, the standard method is modified to achieve higher spatial resolution (1.3 × 1.3 × 5 mm) by acquiring a three-dimensional volume during free-breathing with ventilatory motion compensated imaging [68].

The figure shows a LGE image with bright signal indicating scar (*arrows*) at the junction of the right superior (RS) and left inferior (LI) pulmonary veins with the LA. The *inset* shows circumferential scarring around the LI pulmonary vein. Ao—aorta.

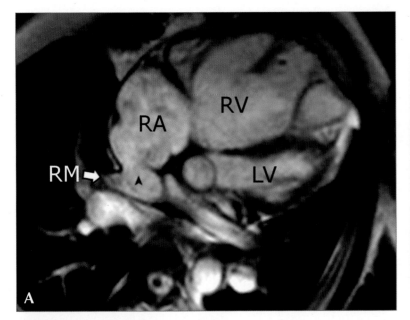

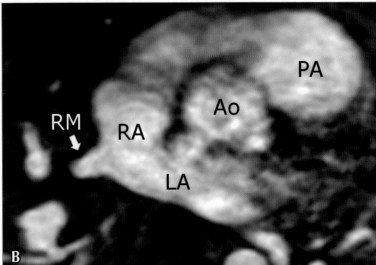

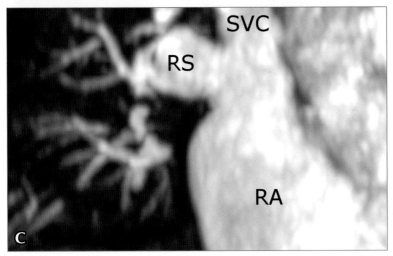

comprising 70% of defects [70]. Ostium primum defects affect the inferior portion of the atrial septum, are usually associated with a cleft mitral valve, and comprise 20% of all defects. Sinus venosus defects, comprising 6% of all defects, affect the superior portion of the atrial septum, often with drainage of the superior vena cava (SVC) into both atria. These defects are frequently associated with partial anomalous pulmonary venous return involving the right-sided pulmonary veins. Coronary sinus defects occur rarely.

These images were obtained in an adult with a sinus venosus atrial septal defect with partial anomalous pulmonary venous return. **A,** Horizontal long-axis steady-state free precession image shows the defect (*arrowhead*). The right middle (RM) pulmonary vein connects at the juncture of the atria. The right atrium (RA) and right ventricle (RV) are markedly enlarged, consistent with chronic volume overload, while the left ventricle (LV) is normal. **B,** Magnetic resonance angiography in the axial plane shows the connection of the RM pulmonary vein to the RA and left atrium (LA) adjacent to the ascending aorta (Ao). The pulmonary artery (PA) is enlarged. **C,** An image in the coronal plane shows the connection of the right superior (RS) pulmonary vein to the junction of the RA and the SVC.

Figure 20-10. Sinus venosus atrial septal defect with partial anomalous pulmonary venous return. Atrial septal defects are common, comprising 10% of all congenital heart disease [69]. There are four major types of atrial septal defect. Ostium secundum defects involve the fossa ovalis and are the most common,

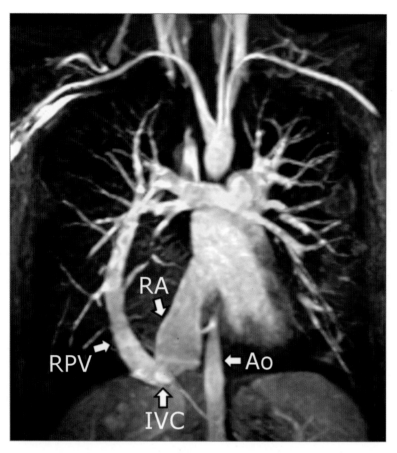

Figure 20-11. Scimitar syndrome. Congenital pulmonary venous anomalies account for 3% of all congenital heart disease and 2% of deaths from congenital heart disease in the first year of life [71]. Anomalous pulmonary venous connections are the most common congenital anomaly [71]. Total anomalous pulmonary venous connection occurs when there is no connection of the pulmonary veins to the left atrium such that all pulmonary venous drainage enters the right atrium (RA). This is necessarily associated with an atrial right to left shunt. Although the mortality rate for symptomatic infants is 80% at 1 year, surgical repair is usually feasible and reduces the mortality rate to less than 25% [71, 72]. In partial anomalous pulmonary venous connection, one or more pulmonary veins, but not all, enter the RA. Surgical repair is usually straightforward. Shown here is an example of the scimitar syndrome, a specific type of partial anomalous connection named after a characteristic chest radiograph finding. A common right pulmonary vein (RPV) drains into the inferior vena cava (IVC) and the RA. This rare syndrome is also associated with anomalous arterial supply of the right lower lobe from the aorta (Ao), dextroposition of the heart, and hypoplasia of the right lung [73]. Congenial pulmonary vein stenosis and atresia occur rarely.

Imaging patients with cardiovascular magnetic resonance (CMR) angiography who have congenital anomalies is a valuable method for determining the pulmonary venous anatomy. CMR angiography is generally able to identify all pulmonary venous anomalies, providing new information in 75% and identifying previously unsuspected anomalies in 30% [74]. (*Courtesy of* A. Powell, MD.)

REFERENCES

1. Feinberg WM, Blackshear JL, Laupacis A, *et al.*: Prevalence, age distribution, and gender of patients with atrial fibrillation. Analysis and implications. *Arch Intern Med* 1995, 155:469–473.

2. Heart Disease and Stroke Statistics — 2004 Update. Dallas, TX: American Heart Association.

3. Benjamin EJ, Wolf PA, D'Agostino RB, *et al.*: Impact of atrial fibrillation on the risk of death: the Framingham Heart Study. *Circulation* 1998, 98:946–952.

4. Wolf PA, Abbott RD, Kannel WB: Atrial fibrillation as an independent risk factor for stroke: the Framingham Study. *Stroke* 1991, 22:983–988.

5. Hauser TH, Pinto DS, Josephson ME, Zimetbaum P: Safety and feasibility of a clinical pathway for the outpatient initiation of antiarrhythmic medications in patients with atrial fibrillation or atrial flutter. *Am J Cardiol* 2003, 91:1437–1441.

6. Hauser TH, Pinto DS, Josephson ME, Zimetbaum P: Early recurrence of arrhythmia in patients taking amiodarone or class 1C agents for treatment of atrial fibrillation or atrial flutter. *Am J Cardiol* 2004, 93:1173–1176.

7. Singh BN, Singh SN, Reda DJ, *et al.*: Amiodarone versus sotalol for atrial fibrillation. *N Engl J Med* 2005, 352:1861–1872.

8. Roy D, Talajic M, Dorian P, *et al.*: Amiodarone to prevent recurrence of atrial fibrillation. Canadian Trial of Atrial Fibrillation Investigators. *N Engl J Med* 2000, 342:913–920.

9. Moore KL: *The Developing Human.* Philadelphia: WB Saunders Co; 1988.

10. Hassink RJ, Aretz HT, Ruskin J, Keane D: Morphology of atrial myocardium in human pulmonary veins: a postmortem analysis in patients with and without atrial fibrillation. *J Am Coll Cardiol* 2003, 42:1108–1114.

11. Arora R, Verheule S, Scott L, *et al.*: Arrhythmogenic substrate of the pulmonary veins assessed by high-resolution optical mapping. *Circulation* 2003, 107:1816–1821.

12. Haissaguerre M, Jais P, Shah DC, *et al.*: Spontaneous initiation of atrial fibrillation by ectopic beats originating in the pulmonary veins. *N Engl J Med* 1998, 339:659–666.

13. Pappone C, Rosanio S, Oreto G, *et al.*: Circumferential radiofrequency ablation of pulmonary vein ostia. A new anatomic approach for curing atrial fibrillation. *Circulation* 2000, 102:2619–2628.

14. Arentz T, von Rosenthal J, Blum T, *et al.*: Feasibility and safety of pulmonary vein isolation using a new mapping and navigation system in patients with refractory atrial fibrillation. *Circulation* 2003, 108:2484–2490.

15. Oral H, Knight BP, Ozaydin M, *et al.*: Segmental ostial ablation to isolate the pulmonary veins during atrial fibrillation: feasibility and mechanistic insights. *Circulation* 2002, 106:1256–1262.

16. Pappone C, Rosanio S, Augello G, *et al.*: Mortality, morbidity, and quality of life after circumferential pulmonary vein ablation for atrial fibrillation: outcomes from a controlled nonrandomized long-term study. *J Am Coll Cardiol* 2003, 42:185–197.

17. Friedman BJ, Waters J, Kwan OL, DeMaria AN: Comparison of magnetic resonance imaging and echocardiography in determination of cardiac dimensions in normal subjects. *J Am Coll Cardiol* 1985, 5:1369–1376.

18. Benjamin EJ, D'Agostino RB, Belanger AJ, *et al.*: Left atrial size and the risk of stroke and death. The Framingham Heart Study. *Circulation* 1995, 92:835–841.

19. Scanavacca MI, D'Avila A, Parga J, Sosa E: Left atrial-esophageal fistula following radiofrequency catheter ablation of atrial fibrillation. *J Cardiovasc Electrophysiol* 2004, 15:960–962.

20. Cummings JE, Schweikert RA, Saliba WI, *et al.*: Assessment of temperature, proximity, and course of the esophagus during radiofrequency ablation within the left atrium. *Circulation* 2005, 112:459–464.

21. Lemola K, Sneider M, Desjardins B, *et al.*: Computed tomographic analysis of the anatomy of the left atrium and the esophagus: implications for left atrial catheter ablation. *Circulation* 2004, 110:3655–3660.

22. Tsao HM, Wu MH, Higa S, *et al.*: Anatomic relationship of the esophagus and left atrium: implication for catheter ablation of atrial fibrillation. *Chest* 2005, 128:2581–2587.

23. Sanchez-Quintana D, Cabrera JA, Climent V, *et al.*: Anatomic relations between the esophagus and left atrium and relevance for ablation of atrial fibrillation. *Circulation* 2005, 112:1400–1405.

24. Monnig G, Wessling J, Juergens KU, *et al.*: Further evidence of a close anatomical relation between the oesophagus and pulmonary veins. *Europace* 2005, 7:540–545.

25. Good E, Oral H, Lemola K, *et al.*: Movement of the esophagus during left atrial catheter ablation for atrial fibrillation. *J Am Coll Cardiol* 2005, 46:2107–2110.

26. Vaziri SM, Larson MG, Lauer MS, *et al.*: Influence of blood pressure on left atrial size. *Hypertension* 1995, 25:1155–1160.

27. Benjamin EJ, D'Agostino RB, Belanger AJ, *et al.*: Left atrial size and the risk of stroke and death: the Framingham Heart Study. *Circulation* 1995, 92:835–841.

28. DiTullio MR, Sacco RL, Sciacca RR, Homma S: Left atrial size and the risk of ischemic stroke in an ethnically mixed population. *Stroke* 1999, 30:2019–2024.

29. Henry WL, Morganroth J, Pearlman AS, *et al.*: Relation between echocardiographically determined left atrial size and atrial fibrillation. *Circulation* 1976, 53:273–279.

30. Sanfilippo AJ, Abascal VM, Sheehan M, *et al.*: Atrial enlargement as a consequence of atrial fibrillation: a prospective echocardiographic study. *Circulation* 1990, 82:792–797.

31. Vaziri SM, Larson MG, Benjamin EJ, Levy D: Echocardiographic predictors of nonrheumatic atrial fibrillation: the Framingham Heart Study. *Circulation* 1994, 89:724–730.

32. The Stroke Prevention in Atrial Fibrillation Investigators. Predictors of thromboembolism in atrial fibrillation: II. Echocardiographic features of patients at risk. *Ann Intern Med* 1992, 116:6–12.

33. Tsang TS, Barnes ME, Bailey KR, *et al.*: Left atrial volume: important risk marker of incident atrial fibrillation in 1655 older men and women. *Mayo Clin Proc* 2001, 76:467–475.

34. Tsang TS, Barnes ME, Gersh BJ, *et al.*: Left atrial volume as a morphophysiologic expression of left ventricular diastolic dysfunction and relation to cardiovascular risk burden. *Am J Cardiol* 2002, 90:1284–1289.

35. Pritchett AM, Jacobsen SJ, Mahoney DW, *et al.*: Left atrial volume as an index of left atrial size: a population-based study. *J Am Coll Cardiol* 2003, 41:1036–1043.

36. Hauser TH, McClennen S, Katsimaglis G, *et al.*: Assessment of left atrial volume by contrast enhanced magnetic resonance angiography. *J Cardiovasc Magn Reson* 2004, 6:491–497.

37. Prince MR, Narasimham DL, Stanley JC, *et al.*: Breath-hold gadolinium-enhanced MR angiography of the abdominal aorta and its major branches. *Radiology* 1995, 197:785–792.

38. Lickfett L, Dickfeld T, Kato R, *et al.*: Changes of pulmonary vein orifice size and location throughout the cardiac cycle: dynamic analysis using magnetic resonance cine imaging. *J Cardiovasc Electrophysiol* 2005, 16:582–588.

39. Syed MA, Peters DC, Rashid H, Arai AE: Pulmonary vein imaging: comparison of 3D magnetic resonance angiography with 2D cine MRI for characterizing anatomy and size. *J Cardiovasc Magn Reson* 2005, 7:355–360.

40. Hauser TH, Yeon SB, McClennen S, *et al.*: Variability in pulmonary vein anatomy during the cardiac cycle. Society for Cardiovascular Magnetic Resonance, 2005.

41. Earls JP, Rofsky NM, DeCorato DR, *et al.*: Breath-hold single-dose gadolinium-enhanced three-dimensional MR aortography: usefulness of a timing examination and MR power injector. *Radiology* 1996, 201:705–710.

42. Wilman AH, Riederer SJ, King BF, *et al.*: Fluoroscopically triggered contrast-enhanced three-dimensional MR angiography with elliptical centric view order: application to the renal arteries. *Radiology* 1997, 205:137–146.

43. Dill T, Neumann T, Ekinci O, *et al.*: Pulmonary vein diameter reduction after radiofrequency catheter ablation for paroxysmal atrial fibrillation evaluated by contrast-enhanced three-dimensional magnetic resonance imaging. *Circulation* 2003, 107:845–850.

44. Lin WS, Prakash VS, Tai CT, *et al.*: Pulmonary vein morphology in patients with paroxysmal atrial fibrillation initiated by ectopic beats originating from the pulmonary veins: implications for catheter ablation. *Circulation* 2000, 101:1274–1281.

45. Wittkampf FH, Vonken EJ, Derksen R, *et al.*: Pulmonary vein ostium geometry: analysis by magnetic resonance angiography. *Circulation* 2003, 107:21–23.

46. Hauser TH, Yeon SB, McClennen S, *et al.*: A method for the determination of proximal pulmonary vein size using contrast-enhanced magnetic resonance angiography. *J Cardiovasc Magn Reson* 2004, 6:927–936.

47. Hauser TH, Yeon SB, McClennen S, *et al.*: Subclinical pulmonary vein narrowing after ablation for atrial fibrillation. *Heart* 2005, 91:672–673.

48. Hauser TH, Essebag V, Baldessin F, *et al.*: Larger pulmonary vein cross-sectional area is associated with recurrent atrial fibrillation after pulmonary vein isolation. *Circulation* 2005, 112(S):II-555.

49. Marine JE, Dong J, Calkins H: Catheter ablation therapy for atrial fibrillation. *Prog Cardiovasc Dis* 2005, 48:178–192.

50. Calkins H: Three dimensional mapping of atrial fibrillation: techniques and necessity. *J Interv Card Electrophysiol* 2005, 13 Suppl 1:53–59.

51. Blom NA, Gittenberger-de Groot AC, Jongeneel TH, *et al.*: Normal development of the pulmonary veins in human embryos and formulation of a morphogenetic concept for sinus venosus defects. *Am J Cardiol* 2001, 87:305–309.

52. Webb S, Kanani M, Anderson RH, *et al.*: Development of the human pulmonary vein and its incorporation in the morphologically left atrium. *Cardiol Young* 2001, 11:632–642.

53. Kato R, Lickfett L, Meininger G, *et al.*: Pulmonary vein anatomy in patients undergoing catheter ablation of atrial fibrillation: lessons learned by use of magnetic resonance imaging. *Circulation* 2003, 107:2004–2010.

54. Ghaye B, Szapiro D, Dacher JN, *et al.*: Percutaneous ablation for atrial fibrillation: the role of cross-sectional imaging. *Radiographics* 2003, 23 Spec No:S19-33; discussion S48–50.

55. Moak J, Moore H, Lee S, *et al.*: Case report: pulmonary vein stenosis following RF ablation of paroxysmal atrial fibrillation: successful treatement with balloon dilation. *J Interv Card Electrophysiol* 2000, 4:621–631.

56. Saad EB, Rossillo A, Saad CP, *et al.*: Pulmonary vein stenosis after radiofrequency ablation of atrial fibrillation: functional characterization, evolution, and influence of the ablation strategy. *Circulation* 2003, 108:3102–3107.

57. Saad EB, Marrouche NF, Saad CP, *et al.*: Pulmonary vein stenosis after catheter ablation of atrial fibrillation: emergence of a new clinical syndrome. *Ann Intern Med* 2003, 138:634–638.

58. Scanvacca M, Kajita L, Vieira M, Sosa E: Pulmonary vein stenosis complicating catheter ablation of focal atrial fibrillation. *J Cardiovasc Electrophysiol* 2000, 1:677–681.

59. Yang M, Akbari H, Reddy GP, Higgins CB: Identification of pulmonary vein stenosis after radiofrequency ablation for atrial fibrillation using MRI. *J Comput Assist Tomagr* 2001, 25:34–35.

60. Arentz T, Jander N, von Rosenthal J, *et al.*: Incidence of pulmonary vein stenosis 2 years after radiofrequency catheter ablation of refractory atrial fibrillation. *Eur Heart J* 2003, 24:963–969.

61. Taylor GW, Kay GN, Zheng X, *et al.*: Pathological effects of extensive radiofrequency energy applications in the pulmonary veins in dogs. *Circulation* 2000, 101:1736-1742.

62. Kluge A, Dill T, Ekinci O, *et al.*: Decreased pulmonary perfusion in pulmonary vein stenosis after radiofrequency ablation: assessment with dynamic magnetic resonance perfusion imaging. *Chest* 2004, 126:428–437.

63. Arentz T, Weber R, Jander N, *et al.*: Pulmonary haemodynamics at rest and during exercise in patients with significant pulmonary vein stenosis after radiofrequency catheter ablation for drug resistant atrial fibrillation. *Eur Heart J* 2005, 26:1410–1414.

64. Qureshi AM, Prieto LR, Latson LA, *et al.*: Transcatheter angioplasty for acquired pulmonary vein stenosis after radiofrequency ablation. *Circulation* 2003, 108:1336–1342.

65. Kim RJ, Wu E, Rafael A, *et al.*: The use of contrast-enhanced magnetic resonance imaging to identify reversible myocardial dysfunction. *N Engl J Med* 2000, 343:1445–1453.

66. Simonetti OP, Kim RJ, Fieno DS, *et al.*: An improved MR imaging technique for the visualization of myocardial infarction. *Radiology* 2001, 218:215-223.

67. Judd RM, Lugo-Olivieri CH, Arai M, *et al.*: Physiological basis of myocardial contrast enhancement in fast magnetic resonance images of 2-day-old reperfused canine infarcts. *Circulation* 1995, 92:1902–1910.

68. Peters DC, Wylie JV, Kissinger KV, *et al.*: Detection of pulmonary vein ablation with high resolution MRI(abstr). *J Cardiovasc Magn Reson* 2006, 8:4-5.

69. Nadas AF, Fyler DC: *Pediatric Cardiology*. Philadelphia: Saunders; 1972.

70. Bedford DE: The anatomical types of atrial septal defect. Their incidence and clinical diagnosis. *Am J Cardiol* 1960, 6:568–574.

71. Krabill KA, Lucas RV: Abnormal pulmonary venous connections. In *Moss and Adams' Heart Disease in Infants, Children and Adolescents*. Edited by Emmanouilides GC, Riemenschneider TA, Allen HD, *et al.* Baltimore: Williams and Wilkins; 1995:838.

72. Lamb RK, Qureshi SA, Wilkinson JL, *et al.*: Total anomalous pulmonary venous drainage. Seventeen-year surgical experience. *J Thorac Cardiovasc Surg* 1988, 96:368–375.

73. Gao YA, Burrows PE, Benson LN, *et al.*: Scimitar syndrome in infancy. *J Am Coll Cardiol* 1993, 22:873–882.

74. Greil G, Powell A, Gildein H, Geva T: Gadolinium-enhanced three-dimensional magnetic resonance aniography of pulmonary and systemic venous anomalies. *J Am Coll Cardiol* 2002, 39:335–341.

21

MR Angiography of the Carotid and Aortic Arch

*Xiaoming Zhang, Carolina Sant'Anna Henry,
Hale Ersoy, Honglei Zhang, and Martin R. Prince*

Contrast-enhanced MR angiography (CE MRA) represents a minimally invasive alternative to traditional methods of angiography for imaging the aortic arch and carotid arteries. MR angiography determines the location and severity of stenotic lesions [1-4]. Vessel wall cardiovascular magnetic resonance (CMR) depicts mural plaque and other abnormalities, identifies plaque components, and measures vessel remodeling whereby a normal lumen may be preserved even though there is abundant plaque because the outer diameter is enlarged [5-8]. CE MRA is viewed upon as a desirable screening method for patients suspected of having vascular disease because of its high accuracy and absence of ionizing radiation or nephrotoxicity at standard gadolinium doses [9-11]. Carotid MR angiography evaluates segments of the artery that ultrasound cannot, including the common carotid origins, in addition to the intracranial portions of the internal carotid arteries, which means it is capable of imaging the entire neurovascular tree from the aortic arch to the intracranial vessels. MR angiography has a significantly better discriminatory power than Doppler ultrasound, especially for the distinction between occlusion versus no occlusion [3,12].

A number of MR angiography techniques can be used for carotid imaging, including two-dimensional time-of-flight (TOF), three-dimensional TOF, black blood spin echo or double inversion recovery with or without electrocardiogram gating, and contrast-enhanced CE MRA [7, 13-18]. Advantages of CE MRA over noncontrast techniques include: higher resolution and signal-to-noise ratio, greater coverage with decreased acquisition time, less motion artifact, decreased sensitivity to the direction of blood flow and blood velocity, and minimal artifacts from cardiac pulsation or respiration. All of these advantages improve diagnostic accuracy in determining the severity and length of a stenosis. However, a combination of techniques for a comprehensive carotid assessment may also be useful, including two-dimensional TOF without gadolinium contrast for localizing the carotid arteries, black blood CMR for direct plaque imaging, and large field-of-view three-dimensional CE MRA for precisely characterizing the carotid lumen from the aortic arch to the circle of Willis. CE MRA may be performed as a series of multiple three-dimensional acquisitions to characterize flow dynamics and eliminate the need for contrast bolus timing.

Common indications for arch and carotid CE MRA include aortic aneurysm, aortic dissection, stroke, vasculitis, upper arm ischemia, or suspected embolic disease. Evaluation of the carotid arteries in patients who suffer from neurologic diseases, such as transient ischemic attacks is also common. Additional indications include when disease in the carotid arteries is suspected, to confirm carotid ultrasound findings, for preoperative mapping of carotid arteries prior to endarterectomy, and for postoperative evaluation.

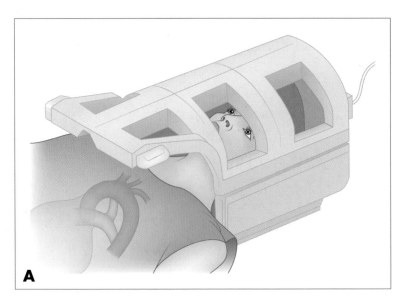

A

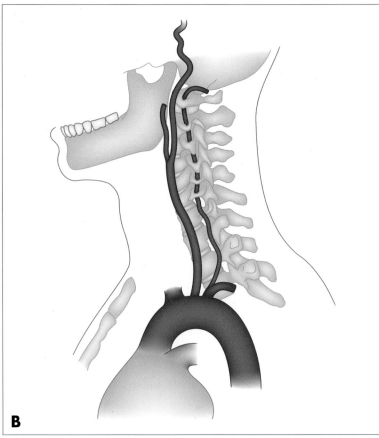

B

Figure 21-1. After confirming the patient is ready to enter the scanner room with no metals in his or her body, start the intravenous line (a 20 or 22 gauge intravenous) in the right arm to avoid filling the left brachiocephalic vein with highly concentrated gadolinium. **A**, A neurovascular coil extending down low enough on the chest to include the aortic arch is essential for simultaneously imaging the carotid origins and bifurcations. If a neurovascular head/neck coil is not available, it may be acceptable to use a body array coil with the elements placed anterior and posterior to the upper chest and neck. **B**, Positioning of the coronal volume for large field-of-view (FOV) three-dimensional contrast-enhanced MR angiography from arch to circle of Willis is illustrated here. Parallel imaging helps by allowing increased FOV or higher resolution while compressing the center of k-space into a shorter period of time to reduce image artifacts.

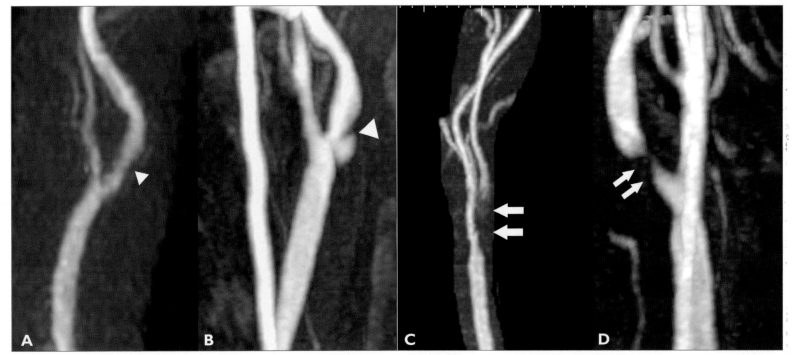

Figure 21-2. Comparison of axial two-dimensional time-of-flight (TOF) and coronal three-dimensional contrast-enhanced MR angiography (CE MRA). Two-dimensional TOF has many artifacts, so it is used primarily as a guide for accurately positioning black blood cardiovascular magnetic resonance and three-dimensional CE MRA. It also serves as a backup in the event that CE MRA fails. Typically, thin (1.5 mm) axial sections are acquired and reformatted at multiple angles. Because of its sensitivity to steady flow distal to severe lesions, two-dimensional TOF reliably detects the "string sign" distal to a severe stenosis. However, two-dimensional TOF is known to easily degrade by excessively slow flow motion, in-plane saturation, and intravoxel dephasing at high-grade stenoses (*arrows*). It often fails to show important luminal features such as plaque ulceration (*arrowhead* on **A**), which is better depicted on three-dimensional CE MRA (*arrowhead* on **B**). The stenotic lumen cannot be directly measured on two-dimensional TOF because flow disturbances create intravoxel signal loss at the stenosis (*arrows* on **C** and **D**).

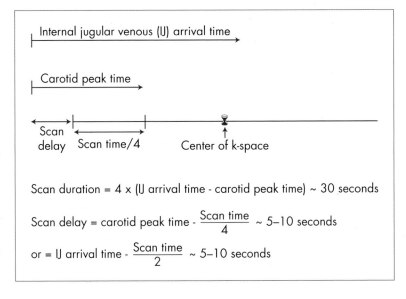

Scan duration = 4 × (IJ arrival time - carotid peak time) ~ 30 seconds

Scan delay = carotid peak time - $\dfrac{\text{Scan time}}{4}$ ~ 5–10 seconds

or = IJ arrival time - $\dfrac{\text{Scan time}}{2}$ ~ 5–10 seconds

Figure 21-3. Calculation of injection timing parameters for carotid MR angiography using sequential ordering of k-space where the center is exactly in the middle of the scan. Optimal implementation of three-dimensional contrast enhanced MR angiography demands accurate timing of the contrast bolus. Data collection needs to coincide with circulation of the gadolinium bolus through the vascular territory under investigation. It is possible to achieve the gadolinium contrast effect with a bolus scan lasting for only one half to two thirds of acquisition time by timing the injection for maximum arterial gadolinium concentration to occur during acquisition of central k-space data. If k-space is mapped centrically or elliptically (*ie*, central k-space data are acquired at the beginning of the scan), scan delay should equal contrast travel time plus an extra 5 or 6 seconds so that data collection does not begin on the leading edge of the bolus.

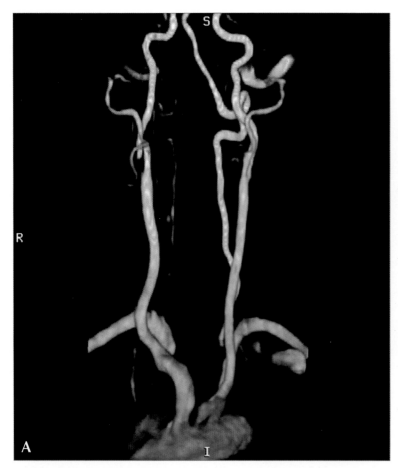

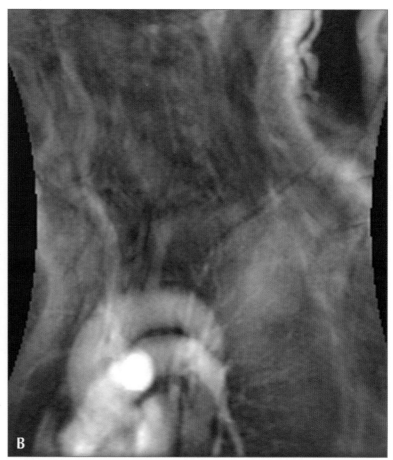

Figure 21-4. **A**, Three-dimensional carotid MR angiography with MR fluoroscopic bolus triggering, and recessed elliptical-centric view order. **B**, MR fluoroscopic triggering includes complex subtraction of an early precontrast mask image to more clearly show early arrival of the contrast bolus to rapidly obtain and reconstruct two-dimensional gradient echo images of the aorta while injecting a gadolinium contrast agent. After starting a three-dimensional contrast-enhanced MR angiography (CE MRA) scan, two-dimensional projection images appear and show the expected location of aortic arch. A 20-mL gadolinium-based contrast agent is injected as a 10-second bolus followed immediately with a 30-mL saline flush. Gadolinium arrival in the right subclavian vein, right side of the heart, pulmonary arteries, left side of the heart, and the aortic arch can be observed. When the agent is seen arriving in the aorta, the operator initiates switching from two-dimensional gradient echo imaging to three-dimensional spoiled gradient echo CE MRA sequence beginning with acquisition of central k-space data. This provides a potentially more reliable way of ensuring acquisition of central k-space data during the moment of peak arterial phase gadolinium concentration. Even better bolus timing occurs when the absolute center of k-space is recessed in from the very beginning of the scan by a few seconds to avoid coinciding with the rising leading edge of the bolus.

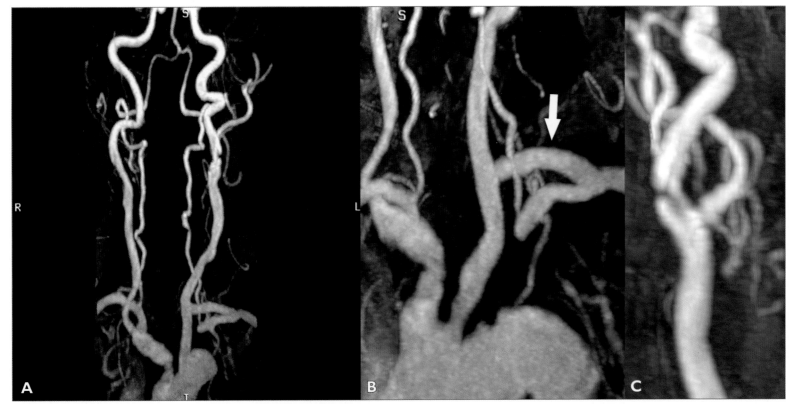

Figure 21-5. Three-dimensional contrast-enhanced MR angiography (CE MRA) of widely patent carotid-to-subclavian bypass graft. Coronal three-dimensional CE MRA volume should cover anteriorly to the carotid arteries, posteriorly to the vertebral and the left subclavian artery origins, superiorly to foramen magnum, and inferiorly to the top of the aortic arch. MR angiography data are postprocessed on a computer work station to obtain reformations and subvolume maximum intensity projections (MIPs) optimized for each carotid artery and the aortic arch. Postprocessing of carotid three-dimensional CE MRA data includes image subtraction, MIP display, volume rendering, and reformatting individual sections. MIP images are typically constructed at 10° intervals to demonstrate the carotid arteries at multiple angles. In addition to MIP displays, images are reformatted at oblique angles as needed to demonstrate carotid bifurcations. Coronal MIP (**A**) and oblique subvolume MIP (**B**) show atherosclerotic disease in great vessel origins with an occluded left subclavian artery, which is reconstituted by a left common carotid to left subclavian bypass graft (*arrow*) and left internal carotid artery (ICA) focal plaque ulceration (**C**). Atherosclerotic disease causes mild narrowing of proximal left common carotid and innominate arteries.

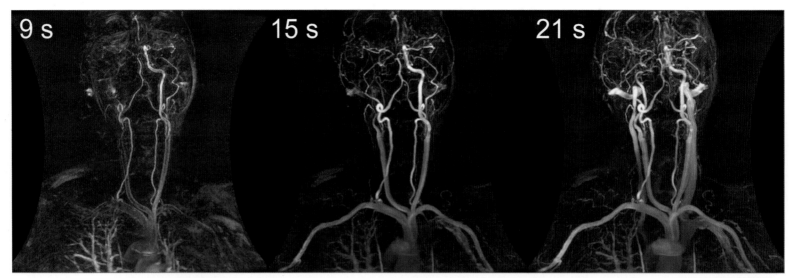

Figure 21-6. Three-dimensional time-resolved contrast enhanced MR angiography (CE MRA) of carotid arteries. Because of the early venous enhancement from rapid transit of gadolinium through the cerebrovascular circulation and because the blood-brain barrier prevents extraction of gadolinium by the brain tissues (unlike in the body), avoiding venous contamination requires meticulous attention to bolus timing details. However, a simpler solution is to acquire time-resolved CE MRA with a new three-dimensional acquisition every 3 to 4 seconds as illustrated in this figure (note only every other image is displayed for this case). Here, three-dimensional time-resolved imaging of contrast kinetics (TRICKS) is used to increase temporal resolution by updating the center of k-space more frequently than the periphery of k-space [19]. Coronal maximum intensity projections through the arch and carotid arteries show pulmonary arteries at 9 seconds, a pure carotid arterial phase at 15 seconds (note the occluded right internal carotid artery), and jugular venous enhancement at 21 seconds. If the time resolve is short enough, it may be possible to perform a time-resolved acquisition without the need for TRICKS view sharing and temporal interpolation. Debates continue about whether it is better to have higher resolution with longer acquisition time and a single phase for maximum detail versus faster, time-resolved acquisitions with limited spatial resolution that may misclassify stenosis severity. Advances in pulse sequence development and coil technology allowing higher and higher parallel imaging factors may soon eliminate the quandary by providing both high temporal and spatial resolution.

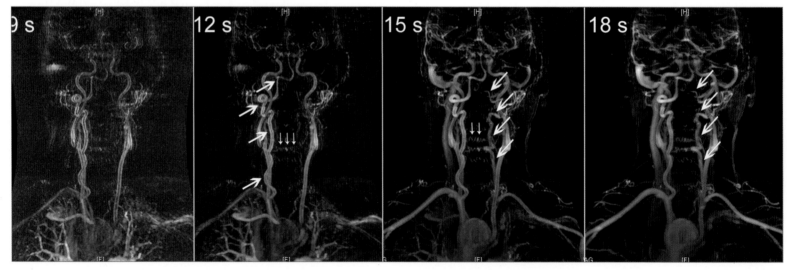

Figure 21-7. Three-dimensional time-resolved imaging of contrast kinetics of subclavian steal syndrome. There is right-sided arch with aberrant left subclavian artery that is occluded at the origin and reconstituted by the enlarged left vertebral artery (*down arrows*) via tortuous corkscrew paravertebral body collateral arteries (*tiny arrows*). The left common carotid artery, right common carotid artery, and right subclavian artery are all widely patent. Time-resolved contrast enhanced MR angiography is particularly useful because it shows the early filling of the right vertebral artery (*up arrows*) and late filling of left vertebral artery (*down arrows*) proving that there is reversal of flow in the left vertebral artery, which is stealing flow from the right vertebral artery. In this case, the patient was only minimally symptomatic which is caused by the severe stenosis of the left vertebral artery superiorly near the basilar artery.

Carotid MR Angiography: Sensitivity and Specificity for Diagnosing Carotid Artery Stenosis

Author	Year	Patients, *n*	Sensitivity, %	Specificity, %
Carotid artery stenosis >70%				
Leclerc *et al.* [20]	1998	27	100	98
Remonda [21]	1998	21 (44*, 18**)		Accuracy = 94%
Carotid artery stenosis >60%				
Jackson [22]	1998	50	85	70
Wintersperger *et al.* [23]	2000	14	100	100
Barbier [24]	2001	29	94-95	89-91
Oberholzer [25]	2001	55	97.7	94
Huston III [26]	2001	50	90	95.5
Randoux [27]	2001	22	93	100
Remonda [28]	2002	120 (73**)		Accuracy = 94%
Lenhart [29]	2002	43	98	86
Butz [30]	2004	50	95.6	90.4
Willinek [31]	2005	50	100	99.3
Carotid artery stenosis >50%				
Wright [32]	2005	81 (51**)	82	97
Fellner [33]	2005	21 (11**)	100	80.6-83.9
D'Onofrio [34]	2006	21		Accuracy = 89%

Number of vessels with correlation.
Number of lesions.

Figure 21-8. Literature on MR angiography sensitivity and specificity for diagnosing significant carotid artery stenosis.

Accuracy of Carotid MR Angiography for Detecting String Sign, Carotid Occlusion, Carotid Aneurysm, and Carotid Plaque Ulceration

Author	Year	Patients, *n*	Accuracy, %
String sign (pseudo occlusion)			
Remonda et al. [21]	1998	21 (44**, 3**)	100
Huston III et al. [26]	2001	50 (6**)	83.3
Remonda et al. [28]	2002	120 (9**)	77.7
Carotid artery occlusion			
Leclerc et al. [20]	1998		27 (54*, 6**)
Remonda et al. [21]	1998	21 (44*, 7**)	100
Sardanelli et al. [35]	1999	30 (114*, 6**)	100
Kollias et al. [36]	1999		20 (40*, 3**)
Serfaty et al. [37]	2000		44 (63*, 2**)
Phan et al. [38]	2001	422 (6**)	100
Remonda et al. [28]	2002	120 (28**)	100
Willinek et al. [31]	2005	50 (35**)	100
Internal carotid artery aneurysm			
Kollias et al. [36]	1999	20 (40*, 2**)	100
Tsuboi et al. [39]	2007	21 (7**)	100
Ulcerated plaque			
Leclerc et al. [20]	1998	27 (108*, 1**)	100
Kollias et al. [36]	1999	20 (40*, 3**)	100
Serfaty et al. [37]	2000	44 (63*, 3**)	
Catalano et al. [40]	2001	37 (74*, 12**)	100
Randoux et al. [27]	2001	22 (44*, 8**)	94

* Number of vessels with correlation.
** Number of lesions.

Figure 21-9. Accuracy of carotid MR angiography for detecting string sign, carotid occlusion, carotid aneurysm, and carotid plaque ulceration.

REFERENCES

1. Ersoy H, Watts R, Sanelli P, *et al.*: Atherosclerotic disease distribution in carotid and vertebrobasilar arteries: clinical experience in 100 patients undergoing fluoro-triggered 3D Gd-MRA. *J Magn Reson Imaging* 2003, 17:545–558.

2. Barth A, Arnold M, Mattle HP, *et al.*: Contrast-enhanced 3-D MRA in decision making for carotid endarterectomy: a 6-year experience. *Cerebrovasc Dis* 2006, 21:393–400.

3. Clevert DA, Johnson T, Michaely H, *et al.*: High-grade stenoses of the internal carotid artery: comparison of high-resolution contrast enhanced 3D MRA, duplex sonography and power Doppler imaging. *Eur J Radiol* 2006, 60:379–386.

4. Layton KF, Huston Jr, Cloft HJ, *et al.*: Specificity of MR angiography as a confirmatory test for carotid artery stenosis: is it valid? *AJR Am J Roentgenol* 2007, 188:1114–1116.

5. Chu B, Phan BA, Balu N, *et al.*: Reproducibility of carotid atherosclerotic lesion type characterization using high resolution multicontrast weighted cardiovascular magnetic resonance. *J Cardiovasc Magn Reson* 2006, 8:793–799.

6. Devuyst G, Piechowski-Jozwiak B, Bogousslavsky J: Arterial wall imaging. *Front Neurol Neurosci* 2006, 21.

7. Koktzoglou I, Chung YC, Carroll TJ, *et al.*: Three-dimensional black-blood MR imaging of carotid arteries with segmented steady-state free precession: initial experience. *Radiology* 2007, 243:220–228.

8. Martin K, Brownfield D, Karmonik C, *et al.*: Short-term tracking of atherosclerosis in operated and unoperated human carotid arteries by high resolution magnetic resonance imaging. *World J Surg* 2007, 31:723–732.

9. Dempsey MF, Condon B, Hadley DM: MRI safety review. *Semin Ultrasound CT MR* 2002, 23:392–401.

10. Dalla-Palma L, Panzetta G, Pozzi-Mucelli RS, *et al.*: Dynamic magnetic resonance imaging in the assessment of chronic medical nephropathies with impaired renal function. *Eur Radiol* 2000, 10:280–286.

11. Morcos SK, Thomsen HS, Webb JA: Contrast-media-induced nephrotoxicity: a consensus report. Contrast Media Safety Committee, European Society of Urogenital Radiology (ESUR). *Eur Radiol* 1999, 9:1602–1613.

12. Borisch I, Horn M, Butz B, *et al.*: Preoperative evaluation of carotid artery stenosis: comparison of contrast-enhanced MR angiography and duplex sonography with digital subtraction angiography. *AJNR Am J Neuroradiol* 2003; 24:1117–1122.

13. Jager HR, Moore EA, Bynevelt M, *et al.*: Contrast-enhanced MR angiography in patients with carotid artery stenosis: comparison of two different techniques with an unenhanced 2D time-of-flight sequence. *Neuroradiology* 2000, 42:240–248.

14. Mitra D, Connolly D, Jenkins S, *et al.*: Comparison of image quality, diagnostic confidence and interobserver variability in contrast enhanced MR angiography and 2D time of flight angiography in evaluation of carotid stenosis. *Br J Radiol* 2006, 79:201–207.

15. Scarabino T, Fossaceca R, Carra L, *et al.*: Actual role of unenhanced magnetic resonance angiography (MRA TOF 3D) in the study of stenosis and occlusion of extracranial carotid artery. *Radiol Med (Torino)* 2003, 106:497–503.

16. Townsend TC, Saloner D, Pan XM, Rapp JH: Contrast material-enhanced MRA overestimates severity of carotid stenosis, compared with 3D time-of-flight MRA. *J Vasc Surg* 2003, 38:36–40.

17. Mani V, Aguiar SH, Itskovich VV, *et al.*: Carotid black blood MRI burden of atherosclerotic disease assessment correlates with ultrasound intima-media thickness. *J Cardiovasc Magn Reson* 2006, 8:529–534.

18. Babiarz LS, Astor B, Mohamed MA, Wasserman BA: Comparison of gadolinium-enhanced cardiovascular magnetic resonance angiography with high-resolution black blood cardiovascular magnetic resonance for assessing carotid artery stenosis. *J Cardiovasc Magn Reson* 2007, 9:63–70.

19. Carroll TJ, Korosec FR, Petermann GM, *et al.*: Carotid bifurcation: evaluation of time-resolved three-dimensional contrast-enhanced MR angiography. *Radiology* 2001, 220:525–532.

20. Leclerc X, Martinat P, Godefroy O, *et al.*: Contrast-enhanced three-dimensional fast imaging with steady-state precession (FISP) MR angiography of supraaortic vessels: preliminary results. AJNR *Am J Neuroradiol* 1998, 19:1405–1413.

21. Remonda L, Heid O, Schroth G: Carotid artery stenosis, occlusion, and pseudo-occlusion: first-pass, gadolinium-enhanced, three-dimensional MR angiography—preliminary study. *Radiology* 1998, 209:95–102.

22. Jackson MR, Chang AS, Robles HA, *et al.*: Determination of 60% or greater carotid stenosis: a prospective comparison of magnetic resonance angiography and duplex ultrasound with conventional angiography. *Ann Vasc Surg* 1998, 12:236–243.

23. Wintersperger BJ, Huber A, Preissler G, *et al.*: MR angiography of the supraaortic vessels. *Radiology* 2000, 40:785–791.

24. Barbier C, Lefevre F, Bui P, *et al.*: Contrast-enhanced MRA of the carotid arteries using 0.5 Tesla: comparison with selective digital angiography. *J Radiol* 2001, 82:245–249.

25. Oberholzer K, Kreitner KF, Kalden P, *et al.*: Contrast-enhanced three-dimensional MR angiography of the carotid artery at 1.0 Tesla compared to i.a. DSA: is the method suitable for the diagnosis of carotid stenosis? *Rofo* 2001, 173:350–355.

26. Huston Jr, Fain SB, Wald JT, *et al.*: Carotid artery: elliptic centric contrast-enhanced MR angiography compared with conventional angiography. *Radiology* 2001, 218:138–143.

27. Randoux B, Marro B, Koskas F, *et al.*: Carotid artery stenosis: prospective comparison of CT, three-dimensional gadolinium-enhanced MR, and conventional angiography. *Radiology* 2001, 220:179–185.

28. Remonda L, Senn P, Barth A, *et al.*: Contrast-enhanced 3D MR angiography of the carotid artery: comparison with conventional digital subtraction angiography. *AJNR Am J Neuroradiol* 2002, 23:213–219.

29. Lenhart M, Framme N, Volk M, *et al.*: Time-resolved contrast-enhanced magnetic resonance angiography of the carotid arteries: diagnostic accuracy and inter-observer variability compared with selective catheter angiography. *Invest Radiol* 2002, 37:535–541.

30. Butz B, Dorenbeck U, Borisch I, *et al.*: High-resolution contrast-enhanced magnetic resonance angiography of the carotid arteries using fluoroscopic monitoring of contrast arrival: diagnostic accuracy and interobserver variability. *Acta Radiol* 2004, 45:164–170.

31. Willinek WA, von Falkenhausen M, Born M, *et al.*: Noninvasive detection of steno-occlusive disease of the supra-aortic arteries with three-dimensional contrast-enhanced magnetic resonance angiography: a prospective, intra-individual comparative analysis with digital subtraction angiography. *Stroke* 2005, 36:38–43.

32. Wright VL, Olan W, Dick B, *et al.*: Assessment of CE-MRA for the rapid detection of supra-aortic vascular disease. *Neurology* 2005, 65:27–32.

33. Fellner C, Lang W, Janka R, *et al.*: Magnetic resonance angiography of the carotid arteries using three different techniques: accuracy compared with intraarterial x-ray angiography and endarterectomy specimens. *J Magn Reson Imaging* 2005, 21:424–431.

34. D'Onofrio M, Mansueto G, Faccioli N, *et al.*: Doppler ultrasound and contrast-enhanced magnetic resonance angiography in assessing carotid artery stenosis. *Radiol Med (Torino)* 2006, 111:93–103.

35. Sardanelli F ZF, Parodi RC, De Caro G: MR angiography of internal carotid arteries: breath-hold Gd-enhanced 3D fast imaging with steady-state precession versus unenhanced 2D and 3D time-of-flight techniques. *J Comput Assist Tomogr* 1999, 23:208–215.

36. Kollias SS, Binkert CA, Ruesch S, Valavanis A: Contrast-enhanced MR angiography of the supra-aortic vessels in 24 seconds: a feasibility study. *Neuroradiology* 1999, 41:391–400.

37. Serfaty JM, Chirossel P, Chevallier JM, *et al.*: Accuracy of three-dimensional gadolinium-enhanced MR angiography in the assessment of extra-cranial carotid artery disease. *AJR Am J Roentgenol* 2000, 175:455–463.

38. Phan T, Huston Jr, Bernstein MA, *et al.*: Contrast-enhanced magnetic resonance angiography of the cervical vessels: experience with 422 patients. *Stroke* 2001, 32:2282–2286.

39. Tsuboi T, Tokunaga K, Shingo T, *et al.*: Differentiation between intradural and extradural locations of juxta-dural ring aneurysms by using contrast-enhanced 3-dimensional time-of-flight magnetic resonance angiography. *Surg Neurol* 2007, 67:381–387.

40. Catalano C, Laghi A, Pediconi F, *et al.*: Magnetic resonance angiography with contrast media in the study of carotid arteries. *Radiol Med (Torino)* 2001, 101:54–59.

22

MR Angiography of the Aorta, Peripheral, and Renal Arteries

Rajiv Agarwal and Scott D. Flamm

Magnetic resonance angiography (MRA) has achieved widespread acceptance as an imaging modality for detailed three-dimensional vasculature evaluation. Compared with traditional radiograph angiography, the distinct advantages of MRA include its noninvasive nature, its lack of radiation exposure, avoidance of potentially nephrotoxic iodinated contrast agents, and its ability to manipulate reconstructed images in oblique three-dimensional planes. The most commonly employed MRA methods include two-dimensional and three-dimensional time-of-flight, phase contrast, contrast-enhanced, and, more recently, noncontrast-enhanced techniques. Each method has its own unique set of advantages and challenges. Currently, contrast-enhanced MRA is the most commonly employed method and involves the administration of gadolinium-chelate to shorten the T1 relaxation time of intraluminal blood. With meticulous attention to timing patterns, high signal intensity can be attained in the vascular region of interest. Recent concerns of nephrogenic systemic sclerosis stemming from use of gadolinium-chelate have triggered substantial advancements in noncontrast-enhanced MRA. Phase contrast imaging provides valuable information on the hemodynamic significance of a vascular stenosis. Forthcoming advances in cardiovascular magnetic resonance hardware and post-processing technologies will continue to propel MRA as a mainstay imaging modality for thorough evaluation of vascular pathology.

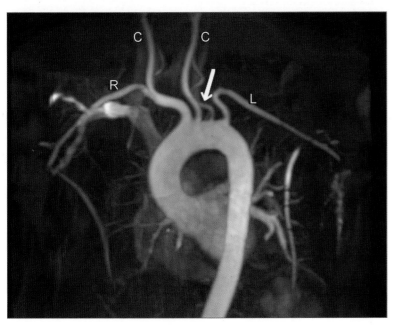

Figure 22-1. Normal thoracic aorta and branches. Contrast-enhanced MRA of a patient with a normal thoracic aorta and arch branch vessels. Note the smooth walls of the aorta and its branch vessels, indicating no significant atherosclerosis. Pictured are the common carotid arteries (C) and left (L) and right (R) subclavian arteries. Incidentally noted is the direct origin of the left vertebral artery (*arrow*) from the aortic arch.

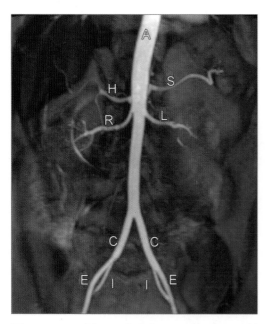

Figure 22-2. Normal abdominal aorta and branches. Contrast-enhanced MRA of a patient with a normal aorta and branch vessels. Note the smooth walls of the aorta (A) and its branch vessels, indicating no significant atherosclerosis. Pictured are the common hepatic artery (H), splenic artery (S), right (R) and left (L) renal arteries, common iliac arteries (C), external iliac arteries (E), and internal iliac arteries (I).

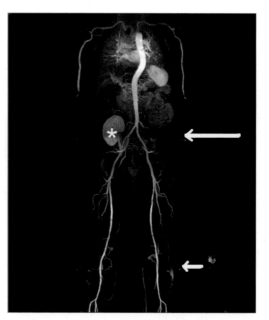

Figure 22-3. Whole body MRA. Three stage contrast-enhanced MRA of a patient with a renal transplant (*see asterisk*). Images of the chest and abdomen are first acquired (*top of image to long arrow*). Subsequently, the table is moved to acquire images of the pelvis and thighs (*long arrow to short arrow*). Finally, the table is moved again to acquire the final set of images of the calves and feet. Each stage of this process can be evaluated individually by the interpreting physician. The entire process involves a single administration of gadolinium chelate and requires meticulous handling of the imaging parameters by an experienced technologist.

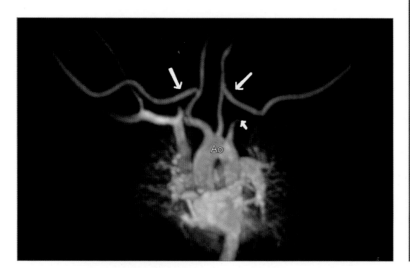

Figure 22-4. Bilateral subclavian artery stenosis. Contrast-enhanced MRA of a patient with Takayasu arteritis with bilateral subclavian artery stenosis. The patient has undergone grafting of bilateral common carotid arteries to brachial arteries. The image shows bilateral grafts (*long arrows*) from the common carotid arteries extending out distally. Also noted is occlusion of the proximal left subclavian artery (*short arrow*). The right subclavian artery occlusion is not seen in this view. Ao—aorta.

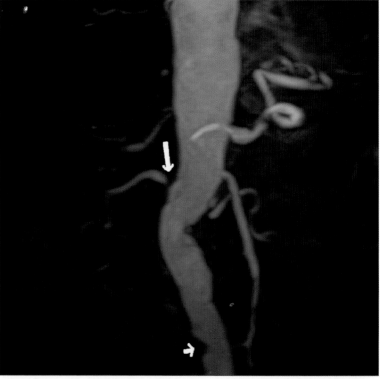

Figure 22-5. Renal artery stenosis. Contrast-enhanced MRA of a patient with azotemia and hypertension with suspicion for renovascular hypertension. The image shows severe stenosis of the right renal artery (*long arrow*). The mid to distal right renal artery is well visualized without evidence for significant disease. Also noted is tapering of the abdominal aorta with areas of eccentric luminal irregularity (*short arrow*), suggestive of atherosclerosis.

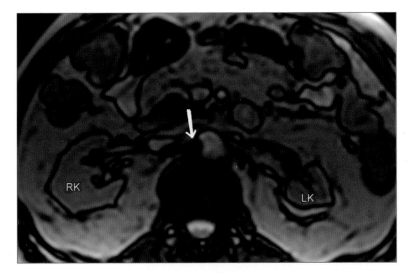

Figure 22-6. Renal artery stenosis. Steady-state free precession axially oriented image of a patient with known severe renal artery stenosis involving the left renal artery and a recently placed stent in the right renal artery. Note that the left kidney (LK) is substantially smaller in size compared with the right kidney (RK). Additionally, susceptibility artifact related to the intravascular stent is present at the proximal right renal artery (*arrow*).

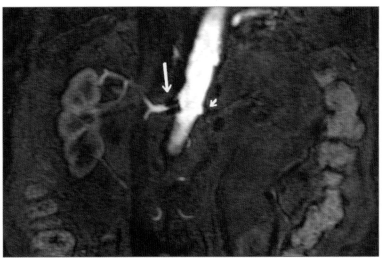

Figure 22-7. Renal artery stenosis. Contrast-enhanced MRA of a patient with a history of intravascular stent placement in the proximal right renal artery. Susceptibility artifact from an intravascular stent is visualized (*long arrow*). The image shows incomplete signal in the area of the stent and full signal distal to the stent. The proximal segment of the stent extends into the lumen of the abdominal aorta. This patient also has occlusion of the left renal artery, as manifested by a "stump" (*short arrow*).

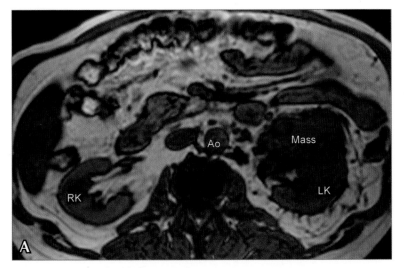

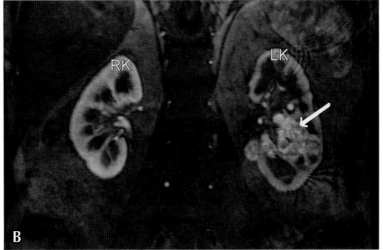

Figures 22-8. Renal cell carcinoma. Images were obtained in a patient with azotemia and hypertension for detection of renal artery stenosis. A hypervascular tumor was incidentally discovered and a diagnosis of renal cell carcinoma was confirmed after excisional biopsy. **A**, A steady-state free precession axial image of the patient showing an irregularly shaped, heterogeneous mass involving the left kidney (LK). The right kidney appears normal in shape and contour. **B**, A contrast-enhanced MRA in the venous phase reveals hypervascularity of the tumor in the LK (*long arrow*). Note the normal architecture and enhancement of the right kidney (RK).

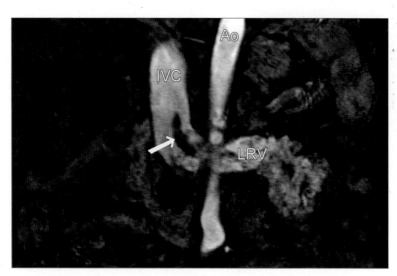

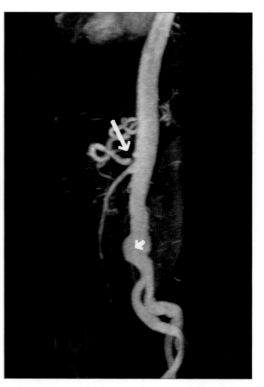

Figure 22-9. Renal vein thrombosis. Venous phase image of contrast-enhanced MRA of a patient with renal cell carcinoma and suspicion of renal vein thrombosis. Note the large signal void (*arrow*) in the left renal vein (LRV) that extends into the inferior vena cava (IVC). A venous phase is obtained following the arterial phase after the administration of gadolinium chelate. This patient was diagnosed with renal cell carcinoma and the signal void was confirmed as thrombus. Ao—aorta.

Figure 22-10. Celiac trunk stenosis. Contrast-enhanced MRA of an elderly patient with postprandial abdominal pain. The proximal segment of the celiac trunk has severe luminal stenosis (*long arrow*), as noted on multiple views. This stenosis was confirmed by selective radiograph angiography. The superior mesenteric artery is widely patent. Incidentally noted is a small, distal infrarenal aneurysm (*short arrow*).

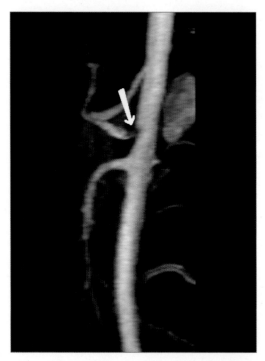

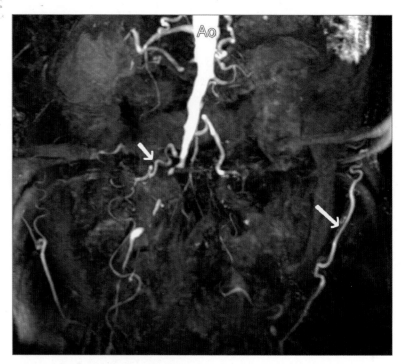

Figure 22-11. Celiac trunk compression by median arcuate ligament. Contrast-enhanced MRA in a young woman with a study performed to assess for renovascular hypertension. The intensity in the proximal segment of the celiac trunk is reduced, suggestive of celiac trunk stenosis (*arrow*). The patient underwent a radiograph angiogram that revealed a widely patent celiac trunk. The cardiac magnetic resonance findings were attributed to extrinsic compression by the median arcuate ligament mimicking celiac trunk stenosis.

Figure 22-12. LeRiche syndrome. Contrast-enhanced MRA in an elderly man with severe claudication. The distal abdominal aorta (Ao) tapers down in caliber and is occluded prior to its bifurcation into the common iliac arteries. Extensive collateral vessels (*arrows*) are noted bilaterally that supply flow into the distal vessels.

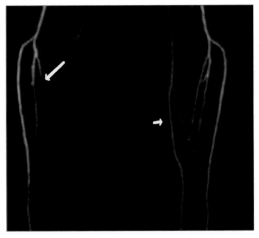

Figure 22-13. Right posterior tibial artery occlusion. Contrast-enhanced MRA of a patient with acute onset of right lower leg pain one day after successful percutaneous placement of an intracoronary artery stent. There is abrupt cessation of contrast opacification of the right posterior tibial artery (*long arrow*). The lack of collateral vessels suggests the subacute or acute nature of this occlusion. There is venous contamination of the left leg (*short arrow*), suggesting a delayed imaging phase. Perfect arterial phase image acquisitions require keen attention to timing to avoid venous contamination. Blood pressure cuffs were used to minimize venous contamination.

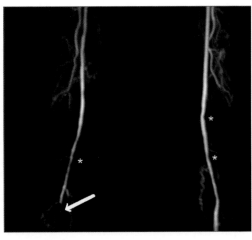

Figure 22-14. Right superficial femoral artery stenosis. Contrast-enhanced MRA of a patient with right leg claudication during daily walks. The right superficial femoral artery is occluded at its distal segment (*arrow*). There are also multiple segments of luminal irregularities in bilateral superficial femoral arteries (*see asterisk*). The patient underwent successful surgical grafting of the right popliteal artery and had complete resolution of his claudication.

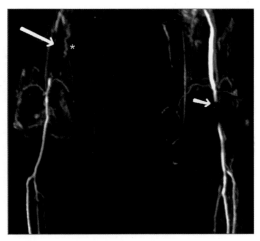

Figure 22-15. Stenoses of right superficial femoral and left popliteal arteries. Contrast-enhanced MRA of an elderly patient with bilateral leg claudication. There is long segment occlusion of the right superficial femoral artery (*long arrow*). There are collateral vessels (*see asterisk*) that reconstitute flow distal to the occlusion. The right popliteal artery is well visualized and enhances normally with gadolinium. There is occlusion of the left popliteal artery (*short arrow*) with reconstitution of the distal popliteal artery via collateral vessels.

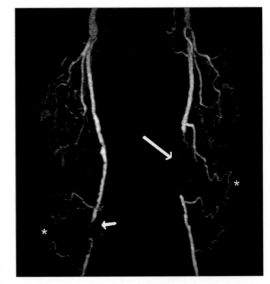

Figure 22-16. Stenoses of bilateral superficial femoral arteries. Contrast-enhanced MR angiogram of a patient with bilateral leg claudication. There is long segment occlusion of the mid left superficial femoral artery (*long arrow*). Note the extensive collateral vessel (*see asterisk*) that reconstitutes the distal left superficial femoral artery. Also, there is short segment occlusion of the distal right superficial femoral artery (*short arrow*) with reconstitution via collateral vessels (*see asterisk*). Luminal irregularities are noted in the right proximal to mid superficial femoral artery consistent with atherosclerotic disease.

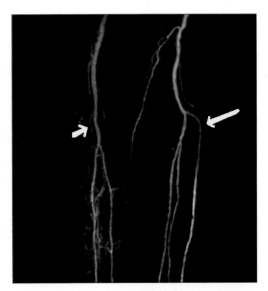

Figure 22-17. Severe diffuse stenoses of the right anterior tibial artery. Contrast-enhanced MRA of an elderly patient with right lower leg pain upon extended walking. The left anterior tibial artery (*long arrow*) is well visualized and is widely patent without significant stenosis. On the other hand, the right anterior tibial artery (*short arrow*) is small in caliber at its proximal segment and then is occluded throughout the rest of its course. There is two-vessel infrapopliteal runoff on the right and three-vessel runoff on the left.

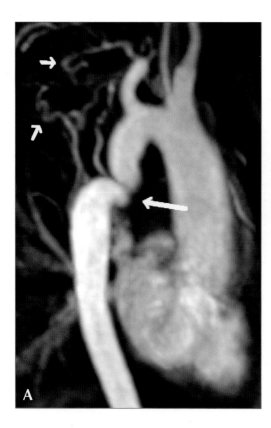

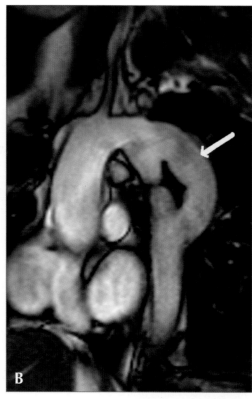

Figures 22-18. Aortic coarctation. A,
Contrast-enhanced MRA of a patient with
aortic coarctation. There is severe, focal
stenosis (*long arrow*) of the descending
thoracic aorta distal to the takeoff of the
left subclavian artery. There are extensive
collateral vessels noted that supply flow to
the descending thoracic aorta distal to the
stenosis. The patient underwent surgical
repair. **B,** Steady-state free precession
image of the same patient after surgical
repair of the aortic coarctation. There
was interval placement of a surgical graft
(*arrow*) that bypasses the area of stenosis in
the proximal descending thoracic aorta.

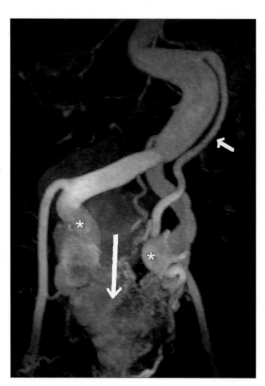

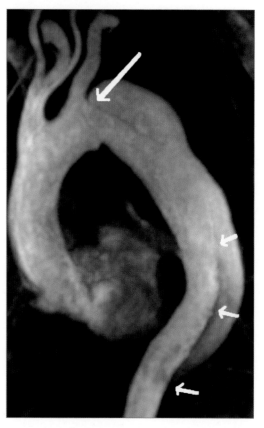

Figure 22-19. Pelvic arteriovenous malformation. Contrast-
enhanced MRA from a patient with a large pelvic arteriovenous
malformation (AVM). The AVM (*long arrow*) is irregularly shaped
and fills rapidly with contrast because of the patient's high cardiac
output of 18 liters per minute as calculated by phase contrast
velocity mapping. The AVM is supplied by many vessels including the prominent inferior mesenteric (*short arrow*) and massively
enlarged bilateral internal iliac arteries (*see asterisk*).

Figure 22-20. Type B aortic dissection. Contrast-enhanced MRA
from a patient with hypertension and clinical suspicion for an aortic
dissection. There is a Type B aortic dissection with the intimal flap
starting immediately distal to the takeoff of the left subclavian
artery (*long arrow*). The intimal flap continues distally (*short arrows*)
and extends to the distal descending thoracic aorta. The proximal to
mid-descending thoracic aorta is dilated. The ascending aorta and
aortic arch are normal in caliber.

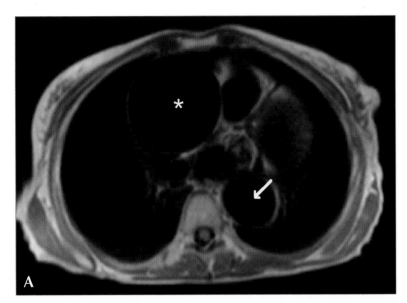

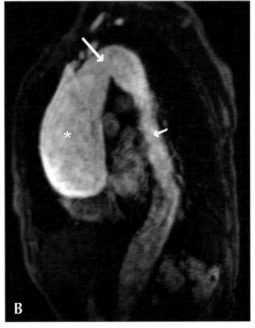

Figure 22-21. Ascending thoracic aorta aneurysm. **A,** Axial black blood image from a patient with a family history of aortic aneurysms and nonspecific chest discomfort. There is aneurysmal dilation (7.4 cm) of the ascending thoracic aorta (*see asterisk*). The visualized descending thoracic aorta (*arrow*) is normal in caliber.

B, Oblique sagittal contrast-enhanced MRA of the same patient revealing aneurysmal dilation of the ascending thoracic aorta (*see asterisk*). Note that the aortic arch (*long arrow*) and descending thoracic aorta (*short arrow*) are normal in caliber. The patient underwent surgical repair and had an uneventful postoperative course.

SUGGESTED READING

1. Zhang H, Maki JH, Prince MR: 3D contrast-enhanced MR angiography. *J Magn Reson Imaging* 2007, 26:816.

2. Prince MR, Yucel EK, Kaufman JA, *et al:* Dynamic gadolinium-enhanced three-dimensional abdominal arteriography. *J Magn Reson Imaging* 1993, 3:877-881.

3. Gozzi M, Amorico MG, Colopi S, et al: Peripheral arterial occlusive disease: role of MR angiography. *Radiol Med (Torino)* 2006, 111:225-237.

4. Czum JM, Corse WR, Ho VB: MR angiography of the thoracic aorta. *Magn Reson Imaging Clin N Am* 2005, 13:41-64.

5. Ersoy H, Zhang H, Prince MR: Peripheral MR angiography. *J Cardiovasc Magn Reson* 2006,8:517-528.

6. Zhang H, Prince MR: Renal MR angiography. *Magn Reson Imaging Clin N Am* 2004,12:487-503.

23

Coronary Artery Imaging

Warren J. Manning

Despite ongoing progress in both primary prevention and early diagnosis, coronary artery disease (CAD) remains the leading cause of death for both men and women in the United States. Catheter-based, invasive radiograph coronary angiography is the clinical "gold standard" for the diagnosis of significant (> 50% diameter stenosis) CAD, with over a million catheter-based radiograph coronary angiograms performed annually in the United States. Although numerous noninvasive tests are available to help discriminate among those with and without significant CAD, up to 35% of patients referred for a diagnostic angiogram in the absence of acute coronary syndrome and prior myocardial infarction are diagnosed with no significant stenoses. Despite the absence of disease, these individuals are exposed to the cost, inconvenience, and potential morbidity of radiograph angiography [1]. Data also suggest that in selected high-risk populations such as those who have aortic valve stenosis, the incidence of subclinical stroke associated with retrograde catheter crossing of the stenotic valve may exceed 20% [2].

Though percutaneous intervention in single vessel CAD is commonly performed, the greatest impact on mortality occurs with mechanical intervention among patients with left main and multivessel CAD. Thus, it is desirable to have a noninvasive method that allows for direct visualization of the proximal/mid native coronary vessels for the accurate identification or exclusion of this disorder.

Over the past decade, coronary CMR has evolved as a preferred clinical alternative to catheter-based radiograph angiography among patients with suspected anomalous CAD and coronary artery aneurysms. In addition, at experienced centers, it has reached sufficient maturity to obviate the need for catheter-based radiograph angiography in the discrimination of ischemic versus nonischemic etiologies for patients with a dilated cardiomyopathy. Coronary cardiovascular magnetic resonance (CMR) has not been studied as a screening test for CAD in asymptomatic or high-risk populations.

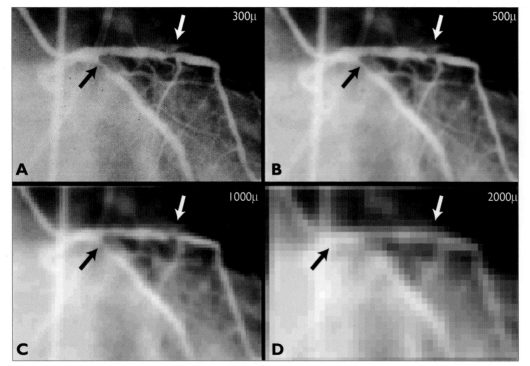

Figure 23-1. A–D, Technical challenges to coronary cardiovascular magnetic resonance [CMR] (and coronary CT angiography) include providing contrast to the intracoronary lumen signal, adequate spatial resolution, and motion suppression from both cardiac and chest wall/diaphragm motion. The coronary artery lumen diameter is only 3 mm to 5 mm. Conventional radiograph angiography is a projection method with high spatial resolution (300 micron). Shown is a conventional radiograph angiogram presented at 300, 500, 1000, and 2000 micron spatial resolutions. Note that the left anterior descending (*white arrow*) and left circumflex (*black arrow*) coronary artery stenoses are easily appreciated at 300 and 500 micron spatial resolution, but less demonstrated at 1000 micron spatial resolution. This suggests that coronary CMR spatial resolution of at least 1000 micron is required. (*Courtesy of* D. Sodickson, MD, PhD.)

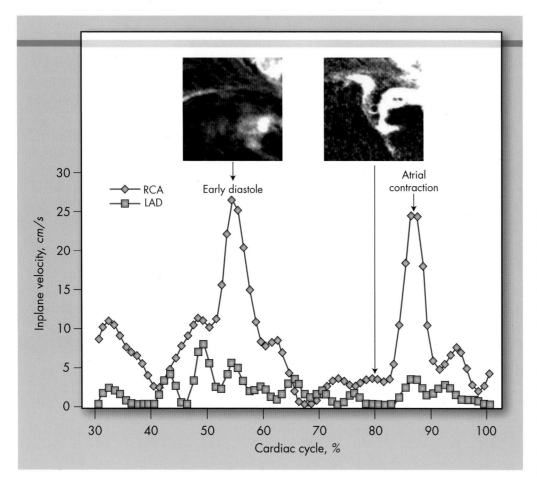

Figure 23-2. Accurate electrocardiogram sampling is imperative for coronary cardiovascular magnetic resonance (CMR) to acquire CMR data during a period of diastasis. Coronary artery in-plane motion varies during the cardiac cycle, with prominent motion during ventricular contraction/relaxation, and after atrial systole. This motion can be appreciated in this graph of in-plane right coronary artery (RCA) and left anterior descending (LAD) coronary artery motion during the cardiac cycle. The x-axis displays time as a percentage of the R-R interval. Note the improved image quality of the RCA cross section when coronary cardiovascular CMR data are acquired during mid diastole as compared with early diastole [3].

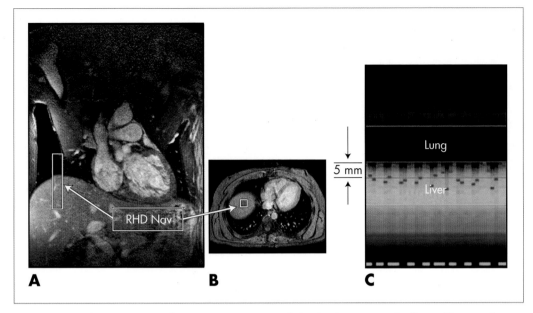

Figure 23-3. Suppression of respiratory motion from its impact on bulk cardiac motion is also important for coronary cardiovascular magnetic resonance (CMR). This can be achieved with sustained breath-holds, respiratory bellows gating, or CMR navigators.

CMR navigators can be considered analogous to an M-mode echocardiogram. Shown are (**A**) coronal and (**B**) transverse thoracic CMR with identification of a navigator through the dome of the right hemidiaphragm (RHD Nav). **C**, Respiratory motion of the lung-diaphragm interface recorded using a two-dimensional selective navigator with the lung (superior) and liver (inferior) interface. The maximum excursion between end inspiration and end expiration in this example is ~11 mm. The broken line in the middle of **C** indicates the position of the lung-liver interface at each R-R interval. Data are only accepted if the lung-liver interface is within the acceptance window of 5 mm. Data acquired with the navigator outside of the window are rejected. Accepted data is indicated by the broken line at the bottom of **C**.

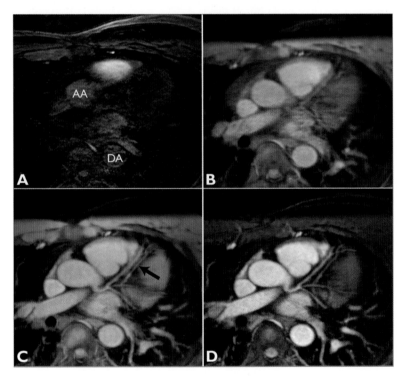

Figure 23-4. Transverse coronary cardiovascular magnetic resonance (CMR) at the level of the left main (LM) and left anterior descending (LAD). **A**, In the absence of cardiac and respiratory gating, note that the ascending aorta (AA) and descending aorta (DA) are visible, but the coronary arteries cannot be seen. **B**, The incremental value of the electrocardiogram trigger with mid-diastolic data acquisition allows for improved visualization of the AA and DA, as well as the right ventricular outflow tract. **C**, Respiratory navigator gating with clear depiction of the LM, LAD, and left circumflex (LCX). The great cardiac vein (*black arrow*) is also seen, lateral to the LAD and extending into the left atrioventricular groove. **D**, T2 prepulse suppresses the signal from the myocardium and deoxygenated blood in the great cardiac vein. Note that coronary CMR does not require a contrast agent. There is natural contrast between the blood flowing in the coronary lumen and surrounding tissue. (*Courtesy of* M. Stuber, PhD.)

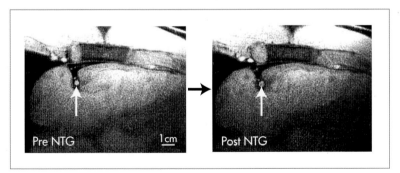

Figure 23-5. A final technical aspect of coronary cardiovascular magnetic resonance (CMR) is the addition of a vasodilator that dilates the coronary arteries and increases coronary blood flow velocity. Sublingual nitroglycerin or isosorbide dinitrate is typically used. As the signal in k-space gradient echo coronary CMR is dependent on inflow of unsaturated spins (blood), the increase in coronary blood flow provided by these agents leads to an increase in signal-to-noise ratio. (*Adapted from* Terachima *et al.* [4].)

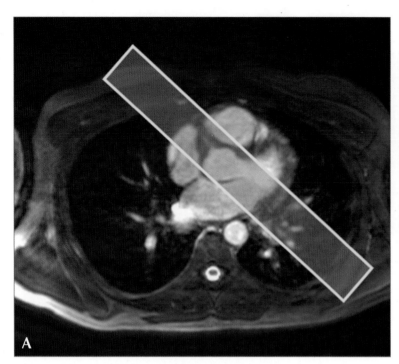

A

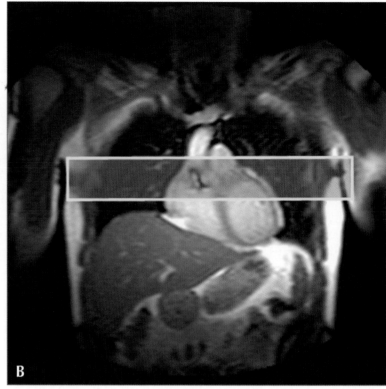

B

Figure 23-6. Although two-dimensional coronary cardiovascular magnetic resonance was the common approach for many years, three-dimensional approaches now dominate because of their superior coverage of coronary anatomy and postprocessing advantages. Shown is a typical orientation for targeted three-dimensional thin slab approach with an oblique three-dimensional slab aligned in the atrioventricular for depiction of the right coronary artery (RCA), left main (LM), and left circumflex (LCX) **A** and an axial three-dimensional slab centered in the take-off of the LM for demonstration of the LM, left anterior descending, LCX, and often the proximal RCA, **B**. Each three-dimensional slab can be 3 cm thick and can contain 12 to 14 slices.

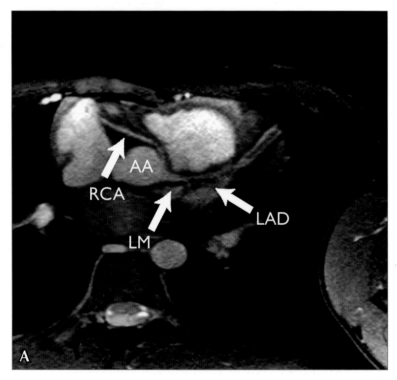

A

Figure 23-7. Using the above method, the major coronary arteries can be defined in the vast majority of subjects. The first clinical application of coronary cardiovascular magnetic resonance was in patients with suspected anomalous coronary artery disease. While coronary artery origins are easily identified in infants and young children with transthoracic echocardiography, this is more difficult as young patients begin to age into adolescence and adulthood. Anomalous coronary artery disease is found in ~ 1% of the population. Fortunately, the majority are of the benign form in which the anomalous segment courses anterior to the pulmonary artery (PA) or posterior to the aorta. In the malignant form, the anomalous segment courses anterior to the aorta and posterior to the PA. **A,** Malignant form of the anomalous right coronary artery (RCA) originating from the left coronary sinus and traversing anteriorly. Ao—aorta; LA—left atrium.

Continued on the next page

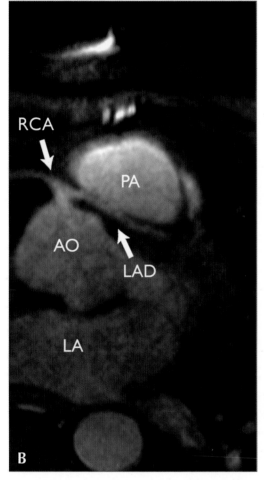

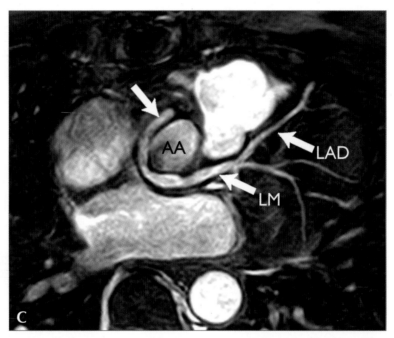

Figure 23-7. *(Continued)* **B**, Malignant form of the anomalous left anterior descending (LAD) originating from the right cusp. **C**, Benign form of anomalous disease with the left main (LM) originating from the right coronary sinus and traversing posterior to the ascending aorta (AA). Data suggest that coronary cardiovascular magnetic resonance is extremely accurate in defining anomalous coronary artery disease [5-7] with the advantage of a nonionizing environment and lack of iodinated contrast. The former issue is particularly important as patients with suspected anomalous coronary artery disease are typically quite young. AA—ascending aorta; LA—left atrium; PA—pulmonary artery.

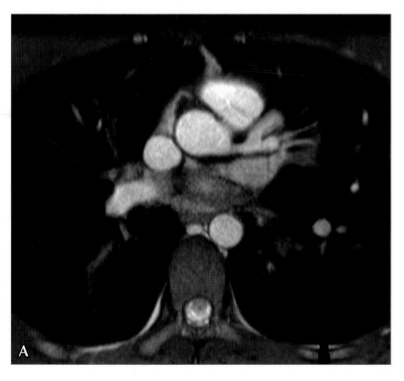

Figure 23-8. Though relatively uncommon, coronary artery aneurysms are also well demonstrated by coronary cardiovascular magnetic resonance (CMR). In the absence of a prior percutaneous intervention, the vast majority of acquired coronary aneurysms are from mucocutaneous lymph node syndrome (Kawasaki disease), a generalized vasculitis of unknown etiology usually occurring in children under 5 years of age, with nearly 20% afflicted children developing coronary artery aneurysms. Among small children, transthoracic echocardiography is usually adequate for diagnosing and monitoring proximal aneurysms, but as with anomalous coronary disease, transthoracic echocardiography is deficient in older and obese children. These young adults are therefore often referred for serial catheter-based radiograph coronary angiography. Coronary CMR data from adolescents and young adults with coronary artery aneurysms have confirmed the high accuracy of coronary CMR for both the identification and the characterization (diameter/length) of these aneurysms [8,9]. **A**, Transverse targeted three-dimensional T2 prepulse coronary CMR of a young man with an aneurysm of the left main, left anterior descending, and ramus intermedius coronary arteries.

Continued on the next page

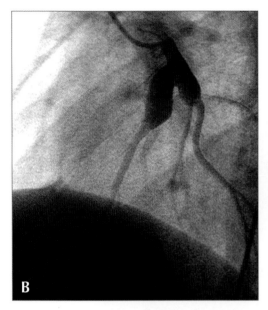

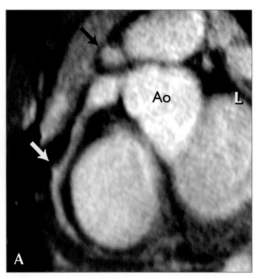

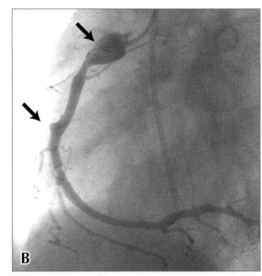

Figure 23-8. *(Continued)* **B**, Corresponding radiograph angiogram, demonstrating good correlation of the coronary cardiovascular magnetic resonance.

Figure 23-9. **A**, Oblique coronary cardiovascular magnetic resonance in a young adult with Kawasaki disease and resultant aneurysm of the proximal and mid- right coronary artery. **B**, Corresponding radiograph angiogram. *(Adapted from* Greil *et al.* [8].) Ao—aorta.

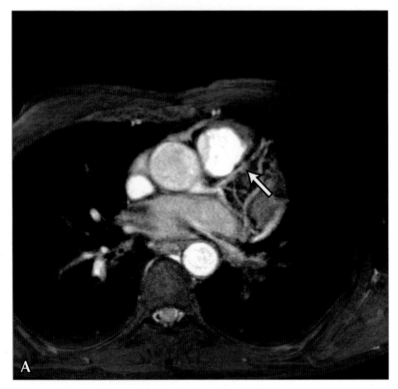

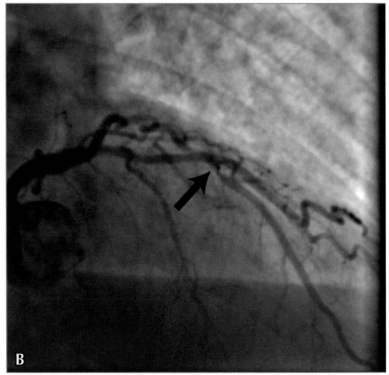

Figure 23-10. Gradient echo coronary cardiovascular magnetic resonance (CMR) sequences demonstrate rapidly moving laminar coronary lumen blood flow as "bright," whereas areas of stagnant flow and/or focal turbulence appear "dark" because of local saturation (stagnant flow) or dephasing (turbulence). **A**, Coronary CMR in a middle-aged man demonstrating a normal left main (LM) and left circumflex, but a severe signal void *(arrow)* in the mid-left anterior descending. **B**, Corresponding radiograph angiogram. A multicenter coronary CMR study in which > 100 subjects underwent coronary CMR prior to their first elective radiograph angiogram demonstrated a good sensitivity of coronary CMR, but relatively low specificity when analyzed on a vessel basis and compared with quantitative radiograph coronary angiography. However, when the data were analyzed for the clinically relevant LM/multivessel disease, coronary CMR had extremely high sensitivity and specificity [10].

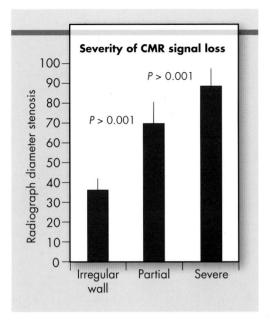

Severity of CMR signal loss

Figure 23-11. While coronary cardiovascular magnetic resonance (CMR) data are not of sufficient spatial resolution to allow for quantitative stenoses, the severity of vessel attenuation appears to correlate with the severity of angiographic diameter stenosis. In addition, the location of the stenosis on coronary CMR correlates well with the anatomic location (distance from the vessel origin) as demonstrated by radiograph angiography. (*Adapted from* Pennell *et al.* [11].)

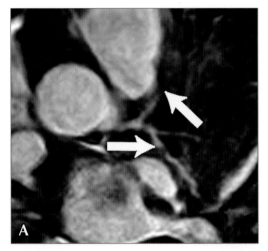

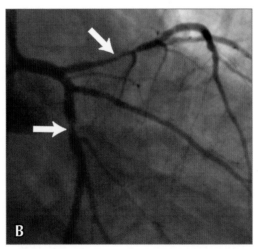

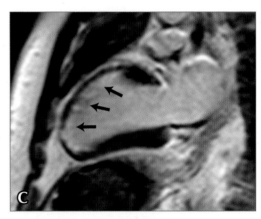

Figure 23-12. While late gadolinium enhancement (LGE) has proven useful in discriminating ischemic from nonischemic etiologies in patients with depressed left ventricular systolic function, up to 25% of patients without coronary artery disease will demonstrate a subendocardial/ischemic pattern. We have found that coronary cardiovascular magnetic resonance (CMR) is particularly helpful for patients presenting with a dilated cardiomyopathy in the absence of clinical infarction [12]. **A**, Coronary CMR demonstrating left anterior descending and left circumflex stenoses in a patient with a dilated cardiomyopathy. **B**, The narrowings are confirmed on the corresponding radiograph angiogram while LGE imaging (**C**) fails to demonstrate any hyperenhancement in the thin anterior wall and suggests a nonischemic etiology. (*Courtesy of* T. Hauser, MD.)

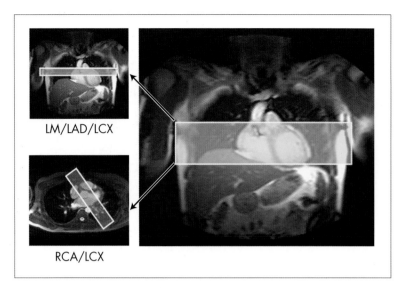

LM/LAD/LCX

RCA/LCX

Figure 23-13. In addition to targeted three-dimensional thin slab gradient echo acquisitions in the atrioventricular groove and axial plane, a "whole heart" acquisition in which a larger volume of data is acquired in the axial plane, somewhat analogous to coronary CT angiogram (CTA), was proposed. Advantages of the "whole heart" coronary cardiovascular magnetic resonance (CMR) acquisition include depiction of more extensive/distal portions of the coronary arteries and a single acquisition that is shorter in total acquisition duration than two targeted three-dimensional acquisitions [13]. Another advantage of the "whole heart" CMR approach is that it greatly facilitates postprocessing reconstructions that are visually attractive. LAD—left anterior descending; LCX—left circumflex artery; LM—left main; RCA—right coronary artery.

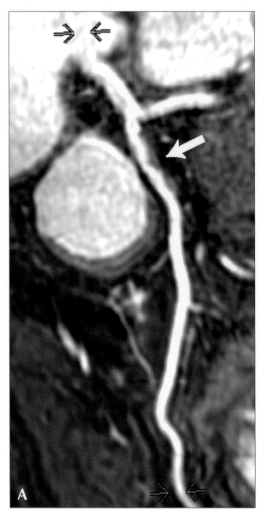

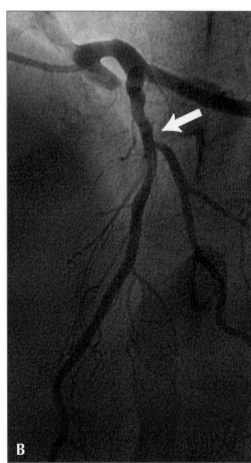

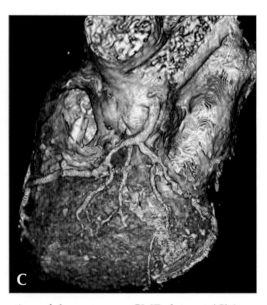

Figure 23-14. An example of whole heart coronary cardiovascular magnetic resonance (CMR) acquisition with steady-state free precession (SSFP). **A**, Curved reconstruction coronary CMR of the left main and left anterior descending (LAD) demonstrating a mild lesion (*arrow*) of the proximal LAD. **B**, Radiograph angiography demonstrating the same lesion (*arrow*) and three-dimensional reconstruction of the coronary CMR dataset (**C**) in which the coronary artery is depicted overlying the epimyocardium. Lesion and artery analysis of single center data suggest that the "whole heart" coronary CMR approach has sensitivity and specificity of ~ 90% [14,15]. (*Courtesy of* Drs. Ichikaswa and Sakuma, MD.)

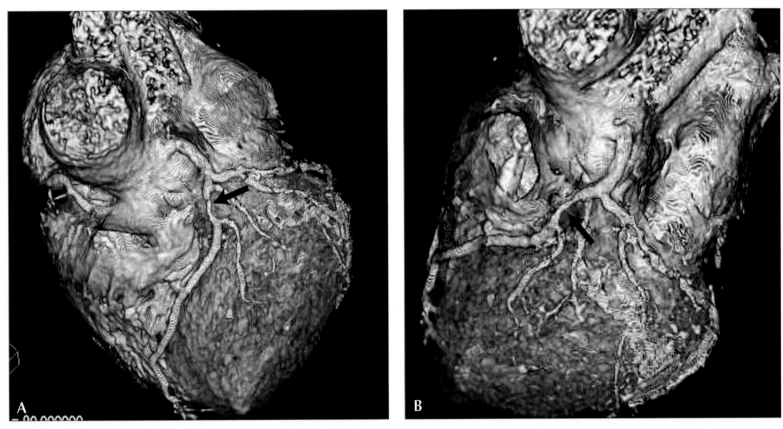

Figure 23-15. **A** and **B**, Whole heart coronary cardiovascular magnetic resonance reconstruction in another patient with a proximal left anterior descending stenosis (*arrow*). (*Courtesy of* H. Sakuma, MD.)

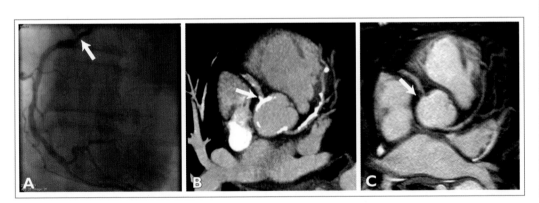

Figure 23-16. One of the limitations of coronary carotid compression tomography (CCT) is the artifact caused by epicardial calcium. **A**, Radiograph angiography, (**B**) coronary CT angiogram (CCT), and (**C**) coronary cardiovascular magnetic resonance (CMR) in a patient with a severe ostial right coronary artery stenosis (*white arrows*). Note the large amount of calcium precludes identification of the ostial lesion on coronary CCT, while the stenosis is well identified by coronary CMR. Data suggest that coronary CMR is superior to 64-slice coronary CCT in patients with high calcium scores [16].

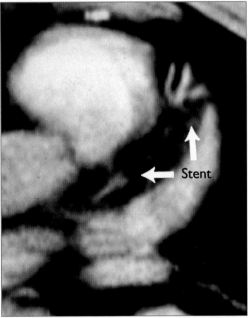

Figure 23-17. While intracoronary stents have proven safe for coronary cardiovascular magnetic resonance (CMR) with no risk for significant heating or displacement, their material leads to local field inhomogeneity and artifact that precludes lumen characterization. Shown is an axial coronary CMR in a patient with a proximal left anterior descending (LAD) stent and widely patent LAD. Note the signal void in the area of the stent that precludes lumen assessment. (*Adapted from* Kramer *et al.* [17].)

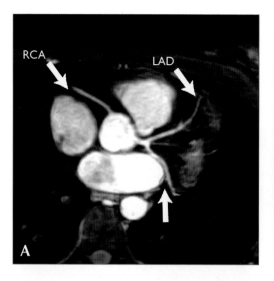

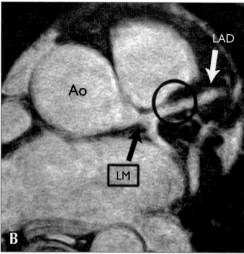

Figure 23-18. The increased signal-to-noise ratio (SNR) afforded by high field (3 T) coronary cardiovascular magnetic resonance (CMR) versus 1.5 T allows for the option of faster acquisitions or high spatial resolution. **A,** Targeted three-dimensional coronary CMR at 1.5 T with 1 × 1 × 3 mm spatial resolution, as compared with targeted three-dimensional coronary CMR at 3 T with 0.35 × 0.35 × 1.5 mm spatial resolution (**B**). Limited data suggest that while there are improvements in SNR, accuracy of coronary CMR at 1.5 T and 3 T is similar [18]. (*Courtesy of* M. Stuber, PhD.) Ao—aorta; LAD—left anterior descending; LM—left main; RCA—right coronary artery.

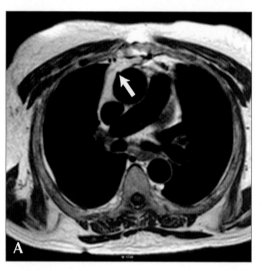

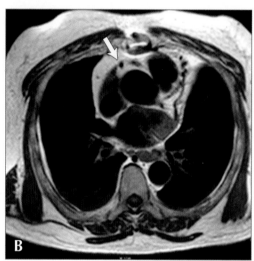

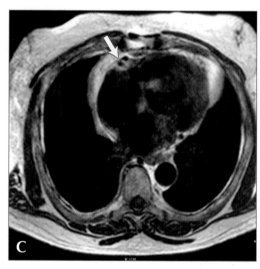

Figure 23-19. Technical imaging impediments of reverse saphenous vein grafts are much less burdensome because of their relatively larger diameter and stationary position within the thorax. Both electrocardiogram-triggered black blood spin echo and bright blood gradient echo methods were described for imaging of these grafts with interpretations of a patent graft if there is evidence of a patent lumen on two contiguous slices. Shown are a series of axial fast spin echo images in a patient with a widely patent reverse saphenous vein graft to the right coronary artery. **A,** Patent ostial graft (*arrow*), (**B**) proximal graft (*arrow*), and (**C**) midportion of the graft (*arrow*).

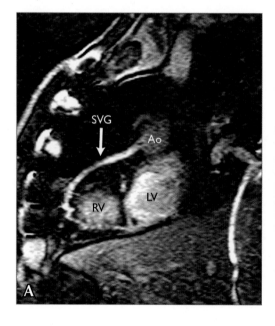

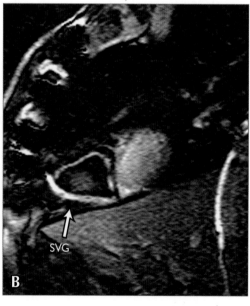

Figure 23-20. **A** and **B,** Both two-dimensional segmented k-space gradient echo and targeted three-dimensional coronary cardiovascular magnetic resonance (CMR) acquisitions may also be used to image the larger diameter coronary artery bypass grafts. Oblique breath hold two-dimensional coronary CMR of a patent saphenous vein bypass graft (SVG). Two adjacent images show the SVG extending from its aortic origin (Ao) to the distal touchdown. LV—left ventricle; RV—right ventricle.

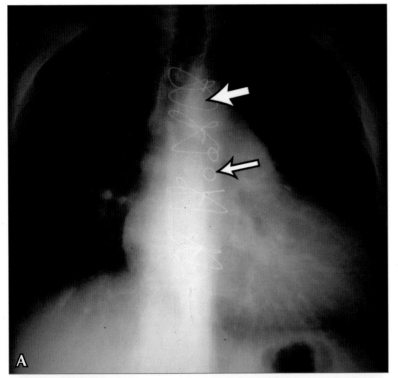

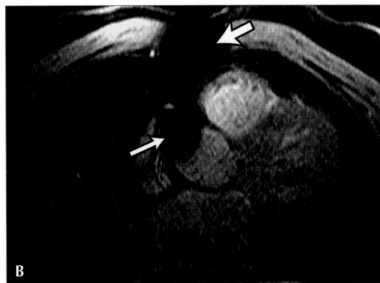

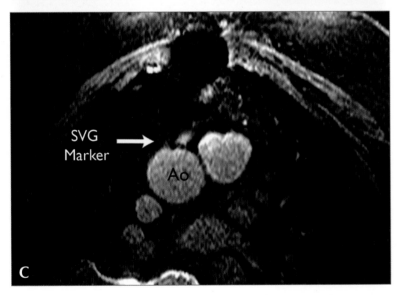

SVG
Marker

Ao

Figure 23-21. **A**, Posterior-anterior chest radiograph in a patient post thoracotomy with both coronary artery bypass graft markers (*long arrow*) and stainless steel sternal wires (*thick arrow*). **B**, Transverse coronary cardiovascular magnetic resonance (CMR) in the same patient. Note the large local artifacts (signal voids) related to the sternal wires (*thick arrow*) and bypass graft markers (*long arrows*). The size of the artifacts are related to the type of graft marker used with stainless steel associated with the largest artifacts. **C**, Barium and tantalum bypass graft markers (*arrow*) result in the smallest artifacts. The size of the artifacts are also reduced with spin-echo/black blood CMR. SVG—saphenous vein graft.

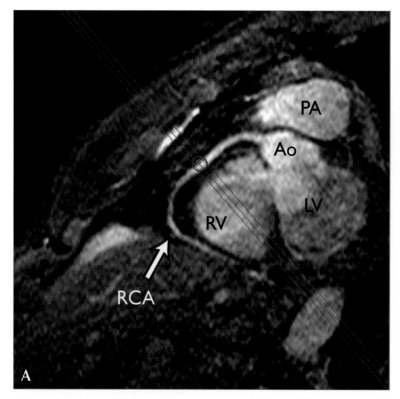

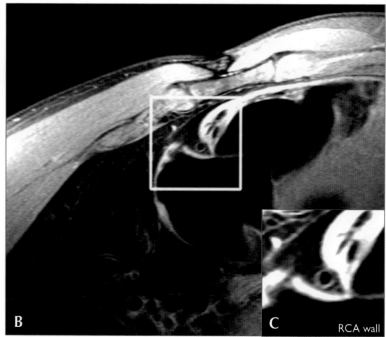

Figure 23-22. A–C, The motion suppression criteria for imaging of the very thin coronary artery wall exceed those of the coronary lumen. In selected patients, dual inversion and other black blood coronary cardiovascular magnetic resonance methods allow for depiction of the coronary wall [19] with demonstration of increased wall thickness in diseased arteries and patients with risk factors [20]. (*Courtesy of* R. Botnar, PhD.) Ao—aorta; LV—left ventricle; PA—pulmonary artery; RV—right ventricle.

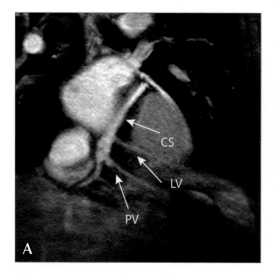

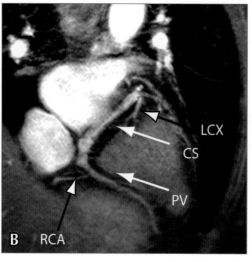

Figure 23-23. In addition to coronary artery imaging, Cardiovascular magnetic resonance (CMR) can also be used to image the coronary veins. Such visualization may assist in characterization of coronary vein acceptance for biventricular pacing for patients with congestive heart failure. Since the T2 prep suppresses signal from deoxygenated blood, a magnetization transfer contrast (MTC) prepulse is preferred [21]. Shown here are examples of coronary sinus (CS) and coronary vein CMR in a patient with favorable coronary vein anatomy (**A**), and a patient without lateral coronary veins to accept a pacing lead (**B**). (*Courtesy of* R. Nezafat, PhD.) CS—coronary sinus; LCX—left circumflex; LV—lateral vein; PV—pulmonary vein; RCA—right coronary artery.

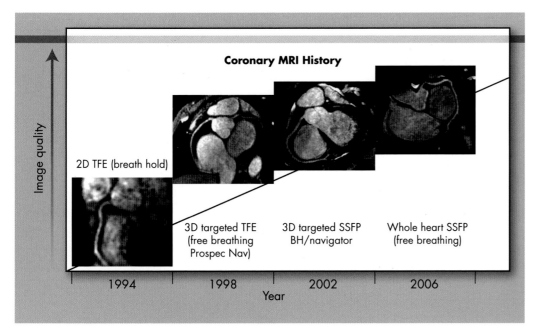

Figure 23-24. Summary of the history of coronary cardiovascular magnetic resonance (CMR) technical developments over the past 15 years. While coronary carotid compression tomography (CCT) methods have depended on hardware advancements (more detectors, fast gantry speed), coronary CMR advances have been software advances (breath hold to navigator; two-dimensional to targeted three-dimensional to whole heart; turbo field echo to steady-state free precession). Each of these advances has led to improved image quality and postprocessing capabilities. Future developments are likely to be related to parallel imaging (faster acquisitions), better motion compensation algorithms, and possibly high field coronary CMR that facilitates faster acquisitions and enhanced spatial resolution. (*Adapted from* M. Kouwenhoven, PhD.) BH—breath hold; SSFP—steady-state free precession; TFE—turbo field echo.

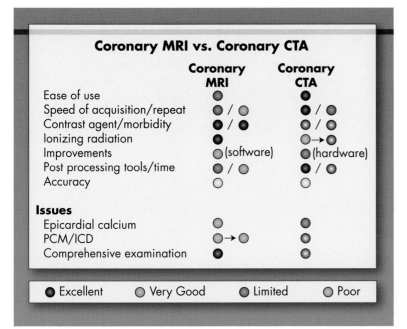

Figure 23-25. "Consumer Reports–style" comparison of coronary cardiovascular magnetic resonance (CMR) and coronary computed tomography (CCT). Coronary CCT acquisitions offer the advantages of ease of implementation, speed of acquisition, and postprocessing tools, while coronary CMR methods offer a nonionizing environment without the need for exogenous contrast agents with superior accuracy in patients with epicardial calcium. The radiation issue is particularly important in younger patients if the first acquisition is not successful (*eg*, inadequate breath hold or motion during coronary CCT breath hold) or if follow-up studies are anticipated. Preliminary data suggest the accuracy of whole heart coronary CMR and 64-slice CCT are similar [22].

References

1. Davidson, CJ, Mark, DB, Pieper, KS, *et al.*: Thrombotic and cardiovascular complications related to nonionic contrast media during cardiac catheterization: analysis of 8,517 patients. *Am J Cardiol* 1990, 65:1481–1484.

2. Omran, H, Schmidt, H, Hackenbroch, M, *et al.*: Silent and apparent cerebral embolism after retrograde catheterisation of the aortic valve in valvular stenosis: a prospective, randomised study. *Lancet* 2003, 361:1241–1246.

3. Kim, WY, Danias, PG, Stuber, M, *et al.*: Impact of bulk cardiac motion on right coronary MR angiography and vessel wall imaging. *J Magn Reson Imaging* 2001, 14:383–390.

4. Terachima M, Meyer CH, Keeffe BG, *et al.*: Noninvasive assessment of coronary vasodilation using magnetic resonance angiography. *J Am Coll Cardiol* 2005, 45:104–110.

5. McConnell MV, Ganz P, Selwyn A, *et al.*: Identification of anomalous coronary arteries and their anatomic course by magnetic resonance coronary angiography. *Circulation* 1995, 92:3158–3162.

6. Post, JC, van Rossum AC, Bronzwaer, *et al.*: Magnetic resonance angiography of anomalous coronary arteries. A new gold standard for delineating the proximal wma course? *Circulation* 1995, 92:3163–3171.

7. Bunce NH, Lorenz CH, Keegan J, *et al.*: Coronary artery anomalies: assessment with free-breathing three-dimensional coronary MR angiography. *Radiology* 2003, 227:201–208.

8. Greil GF, Stuber M, Botnar RM, *et al.*: Coronary magnetic resonance angiography in adolescents and young adults with Kawasaki disease. *Circulation* 2002, 105:908–911.

9. Mavrogeni S, Papadopoulos G, Douskou M, *et al.*: Magnetic resonance angiography is equivalent to Radiograph coronary angiography for the evaluation of coronary arteries in Kawasaki disease. *J Am Coll Cardiol* 2004, 43:649–652.

10. Kim WY, Danias PG, Stuber M, *et al.*: Coronary magnetic resonance angiography for the detection of coronary stenoses. *N Engl J Med* 2001, 345:1863–1869.

11. Pennell DJ, Bogren HG, Keegan J, *et al.*: Assessment of coronary artery stenosis by magnetic resonance imaging. *Heart* 1996, 75:127–133.

12. Hauser TH, Yeon SB, Appelbaum E, *et al.*: Discrimination of ischemic vs. non-ischmemic cardiomyopathy among patients with heart failure using combined coronary MRI and delayed enhancement MR [abstr]. *J Cardiovasc Magn Reson* 2005, 7:94.

13. Weber OM, Martin AJ, Higgins CB: Whole-heart steady-state free precession coronary artery magnetic resonance angiography. *Magn Reson Med* 2003, 50:1223–1228.

14. Sakuma H, Ichikawa Y, Suzawa N, *et al.*: Assessment of coronary arteries with total study time of less than 30 minutes using whole-heart coronary MR angiography. *Radiology* 2005, 237:316–321.

15. Sakuma H, Ichikawa Y, Chino S, *et al.*: Detection of coronary artery stenosis with whole-heart coronary magnetic resonance angiography. *J Am Coll Cardiol* 2006, 48:1946–1950.

16. Liu X, Zhao X, Huang J, Francois CJ, *et al.*: Comparison of 3D free-breathing coronary MR angiography and 64-MDCT angiography for detection of coronary stenosis in patients with high calcium scores. *Am J of Roentgenol* 2007, 189:1326–1332.

17. Kramer CM, Rogers WJ, Jr, Pakstis DL: Absence of adverse outcomes after magnetic resonance imaging early after stent placement for acute myocardial infarction: a preliminary study. *J Cardiovasc Magn Reson* 2000, 2:257–261.

18. Hackenbroch JCMR 2005.

19. Kim WY, Stuber M, Boernert P, Kissinger KV *et al*: Three-dimensional black-blood cardiac magnetic resonance coronary vessel wall imaging demonstrates positive arterial remodeling in patients with nonsignificant coronary artery disease. *Circulation* 2002, 106:296–299.

20. Astrup A, Kim WY, Tarnow L, *et al.*: Left ventricular function, mass, and volumes in type 1 diabetic patients—relation to NT-proBNP. *Diabetes Care* 2008, Feb 5 [Epub ahead of print].

21. Nezafat R, Han Y, Peters DC, *et al.*: Magnetic Resonance Coronary Vein Imaging: Sequence, Contrast and Timing. *Magn Reson Med* 2007, 58:1196–1206.

22. Pouleur AC, de Waroux JB, Kefer J, *et al.*: Head-to-head comparison of whole-heart coronary MR and 40/64 slice multidetector-CT angiography for detection of coronary artery stenosis. *Circulation* 2007, 116:510–511.

24

CMR Spectroscopy

Stefan Neubauer

Cardiovascular magnetic resonance (CMR) imaging relies on the ^{1}H nucleus in water (H_2O) and fat (-CH_2- and -CH_3 groups) molecules as a signal source. While this technique has had a major clinical impact in recent years regarding the assessment of cardiac anatomy, function, perfusion, and viability, it offers little insight into the biochemical state of cardiac tissue. In contrast, CMR spectroscopy enables physicians to study many other MR-visible nuclei contained in various metabolites of major relevance to the most important forms of cardiac disease, ischemic heart disease, and heart failure. CMR spectroscopy is unique, because it is the only available method for the noninvasive assessment of cardiac metabolism without the need for external radioactive tracers. Theoretically, many clinical questions can be answered with CMR spectroscopy, as will be discussed in this chapter. However, the low temporal and spatial resolution of CMR spectroscopy has thus far prevented its widespread use in clinical practice. To date, CMR spectroscopy remains a "noisy" technique, which, in research studies, can give important insight into the pathophysiological role of cardiac metabolism, by detecting biochemical differences between groups (*eg*, normal vs. diseased, or before vs. after treatment). However, its large measurement variability currently precludes the use of CMR spectroscopy for the reliable assessment of individual patients. Nevertheless, this chapter will describe the fundamental advantages and opportunities provided by CMR spectroscopy, summarize the major clinical results obtained thus far, and offer a vision for the future of this versatile clinical research tool. Comprehensive reviews of the subject are available elsewhere [1-6].

CMR Spectroscopy: Opportunities and Challenges

Opportunities	Challenges
The only noninvasive, nonradiation method for the study of cardiac metabolism [2,5]	Technically complex. Some additional CMR hardware and software required. Team of specialist experts required.
Highly versatile—many aspects of cardiac metabolism can be studied	Low signal-to-noise ratio and, thus, low spatial and temporal resolution. Compared with CMR Imaging, 105–106 times less sensitive
When combined with CMR Imaging, CMR spectroscopy offers unique pathophysiologic insight into the interrelations amongst cardiac function, perfusion, oxygenation, and metabolism	Long scanning times in the magnet (30–60 min); difficult for seriously ill patients
Uses intrinsic MR signal contrast, no external contrast agent needed	Difficult to image the inferior wall (very low signal due to greater distance from surface coil)
CMR spectroscopy is true molecular imaging without the need for specific external molecular imaging probes	Large data variability (~15%) at 1.5 T. Suitable to detect group differences in adequately powered studies, not yet suitable for reliable assessment of individual patients
	Discrepant normal values among different CMR spectroscopy centers, due to differences in methodology

Figure 24-1. The table summarizes the unique capabilities of Cardiovascular magnetic resonance (CMR) spectroscopy and the reasons why this method has not yet found its way into clinical practice. If these difficulties are overcome, CMR spectroscopy could be a highly attractive diagnostic tool, as will be further outlined in this chapter.

CMR SPECTROSCOPY: THE FOUNDATIONS

Nuclei of Interest for CMR Spectroscopy

Nucleus	Natural abundance	Relative MR sensitivity	Myocardial tissue concentrations	Metabolic information
^{1}H	99.98%	100%	H_2O 110 M; up to ~ 90 mM (CH3-^{1}H of creatine)	Creatine, lactate, (deoxy-), lipids, myoglobin, taurine, etc.
^{13}C	1.10%	1.60%	Labeled compounds, several Mm	Intermediary metabolism (glucose, fatty acids, etc.)
^{23}Na	100%	9.30%	10 mM (intracellular); 140 mM (extracellular)	Total, intracellular, extracellular sodium
^{31}P	100%	6.60%	Up to ~ 18 mM (PCr)	High-energy phosphates, inorganic phosphate, intracellular pH

Figure 24-2. Major nuclei of interest for cardiovascular magnetic resonance spectroscopy. Natural abundance is high for all except ^{13}C. For ^{13}C-MRS (MR spectroscopy), the heart is therefore supplied with external ^{13}C-labeled compounds (eg, 1-^{13}C-glucose). The relative CMR sensitivity of nonproton nuclei is 1 to 2 magnitude orders lower, and myocardial tissue concentrations ~4 orders of magnitude lower, compared with ^{1}H-MRI. These factors combine so that the resolution of ^{31}P-MR spectroscopy is ~5 to 6 orders of magnitude lower than CMR Imaging. The major metabolites detectable by CMR spectroscopy are also listed for each nucleus.

Methodological Requirements for CMR Spectroscopy

Same hardware as CMR imaging: 1.5 or 3 T magnets for the study of humans, ultra-high field (7–18 T) magnets for experimental studies (eg, isolated heart, in vivo rodents)

Additional hardware requirements: broadband radiofrequency transmitter to excite nonproton nuclei, nucleus-specific MR coils (eg, ^{31}P-coil). Additional software requirements: dedicated CMR spectroscopy acquisition sequences, CMR spectroscopy postprocessing and data analysis

Patients are studied in prone position to bring the heart closer to the surface coil and minimize the effects of respiratory motion

The CMR signal, the FID, is converted into an MR spectrum by "Fourier transformation"

A large number of acquisitions have to be signal-averaged to yield an MR spectrum with sufficient signal-to-noise ratio

In vivo studies require localization methods, such as DRESS, ISIS, or 3D-CSI, to obtain signal from a voxel positioned with the heart muscle, and to avoid skeletal muscle (chest wall) signal contamination [5]. Initially, [1]H-CMR images are obtained to enable the positioning of the ^{31}P-voxels.

MR spectra have to be corrected for partial saturation, because the T_1 of phosphocreatine is longer than the T_1 of ATP.

At 1.5 T, ^{31}P-MRS voxel sizes are 20–70 mL, acquisition time is 20–45 min, variability of measurements is ~15% [7]

Figure 24-3. Methodologic requirements for cardiovascular magnetic resonance (CMR) spectroscopy. Fourier transformation converts the free induction decay (FID), which relates time and signal intensity, to an MR spectrum, which relates MR frequency and signal intensity. CSI—chemical shift imaging; DRESS—depth-resolved surface coil spectroscopy; ISIS—image-selected in vivo spectroscopy.

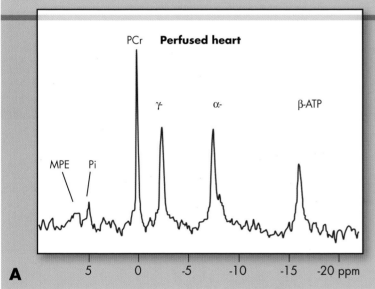

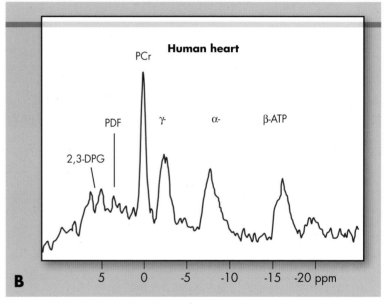

Figure 24-4. Experimental (**A**) and human (**B**) cardiac ^{31}P-MR spectra. ATP has three ^{31}P-atoms (γ, α, β) and is the direct energy source for myofibrillar contraction. Phosphocreatine (PCr; sometimes also abbreviated as CP) is the major energy storage and transport compound in heart. Inorganic phosphate (Pi) is the degradation product of ATP. This resonance obscures the Pi and MPE resonances in human cardiovascular magnetic resonance (CMR) spectra. The area under each resonance is proportional to the concentration of each metabolite in the heart. Experimentally, absolute quantification (in mmol/L) is easily achieved by comparison with a ^{31}P-standard of known concentration [4]. Human CMR spectra are usually quantified in relative terms by calculating the PCr/ATP (area) ratio. The PCr/ATP ratio is a powerful index of the energetic state of the heart [8]. It decreases whenever oxygen demand outstrips oxygen supply (such as in ischemia), or when the total creatine pool of the heart decreases (such as in heart failure). Absolute metabolite quantification is feasible in human CMR spectroscopy, but is technically highly demanding (see Bottomley [5] and Beer et al. [9] for further details). Experimental CMR spectra also allow quantification of intracellular pH, from the frequency (chemical shift) difference of the PCr and Pi resonances, which is pH sensitive. MPE—monophosphate esters, mainly glycolysis metabolites and adenosine monophosphate. 2,3-DPG—2,3-diphosphoglycerate, arising from the presence of blood (blood contamination because of large voxel sizes) in the spectroscopic voxel. PDE—phosphodiesters, mainly membrane and serum phospholipids. ppm—parts per million, a measure of relative CMR frequency.

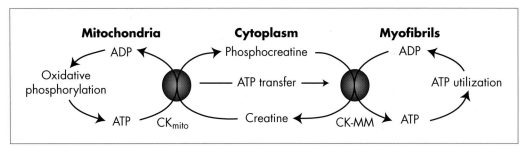

Figure 24-5. Participation of ATP and phosphocreatine (PCr) in the *creatine kinase energy shuttle*. At the site of ATP production, the mitochondria, the high-energy phosphate bond is transferred from ATP to creatine, yielding PCr and ADP. This reaction is catalyzed by the mitochondrial creatine kinase isoenzyme. PCr diffuses through the cytoplasm to the site of ATP usage, the myofibrils, where the back reaction occurs, catalyzed by the myofibrillar-bound ATP is thus reformed and is used for contraction. Free creatine then diffuses back to the mitochondria [10]. (*From* Lardo *et al.;* with permission.) MM—creatine kinase isoenzyme.

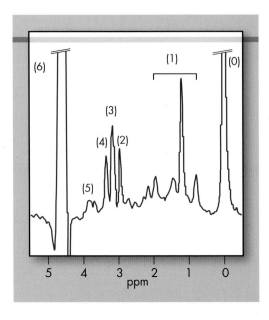

Figure 24-6. Experimental ^{1}H-CMR spectrum from a perfused heart showing multiple resonances: (0) reference solution (TSP = trimethyl silyl propionic acid); (1) lipids (CH$_3$- and -CH$_2$- groups); (2) creatine; (3) taurine, carnitine; (4) taurine, carnitine; (5) creatine; (6) H$_2$O. Furthermore, in a ^{1}H-CMR spectrum, a resonance of about 73 ppm (not shown here) appears, corresponding to deoxymyoglobin; this allows to detection and quantification of myocardial deoxygenation. Technical challenges for ^{1}H-MRS include the need for suppression of the strong ^{1}H signal from water and the complexity of ^{1}H-spectra with overlapping resonances, many of which remain to be characterized. In principle, however, ^{1}H-MRS has a higher sensitivity than ^{31}P-MRS, because the relative MR sensitivity of ^{1}H is ~15 times higher than that of ^{31}P (*see* Fig. 24-2). (*Courtesy of* J. Schneider, MD, Oxford University.)

ISCHEMIC HEART DISEASE

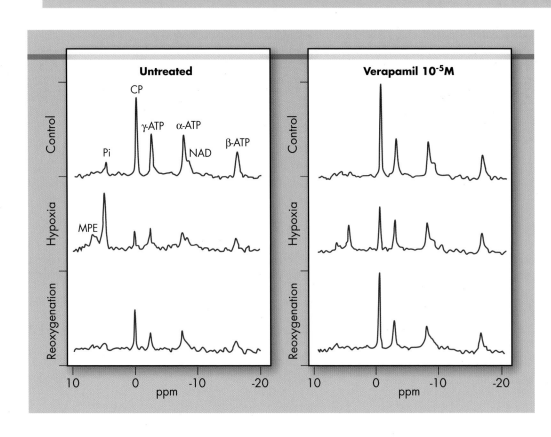

Figure 24-7. Changes of cardiac high-energy phosphate metabolism in an acute experimental setting of hypoxia. ^{31}P-CMR spectra from an untreated perfused heart and a heart treated with verapamil during control, at the end of 30 minutes of oxygen deprivation (hypoxia), and at the end of 30 minutes of reperfusion, demonstrating changes in cardiac energy metabolism. After 30 minutes of hypoxia, ATP resonances are reduced by ~ 50%, phosphocreatine by ~ 80%, and inorganic phosphate and monophosphate esters (MPEs) have increased. During reoxygenation, inorganic phosphate shows full, phosphocreatine partial, and ATP no recovery. When hearts are pretreated with a Ca^{++}-antagonist, changes in energetics are attenuated. Verapamil protects hearts from the effects of hypoxic injury [11]. CP—creatine phosphate, a term synonymous with phosphocreatine; NAD—nicotine adenine dinucleotide. (*From* Neubauer *et al.* [11]; with permission.)

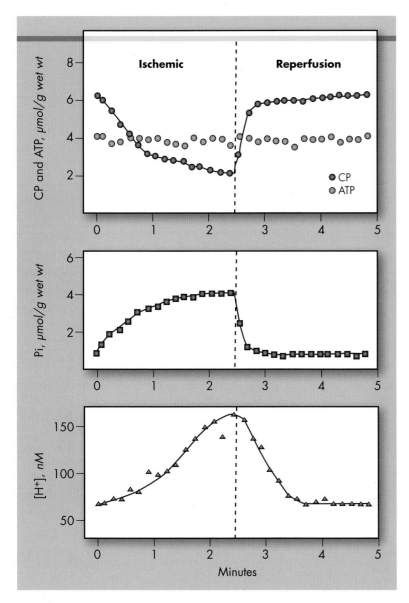

Figure 24-8. Changes of cardiac high-energy phosphate metabolism over the first few minutes of ischemia. Isolated perfused heart model, total, global, normothermic ischemia. Changes of energetics after the onset of ischemia occur extremely rapidly [12]. The decrease of phosphocreatine (CP) and the increase of inorganic phosphate (Pi) are among the earliest metabolic responses, changing within seconds after the onset of ischemia. ATP and intracellular pH$_i$ decrease much more slowly, only after several minutes. In this study, a temporal resolution of 12 s was achieved by summing spectra from several experiments. Thus, the parameters measured by cardiovascular magnetic resonance spectroscopy can detect myocardial ischemia within seconds after its onset. (*From* Clarke *et al.* [12]; with permission.)

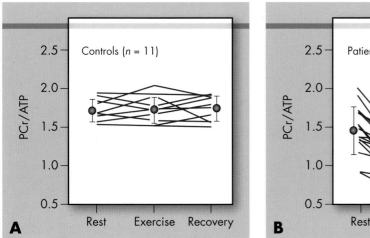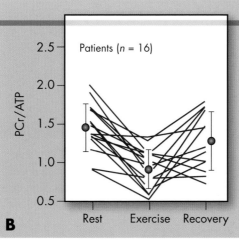

Figure 24-9. Myocardial phosphocreatine/adenosine triphosphate (PCr/ATP) ratios at rest, during handgrip exercise, and recovery in healthy individuals (controls) (**A**) and in patients with stenosis of the left anterior descending coronary artery or of the left main stem (**B**) [13]. Handgrip exercise lead to a 30% to 35% increase of the cardiac rate-pressure product. At this moderate level of stress, the cardiac PCr/ATP ratio decreased in patients but not in healthy subjects.

The figure illustrates the principle of a biochemical stress test in patients with coronary artery disease. However, to become a clinically practical procedure, similar measurements would have to be achieved with high spatial resolution (*ie*, as true metabolic imaging) and high temporal resolution (*ie*, during a graded stepwise exercise protocol). Such a test might allow us in the future to determine the "phosphocreatine threshold" as the maximum workload at which energy metabolism remains unchanged. This threshold might then be used to test the efficacy of antianginal medication or of interventional/surgical revascularization procedures. (*From* Weiss *et al.* [13]; with permission.)

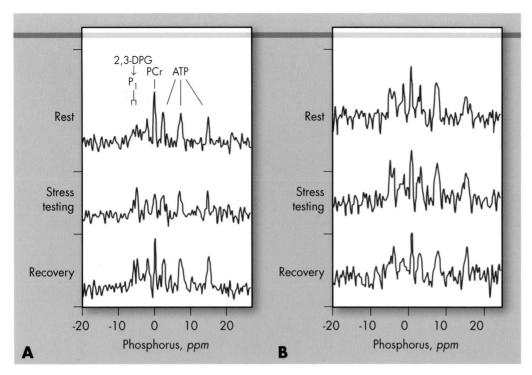

Figure 24-10. The pathophysiologic mechanisms of exercise-induced chest pain in women with normal coronary arteries are being debated, but microvascular dysfunction and resulting tissue ischemia in the absence of macroscopic coronary stenoses are a likely explanation. Buchthal *et al.* [14] showed that in seven of 35 women with chest pain and normal coronary arteries, the phosphocreatine/adenosine triphosphate (PCr/ATP) ratio decreased by 29% ± 5% during handgrip exercise. The figure shows two examples (**A** and **B**) of ^{31}P-MR spectroscopy in women with chest pain and absence of significant coronary artery stenoses. One woman (**A**) showed a significant decrease (27%) in the PCr/ATP ratio during stress testing, whereas the second woman (**B**) did not. These findings provide direct evidence of exercise-induced myocardial ischemia in a subgroup of women with chest pain and normal coronary arteries. ^{31}P-CMR spectroscopy stress testing may contribute to the diagnosis and to monitoring of treatment in this ubiquitous condition.(*From* Buchthal *et al.* [14]; with permission.)

CMR Spectroscopy for Ischemia, Scar, and Viability

CMR spectroscopy-detectable metabolite	Ischemia	Scarred	Stunning/hibernation
ATP (^{31}P-CMR spectroscopy)	↓	↓↓	↔
PCr (^{31}P-CMR spectroscopy)	↓	↓↓	↔ or ↓
pHi (^{31}P-CMR spectroscopy)	↓	↔	↔ or ↓
Na$^+$ (^{23}Na-CMR spectroscopy)	↑	↑	↔
Total creatine (^{1}H-CMR spectroscopy)	↔	↓↓	↔
Deoxymyoglobin (^{1}H-CMR spectroscopy)	↑	↔	↔

Figure 24-11. In experimental studies, ischemic, nonviable scarred, and stunned/hibernating myocardium can be identified by a combination of ^{31}P-, ^{23}Na-, and ^{1}H-CMR spectroscopy measurements, as each of these conditions is characterized by a unique combination of metabolic changes detectable by MRS. With technical progress, a similar approach may be possible for patients in the future. PCr—phosphocreatine; pH—hydrogen ion concentration.

Role of Cardiac Metabolism and the Potential Role of CMR Spectroscopy in Heart Failure

Cardiac energy metabolism is deranged in the failing heart and is a key player in the pathophysiology of contractile dysfunction [8]

^{31}P- and ^{1}H-CMR spectroscopy studies have demonstrated altered cardiac energy metabolism in experimental and clinical studies of heart failure. The extent of energetic derangement correlates with clinical status, systolic and diastolic function, and predicts prognosis [15-18]

Medical therapy that optimizes cardiac energy metabolism is one of the most promising new strategies for the treatment of heart failure [8,20]

CMR spectroscopy, combined with CMR Imaging, can monitor the energetic and functional response of the failing heart to established and new forms of therapy

It is possible that the early energetic response of the failing heart to new pharmacological therapy predicts the long-term outcome. If this were the case, CMR spectroscopy measurements of cardiac energetics would greatly speed up the development of new forms of heart failure therapy

Figure 24-12. Role of cardiac energy metabolism and the potential role of cardiovascular magnetic resonance in heart failure.

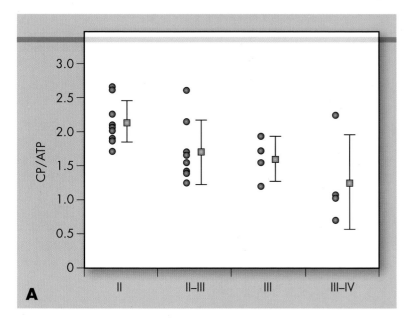

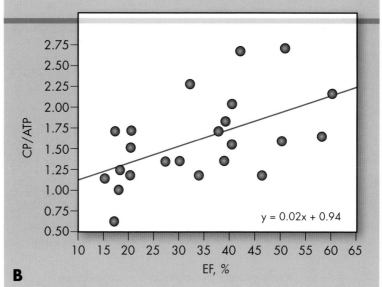

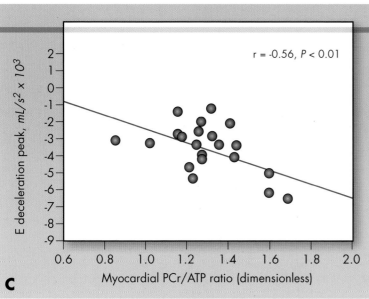

Figure 24-13. Derangement of cardiac energetics in heart failure and correlation with clinical and functional indices. **A,** In patients with dilated cardiomyopathy, the myocardial phosphocreatine/adenosine triphosphate ratio (CP/ATP) declines with increasing clinical severity of heart failure (New York Heart Association class II-IV) [20]. **B,** In the same patients, the myocardial PCr/ATP ratio correlates (r = 0.54, P <0.01) with left ventricular ejection fraction (EF) [16]. **C,** In patients with diastolic heart failure due to hypertensive heart disease, the PCr/ATP ratio correlates with diastolic function, measured as the E deceleration peak [18]. (*Courtesy of Dr H. Lamb, Leiden University, the Netherlands.*) DCM—dilated cardiomyopathy; 2,3-DPG—2,3-diphosphoglycetate.

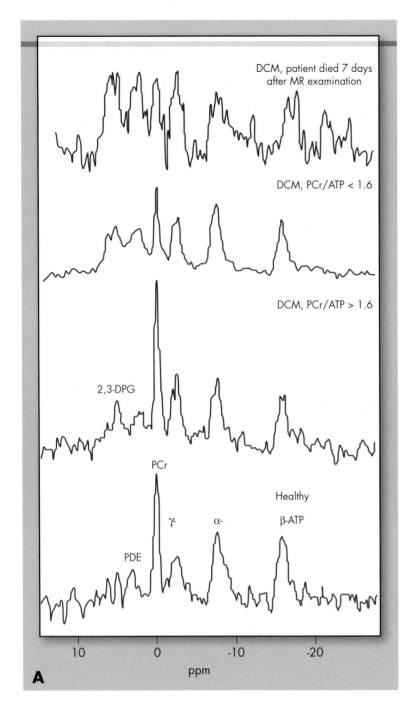

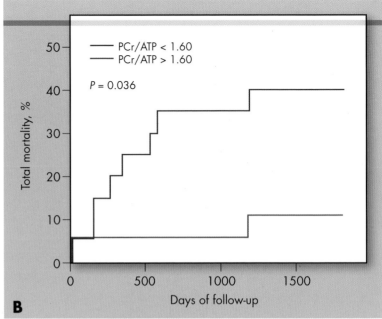

Figure 24-14. Cardiac energetics predict prognosis in heart failure. **A,** Cardiac ³¹P-MR spectra, from *bottom* to *top*: volunteer, dilated cardiomyopathy (DCM) with normal phosphocreatine/adenosine triphosphate (PCr/ATP) ratio, DCM with reduced PCr/ATP ratio, DCM with severely reduced PCr/ATP ratio; this patient died 7 days after the cardiovascular magnetic resonance examination. **B,** Kaplan-Meier life table analysis for total mortality of DCM patients divided into two groups split by the myocardial PCr/ATP ratio (< 1.60 vs. > 1.60). Patients with an initially low PCr/ATP ratio had increased mortality over the mean study period of 2.5 years. In this study, the PCr/ATP ratio was a stronger predictor of mortality than functional (ejection fraction) or clinical (New York Heart Association class) indices. (*From* Neubauer *et al.* [17]; with permission.) 2,3-DPG—2,3-diphosphoglycetate; PDE—phosphodiesters; γ-, α-, and β-P-atom of ATP.

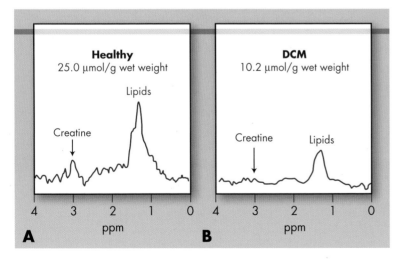

Figure 24-15. A, ¹H-CMR spectroscopy from the interventricular septum of a healthy subject (evident on fig.). The total creatine resonance is seen at 3.0 ppm. The creatine concentration is 25.0 μmol/g wet weight. A lipid resonance is seen at 0.9 to 1.4 ppm. **B,** ¹H-CMR spectrum from a patient with dilated cardiomyopathy (DCM). A much lower creatine peak is observed (10.2 μmol/g wet weight). This study showed that ¹H-CMR spectroscopy can detect the depletion of the myocardial creatine pool in heart failure. If combined with ³¹P-CMR spectroscopy, the method should in the future allow the calculation of the myocardial free ADP concentration. This is important, because an increased free ADP concentration inhibits contractile function even if ATP levels remain relatively normal (*see* Neubauer [8] for a full explanation of the topic). (*From* Nakae *et al.* [21]; with permission.)

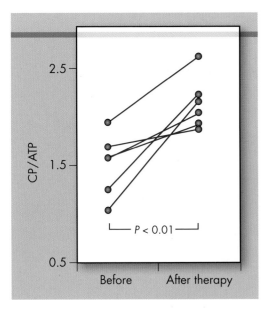

Figure 24-16. Phosphocreatine/adenosine triphosphate (CP/ATP) ratios in six patients with dilated cardiomyopathy before and after 12 ± 6 weeks of drug therapy, including angiotensin-converting-enzyme inhibitors, diuretics and, in four of six patients, β-receptor blockers. There was a significant increase of the PCr/ATP ratio in each patient (* $P < 0.01$). The improvement of cardiac energy metabolism occurred in parallel to clinical recompensation. (*From* Neubauer *et al.* [20]; with permission.)

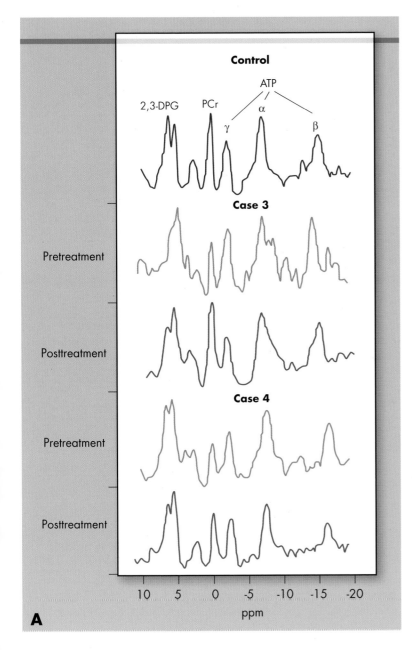

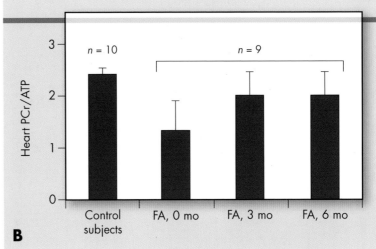

Figure 24-17. Therapy monitoring by ^{31}P-CMR spectroscopy. Friedreich's ataxia (FA) is a hereditary disease with deficiency of the mitochondrial protein frataxin. Frataxin deficiency leads to reduced mitochondrial respiration and increased free radical damage. Patients were treated with antioxidants (coenzyme Q, vitamin E) for 6 months. **A**, ^{31}P-CMR spectra of a control subject and of two patients. Before treatment, the phosphocreatine/adenosine triphosphate (PCr/ATP) ratio is reduced. After treatment, the PCr/ATP ratio has returned toward normal. **B**, The beneficial effect is achieved after 3 months and is maintained at 6 months. While not in patients with heart failure, this study illustrates how ^{31}P-CMR spectroscopy may in the future be used to monitor the energetic effect of novel forms of heart failure therapy. (*From* Lodi *et al.* [22]; with permission.)

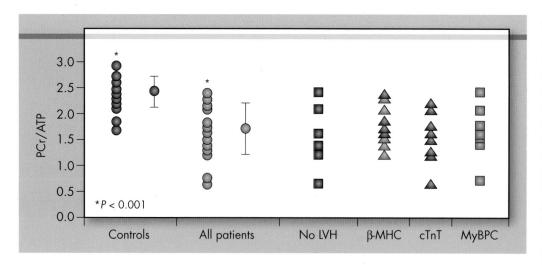

Figure 24-18. Phosphocreatine/adenosine triphosphate (PCr/ATP) ratios in control subjects and in patients with hypertrophic cardiomyopathy (HCM). Similar reductions of the PCr/ATP ratio are observed in HCM, across a range of specific mutations and independent of the presence of left ventricular hypertrophy (*ie*, also in genotype positive, phenotype negative gene carriers). These and other findings have led to the paradigm that the common pathophysiologic mechanism for all forms of HCM is energetic derangement [24]. (Figure *from* Crilley J *et al.* [23]; with permission.) β-MHC—β-myosin heavy chain; cTnT—cardiac troponin T; MyBPC—myosin binding protein C.

DIABETES

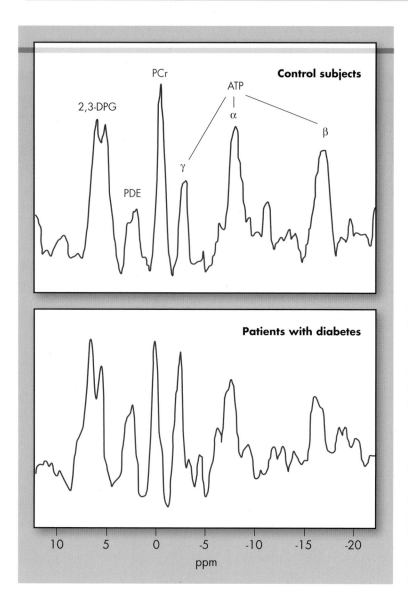

Figure 24-19. Derangement of cardiac energy metabolism in patients with type II diabetes mellitus. These patients had normal cardiac function on echocardiography. Typical cardiac ^{31}P CMR spectra from a normal control subject (*top*) and a patient with type II diabetes (*bottom*), showing a lower phosphocreatine/adenosine triphosphate (PCr/ATP) ratio in the patient. On average, in diabetic patients, the PCr/ATP ratio was reduced by 35%. Correlation of energetic derangement with fatty acid and glucose metabolism. Cardiac high-energy phosphate levels, expressed as the PCr/ATP ratio, correlated negatively with the plasma free fatty acid concentrations ($r^2 = 0.32$, $P = 0.01$) for all subjects and correlated positively with the plasma glucose concentrations ($r^2 = 0.55$, $P = 0.05$) for the patients with type II diabetes, but there was no correlation for healthy control subjects. The data show that derangement of cardiac energetics occurs early in diabetes, and may predispose the heart to failure, a possible explanation for the increased incidence of heart failure in these patients. (*From* Scheuermann-Freestone, *et al.* [25]; with permission.) 2,3-DGP—2,3-diphosphoglycerate; PDE—phosphodiesters; PCr—phosphocreatine; α, β, and γ—the three phosphate groups of ATP.

Outlook: CMR Spectroscopy

Technical developments	Clinical application
Improved spatial resolution. Goal: 5 mL for ^{31}P-MRS, 1 mL for ^{1}H-MRS. True metabolic imaging based on American Heart Association 17 segment model, including inferior wall	Measurement of novel energetic parameters, such as free ADP and creatine kinase reaction velocity and resolution, will yield novel insights into the true role of cardiac energetics in heart disease [26]
Improved temporal resolution. Goal: 2 min for ^{31}P-MRS, to enable MRS stress testing during a graded exercise protocol	With improved measurement accuracy, assessment of individual patient changes, rather than only assessment of patient group differences, will become feasible
Improved reproducibility. Goal: Reduction of within-subject measurement variability from currently 10%–15% to <5%	Evaluation of the functional and metabolic effects of new forms of heart failure therapy. If energy metabolism can be established as a surrogate endpoint for mortality, then development of new treatments could be sped up
Combined ^{31}P-/1H-MRS will yield measurements of free ADP concentration	Derangement of cardiac energy metabolism as a predictor of prognosis in heart failure
Standardization of MRS methods among MRS centers and vendors, a necessary requirement for MRS multicenter studies	Noninvasive phenotyping of cardiomyopathies by their metabolic profile
Potential solutions: Increased static magnetic field strength (7T and higher), phased array MRS coils, novel MRS sequence design	Energetic derangement as a guide for determining the optimal time point for valve replacement, eg, in aortic stenosis

Figure 24-20. Future developments and clinical potential of cardiovascular magnetic resonance (CMR) spectroscopy. The table provides suggestions for technical advances that may, in the coming years, allow development of CMR spectroscopy as a clinically practical diagnostic tool, and summarizes potential future areas of clinical applications. Such clinical indications for CMR spectroscopy will need to be established in the future, after adequate methodology is available.

REFERENCES

1. Pohost GM, Meduri A, Razmi RM, *et al.*: Cardiac MR spectroscopy in the new millennium. *Rays* 2001, 26:93–107.

2. Neubauer S: Cardiac magnetic resonance spectroscopy: potential clinical applications. *Herz* 2000, 25:452–460.

3. Neubauer S: Cardiac magnetic resonance spectroscopy. *Curr Cardiol Rep* 2003, 5:75–82.

4. Ingwall JS: Phosphorus nuclear magnetic resonance spectroscopy of cardiac and skeletal muscles. *Am J Physiol* 1982, 242:H729–744.

5. Bottomley PA: MR spectroscopy of the human heart: the status and the challenges. *Radiology* 1994, 191:593–612.

6. Beyerbacht HP, Vliegen HW, Lamb HJ, *et al.*: Phosphorus magnetic resonance spectroscopy of the human heart: current status and clinical implications. *Eur Heart J* 1996, 17:1158–1166.

7. Lamb HJ, Doornbos J, den Hollander JA, *et al.*: Reproducibility of human cardiac 31P-NMR spectroscopy. *NMR Biomed* 1996, 9:217–227.

8. Neubauer S.: The failing heart: an engine out of fuel. *N Engl J Med* 2007, 356:1140–1151.

9. Beer M, Seyfarth T, Sandstede J, *et al.*: Absolute concentrations of high-energy phosphate metabolites in normal, hypertrophied, and failing human myocardium measured noninvasively with (31)P-SLOOP magnetic resonance spectroscopy. *J Am Coll Cardiol* 2002, 40:1267–1274.

10. Wallimann T, Wyss M, Brdiczka D, *et al.*: Intracellular compartmentation, structure and function of creatine kinase isoenzymes in tissues with high and fluctuating energy demands: the 'phosphocreatine circuit' for cellular energy homeostasis. *Biochem J* 1992, 281:21–40.

11. Neubauer S, Ingwall JS: Verapamil attenuates ATP depletion during hypoxia: 31P NMR studies of the isolated rat heart. *J Mol Cell Cardiol* 1989, 21:1163–1178.

12. Clarke K, O'Connor AJ, Willis RJ: Temporal relation between energy metabolism and myocardial function during ischemia and reperfusion. *Am J Physiol* 1987, 253:H412–421.

13. Weiss RG, Bottomley PA, Hardy CJ, *et al.*: Regional myocardial metabolism of high-energy phosphates during isometric exercise in patients with coronary artery disease. *N Engl J Med* 1990, 323:1593–1600.

14. Buchthal SD, den Hollander JA, Merz CN, *et al.*: Abnormal myocardial phosphorus-31 nuclear magnetic resonance spectroscopy in women with chest pain but normal coronary angiograms. *N Engl J Med* 2000, 342:829–835.

15. Neubauer S, Newell JB, Ingwall JS: Metabolic consequences and predictability of ventricular fibrillation in hypoxia. A 31P- and 23Na-nuclear magnetic resonance study of the isolated rat heart. *Circulation* 1992, 86:302–310.

16. Neubauer S, Horn M, Pabst T, *et al.*: Contributions of 31P-magnetic resonance spectroscopy to the understanding of dilated heart muscle disease. *Eur Heart J* 1995, 16 (Suppl O):115–118.

17. Neubauer S, Horn M, Cramer M, *et al.*: Myocardial phosphocreatine-to-ATP ratio is a predictor of mortality in patients with dilated cardiomyopathy. *Circulation* 1997, 96:2190–2196.

18. Lamb HJ, Beyerbacht HP, van der Laarse A, *et al.*: Diastolic dysfunction in hypertensive heart disease is associated with altered myocardial metabolism. *Circulation* 1999, 99:2261-2267.

19. Ingwall JS, Weiss RG: Is the failing heart energy starved? On using chemical energy to support cardiac function. *Circ Res* 2004, 95:135–145.

20. Neubauer S, Krahe T, Schindler R, *et al.*: 31P magnetic resonance spectroscopy in dilated cardiomyopathy and coronary artery disease. Altered cardiac high-energy phosphate metabolism in heart failure. *Circulation* 1992, 86:1810–1818.

21. Nakae I MK, Omura T, Yabe T, *et al.*: Proton magnetic resonance spectroscopy can detect creatine depletion associated with the progression of heart failure in cardiomyopathy. *J Am Coll Cardiol* 2003, 42:1587–1593.

22. Lodi R, Hart PE, Rajagopalan B, *et al.*: Antioxidant treatment improves in vivo cardiac and skeletal muscle bioenergetics in patients with Friedreich's ataxia. *Ann Neurol* 2001, 49:590–596.

23. Crilley JG, Boehm EA, Blair E, *et al.*: Hypertrophic cardiomyopathy due to sarcomeric gene mutations is characterized by impaired energy metabolism irrespective of the degree of hypertrophy. *J Am Coll Cardiol* 2003, 41:1776–1782.

24. Ashrafian H, Redwood C, Blair E, *et al.*: Hypertrophic cardiomyopathy: a paradigm for myocardial energy depletion. *Trends Genet* 2003, 19:263–268.

25. Scheuermann-Freestone M, Madsen PL, Manners D, *et al.*: Abnormal cardiac and skeletal muscle energy metabolism in patients with type 2 diabetes. *Circulation* 2003, 107:3040–3046.

26. Smith CS, Bottomley PA, Schulman SP, *et al.*: Altered creatine kinase adenosine triphosphate kinetics in failing hypertrophied human myocardium. *Circulation* 2006, 114:1151–1158.

25

Interventional CMR

Elliot R. McVeigh and Robert J Lederman

During the last decade, steady progress was made to make cardiovascular magnetic resonance (CMR) an effective method for guiding interventional therapy. The ability to observe target tissues in great detail and to measure the response of those tissues for therapeutic treatment makes CMR an attractive modality. Realtime imaging methods have made it possible to make high quality images without gating or averaging multiple acquisitions—a necessary characteristic for guiding devices and observing therapy. Also, some laboratories and companies are developing devices which are visible in CMR either through active coils mounted onto the devices, or using passive properties of the devices. The benefits of using CMR are manifold: no ionizing radiation is needed, soft tissue contrast is available, nephrotoxic radiocontrast in not needed, heavy radiograph–protective lead aprons are not needed, and functional imaging of treated tissues such as flow and perfusion is available immediately. Development of techniques for CMR guided therapies may give us the opportunity to develop novel procedures that are not possible with any other imaging technique.

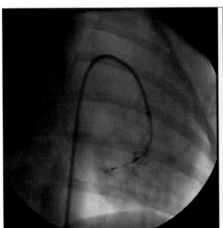 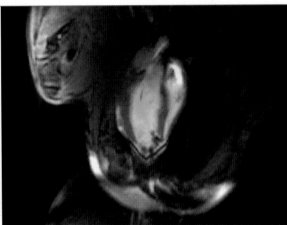

Figure 25-1. A comparison of radiograph and realtime cardiovascular magnetic resonance (CMR) guidance of a catheter-based myocardial injection system, the Boston Scientific Stiletto (Boston Scientific, Natick, MA). The catheter is positioned retrograde across the aortic valve. While the spatial and temporal resolution of radiograph guidance is higher, CMR depicts the target soft tissue and function to facilitate targeting, as well as intramyocardial retention and dispersion of injected material. In this case, iron-labeled stromal cells are injected in and around an apical myocardial infarction.

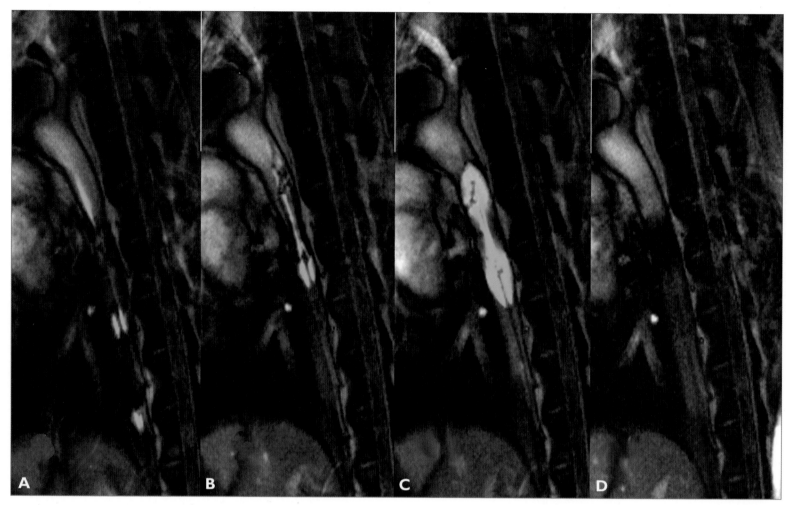

Figure 25-2. Real-time cardiovascular magnetic resonance delivery and implantation of a balloon expandable platinum stent in a pig model of aortic coarctation. Simultaneous device and tissue imaging allows the operator to directly and immediately observe the impact of stent deployment on the target lesion [1]. **A**, Advancing balloon/stent over "active" guidewire. **B**, Positioning into coarctation. **C**, Balloon inflation. **D**, "Shielding" artifact darkens aorta after balloon and guidewire are withdrawn.

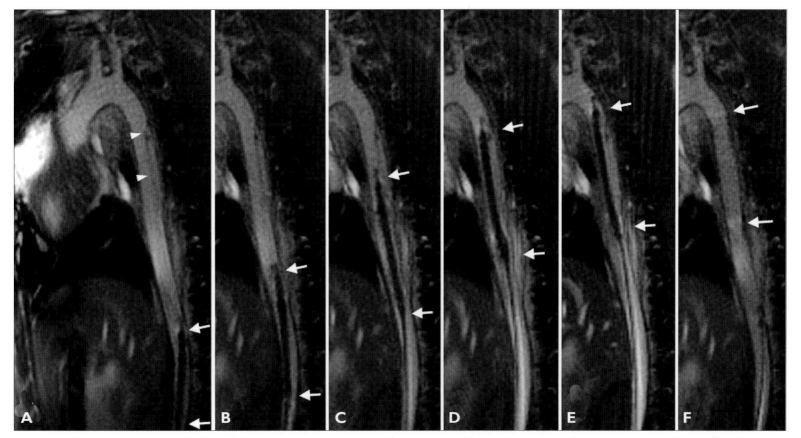

Figure 25-3. Advancement of the stent-graft delivery system (*arrows*) up to the level of the dissection (*arrowheads*) under realtime cardiovascular magnetic resonance (CMR) guidance (**A-F**). CMR fluoroscopy was based on an interactive realtime steady-state free precession sequence with radial k-space filling during free breathing and without cardiac triggering. Realtime radial projection images with a frame rate of 7 frames per second were reconstructed and displayed without detectable image reconstruction delay.

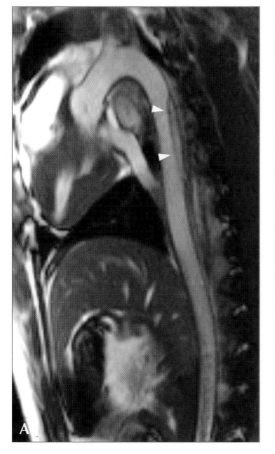

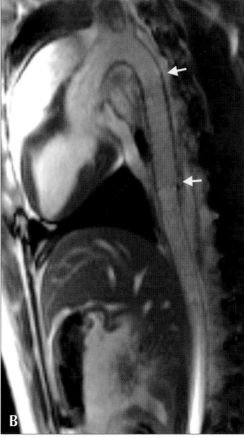

Figure 25-4. Pre and post interventional cardiovascular magnetic resonance (CMR) evaluation. **A**, Preinterventional high-resolution CMR in the parasagittal orientation showing the dissection flap (*arrowheads*) in the proximal descending thoracic aorta. **B**, Corresponding postinterventional CMR demonstrating correct position of the stent-graft (*arrows*) with complete coverage of the dissection. Steady-state precession retro imaging was acquired with electrocardiogram gating and retrospective image reconstruction within one breath hold in parasagittal and in axial orientation. Image acquisition time was 15 seconds for a single slice. (*Courtesy of* Holger Eggebrecht, MD, and Harald H. Quick, PhD, University Hospital Essen, Essen, Germany.)

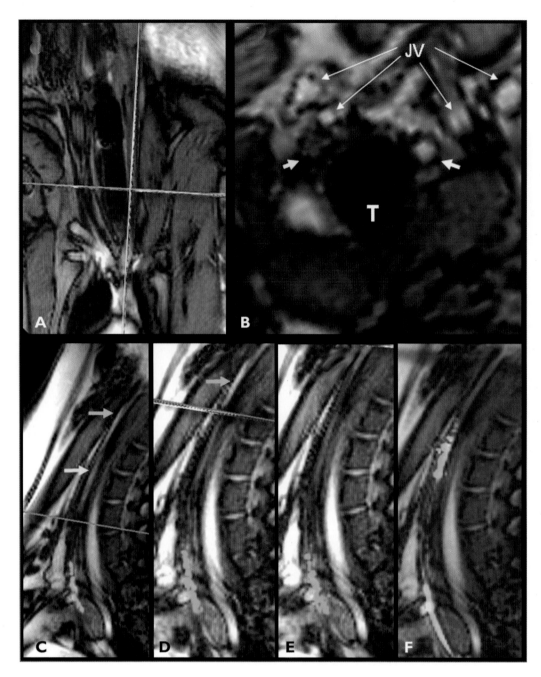

Figure 25-5. Traversing chronic total occlusions (CTO) with active guidewire and catheter. **A**, Realtime, interleaved, multiplanar cardiovascular magnetic resonance of coronal, sagittal and transverse slices through occluded left carotid artery (LCA) showing tip position of active CTO guidewire. **B**, Transverse slice demonstrates right carotid artery (*white arrow*) and occluded LCA (*yellow arrow*). The active CTO wire tip (*red*) is seen entirely within the LCA lumen. **C**, Sagittal view of the occluded LCA (*yellow arrow*). The active wire (*red*) and catheter (*green*) are visualized proximally in the occluded LCA. The transverse slice (**B**) is continually translated cranially in advance of the CTO wire tip. **D**, The active wire is advanced through the remaining CTO into the patent distal LCA [2]. **E**, The active catheter is tracked over the fixed wire into the distal patent LCA. **F**, 5×100 mm angioplasty balloon inflated with gadolinium-dilute diethylenetriamine pentaacetic acid over active delivery wire (*green*). JV—external and internal jugular veins; T—trachea.

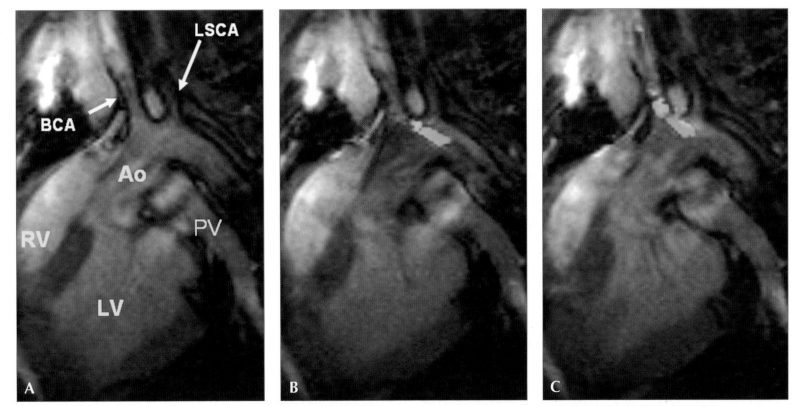

Figure 25-6. Navigating the aorta and its branches using "active" catheter devices under realtime cardiovascular magnetic resonance. **A,** Active guidewire entering and moving retrograde through the descending aorta (Ao). **B,** Active guidewire positioned in the ascending aorta, used to deliver an active catheter to the origin of the brachiocephalic artery (BCA) [2]. **C,** The active guidewire and catheter, respectively, are advanced into the BCA. LSCA—left subclavian artery; LV—left ventricle; PV—pulmonary vein; RV—right ventricle.

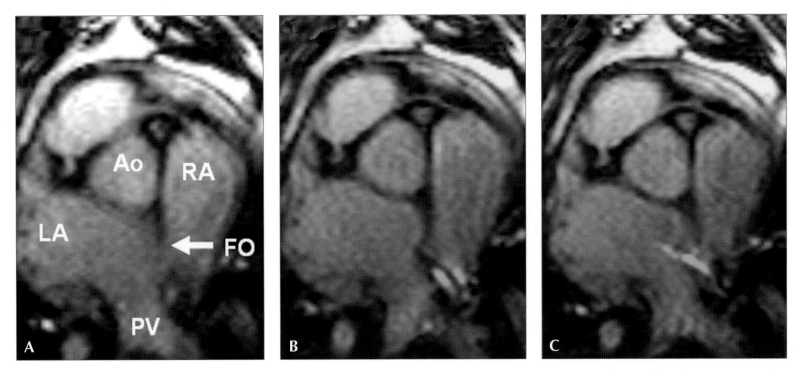

Figure 25-7. Atrial septal puncture under realtime cardiovascular magnetic resonance (CMR) in a healthy pig. The Brockenbrough puncture needle was modified to serve as a CMR antenna (receiver coil) [3]. **A,** The chambers. **B,** Tenting of the foramen ovale while pressure is applied with the "active" Brockenbrough needle. **C,** The needle immediately after crossing into the left atrium. Ao—aorta; FO—fossa ovalis (*white arrow*); LA—left atrium; PV—pulmonary vein; RA—right atrium.

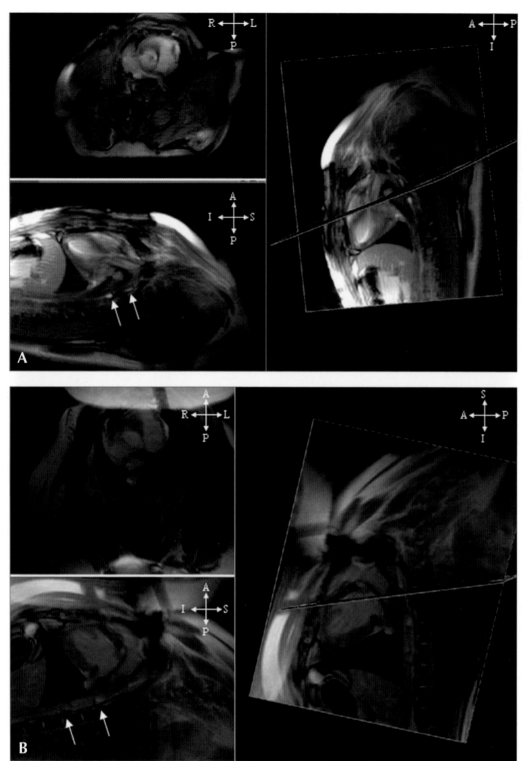

Figure 25-8. A comparison of "passive" (**A**) and "active" (**B**) catheter navigation under realtime cardiovascular magnetic resonance. Each panel shows simultaneous multislice axial (*upper left*), sagittal (*lower left*), and three-dimensional rendered (*right*) display of a platinum stent deployed to treat aortic coarctation in a pig [1]. The stent delivery balloon is filled with dilute gadolinium to make it visible (*arrows*). Using the active guidewire technique dramatically enhances visibility of the devices, thereby simplifying the procedure. Orientation icons: S = superior, I = inferior, A = anterior, P = posterior, L = left, and R = right.

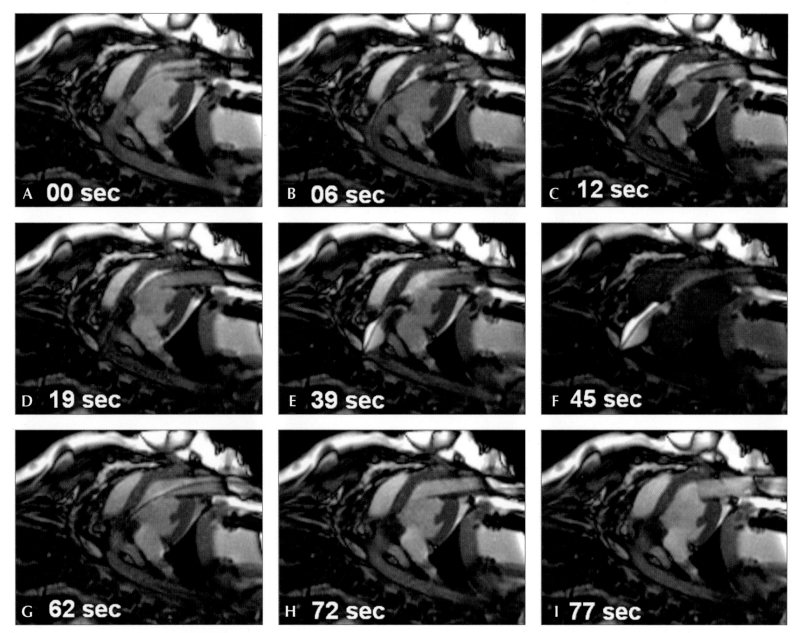

Figure 25-9. Selected frames from the realtime cardiovascular magnetic resonance (CMR) displayed within the scan room, showing the deployment of the prosthetic valve. **A,** A guidewire is advanced through the trocar across the native aortic valve. **B,** The prosthetic valve is advanced to the end of the trocar. **C,** The prosthetic valve is advanced into position in the left ventricular outflow track. **D,** The prosthetic valve is inserted across the native valve and aligned with the coronary ostia and the aortic annulus (**E**), and a balloon filled with a gadolinium- dilute diethylenetriamine pentaacetic acid CMR contrast agent is used to expand the prosthetic valve. **F,** Interactive saturation is used to enhance visualization of the extent of balloon inflation. **G,** The balloon is taken down and pulled back through the trocar. **H,** The guidewire is removed. **I,** The delivery device is removed from the trochar. The total time of this sequence of pictures is 77 seconds. (Also, *see* the movie in the NHLBI archive: http://imagegallery.nhlbi.nih.gov/mcveighe/mrm1.html). (From McVeigh *et al.*, [4]; with permission.)

REFERENCES

1. Raval AN, Telep JD, Guttman MA, *et al.*: Real-time MRI-guided stenting of aortic coarctation with commercially available catheter devices in swine. *Circulation* 2005, 112:699–706.

2. Raval AN, Karmarkar PV, Guttman MA, *et al.*: Real-time MRI-guided endovascular recanalization of chronic total arterial occlusion in a swine model. *Circulation* 2006, 113:1101–1107.

3. Raval AN, Karmarkar PV, Guttman MA, *et al.*: Real-time MRI-guided atrial septal puncture and balloon septostomy in swine. *Catheter Cardiovasc Interv* 2006, 67:637–643.

4. Horvath KA, Li M, Mazilu D, *et al.*: Real-time Magnetic Resonance Imaging Guidance for Cardiovascular Procedures. *Magn Reson Med* 2006, 56:958–964.

26

CHAPTER

High-Field CMR

Matthias Stuber, Nael Osman, Michael Schar, and Robert G. Weiss

In cardiovascular magnetic resonance (CMR) and magnetic resonance spectroscopy (MRS), the available signal-to-noise ratio (SNR) is directly related to the strength (B_0) of the static magnetic field. Thus, improved SNR is expected for CMR/MRS by using magnets with higher magnetic field strength. A higher SNR can result in abbreviated scanning times, a higher spatial, temporal, or spectral resolution, or in any combination of the above. This may ultimately result in an improved diagnostic value of CMR in general, where new areas of innovation are likely to emerge.

However, challenges at higher magnetic field strength include increased susceptibility artifacts at tissue borders (= distortion of the main magnetic field or B_0 inhomogeneity), more rapid signal decay after radiofrequency (RF) excitation (reduced T2*), increased longitudinal relaxation times (T1), RF field distortions and RF transmit field (B1) inhomogeneity [1-4]. In addition, problems associated with increased RF deposition and reliable R-wave triggering in the presence of an amplified magneto-hydro-dynamic effect have to be addressed [5].

Despite the above-mentioned challenges, recent progress in the areas of hardware and software development, and the adaptation of 3 T specific pulse sequences over the past 2 to 3 years have made it possible to implement CMR on commercial whole body 3 T systems [5-7]. As a result, outstanding image quality can now be obtained for most cardiovascular applications. While contemporary results obtained with this new technology are presented in this chapter, studies are now needed that identify distinct advantages and shortcomings for CMR at 3 T.

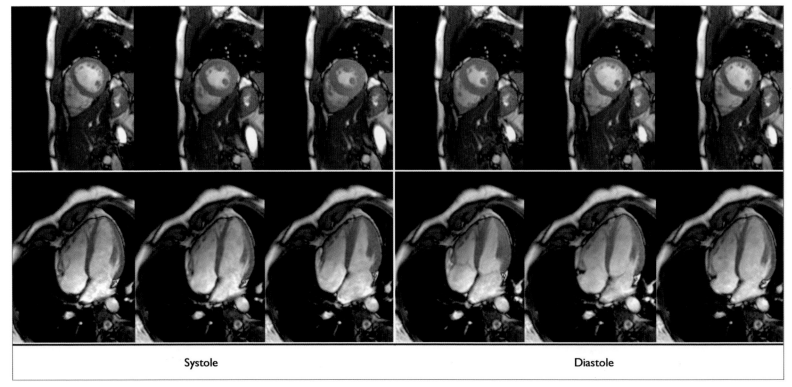

Systole   Diastole

Figure 26-1. Imaging of ventricular function. For the measurement of left ventricular (LV) volume, mass, ejection fraction, and wall thickening, steady-state free precession (SSFP) imaging is the current method of choice at 1.5 T because of the excellent signal-to-noise properties and the exquisite contrast between the ventricular blood pool and the myocardium. This technique relies upon the use of relatively large radiofrequency (RF) excitation angles and a short period of time in-between RF excitations (= repetition time (TR)). At 3 T, such high RF excitation angles and short TR cannot easily be used because of specific absorption rate constraints. To operate this imaging sequence within safety limits, the TR has to be increased and the RF excitation angles have to be reduced. However, this affects the contrast in the images and magnetic field distortions at tissue borders lead to stronger artifacts. Nevertheless, with the use of advanced shimming hardware and software, these artifacts can be minimized and SSFP functional imaging of the heart can be performed successfully at 3 T [7]. Selected systolic and diastolic cine frames from a healthy adult subject obtained in a mid-ventricular short axis orientation are displayed together with the corresponding 4-chamber views. The temporal resolution of this acquisition is 20 ms, and the spatial resolution 1.3×1.6×8 mm³. With parallel imaging, these images are acquired in a breath-hold of ~14 seconds [8].

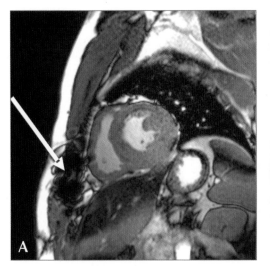 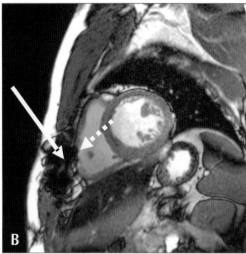

Figure 26-2. 3 T cardiovascular magnetic resonance. Imaging of left ventricular systolic function in a patient after bypass surgery: end-systolic (**A** and **C**) and end-diastolic (**B** and **D**) images obtained in a patient after bypass surgery.

Continued on the next page

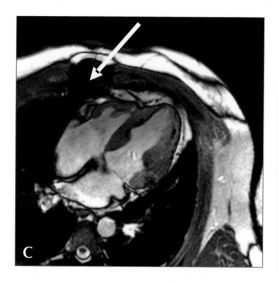 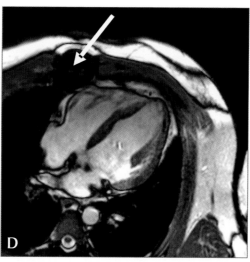

Figure 26-2. *(Continued)* A short axis view (**A** and **B**) is displayed together with a four-chamber view (**C** and **D**). Note the high visual contrast between the ventricular blood pool and the myocardium. In the region of the *solid arrow*, artifacts induced by the sternal wires are visible. While these artifacts lead to main magnetic field distortions, higher-order volumetric shimming can be used to minimize adverse effects on image quality [7]. A residual artifactual signal void in the area of the right ventricle (*dotted arrow*) is still visible. The temporal resolution of this acquisition is 20 ms, and the spatial resolution $1.3 \times 1.6 \times 8$ mm^3. With parallel imaging, these images are acquired in a breath-hold of ~14 seconds [8].

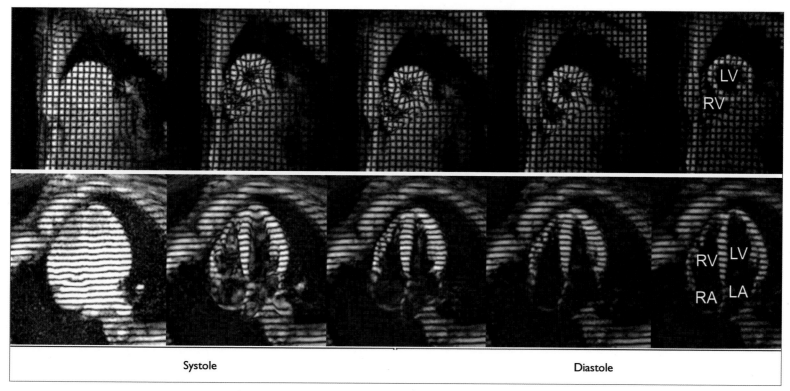

Systole   Diastole

Figure 26-3. Cardiovascular magnetic resonance (CMR) imaging of local myocardial function using tissue tagging. Using conventional CMR as shown in Figures 26-1 and 26-2, ventricular volume, mass, ejection fraction and wall thickening can be measured. However, due to the absence of natural landmarks and internal structures of the left ventricle, quantification of local myocardial motion properties (deformation or strain) is not possible. Therefore, myocardial tagging was developed in the late 1980s [9-10]. At 1.5 T, T1-related fading of the tags restricts quantification of tissue properties mainly to the systolic phase of the cardiac cycle. At 3 T, T1 is prolonged thereby supporting tag persistence. In the short axis (*upper row*) and four-chamber (*lower row*) images, an excellent tagging contrast is obtained for both systole and diastole. Therefore, quantification of both local systolic and diastolic motion properties of the heart is facilitated at 3 T. The images were acquired with a spatial resolution of $1.7 \times 1.7 \times 9$ mm^3 and a temporal resolution of 23 ms. Using spiral imaging, the images are acquired during a breath-hold of ~19 seconds [11]. LA—left atrium; RA—right atrium; RV—right ventricle.

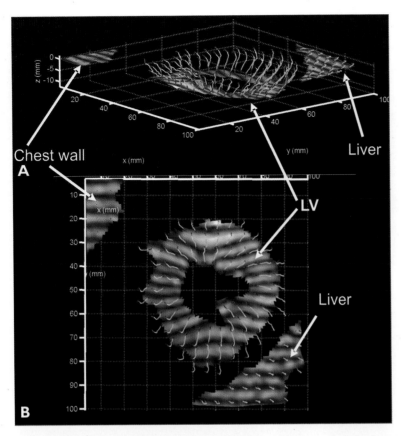

Figure 26-4. Imaging of local three-dimensional motion of the heart. For the display and measurement of three-dimensional myocardial motion, complex acquisition schemes using orthogonal image acquisition planes with subsequent spatial coregistration were needed, or lengthy three-dimensional acquisitions were necessary [12,13]. However, with a more recent technical development at 3 T (zHARP), local three-dimensional displacement of any material point of the myocardium can be extracted from a two-dimensional slice [14]. In **A**, the systolic three-dimensional displacement vectors of a midventricular short axis are shown starting in *red* (diastole) and ending in *purple* (systole). Note that there is minimal displacement in the liver and no displacement at the level of the chest wall as expected. In **B**, the same situation is visualized from a different angle.

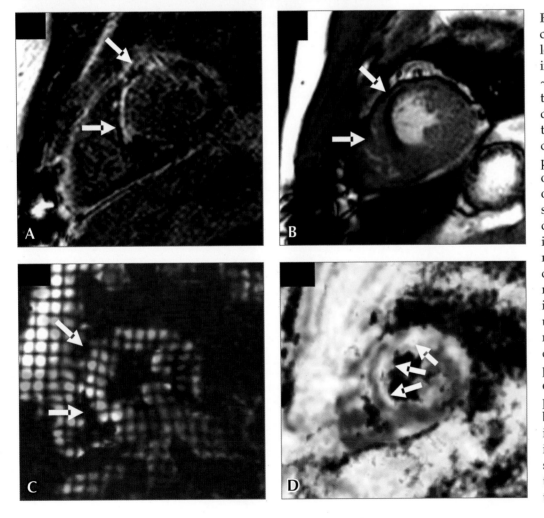

Figure 26-5. Comprehensive cardiovascular magnetic resonance imaging of the left ventricle (LV) in a patient with an infarct. **A**, Late gadolinium enhancement ~15 min after the intravenous administration of gadolinium shows a subendocardial infarct (crescent of positive signal in the anterior-septal wall, *arrows*). On the corresponding short axis steady-state free precession (SSFP) image in **B**, eccentricity of the LV with wall thinning in the region of the infarct is observed (*arrows*). In the same area, hypokinesia is seen on the SSFP cine images (*not shown*). The tagged image in **C** that was analyzed with HARP shows reduced local contractility (*green*) when compared with normal contraction in remote areas (*blue*) [15]. **D**, A SENC image is shown [16,17]. SENC is based on a stimulated echo method with which systolic myocardial strain in the through-plane direction can be quantified on a pixel-by-pixel basis [17]. While the use of stimulated echoes carries a 50% Signal-to-noise ratio penalty, this relative loss can be recovered by using 3 T in conjunction with a spiral imaging readout [18]. On the SENC image in **D**, *orange* refers to a high through-plane strain and *yellow* to a reduced strain. Note the reduced strain values in the region of the infarct (*arrows*).

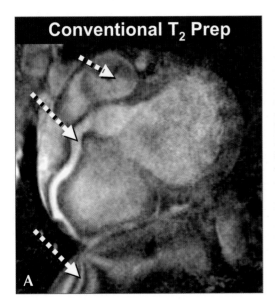

Conventional T₂ Prep

A

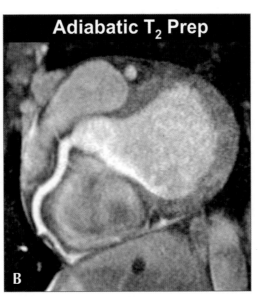

Adiabatic T₂ Prep

B

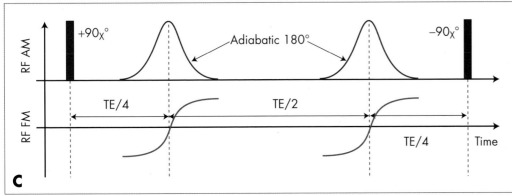

C

Figure 26-6. Adiabatic T_2 Prep for contrast generation in coronary cardiovascular magnetic resonance (CMR). **A** and **B**, Three T coronary CMR obtained in a healthy adult subject [19]. These images were acquired during free breathing using realtime navigator technology for respiratory motion suppression and a T_2 Prep for contrast enhancement between the blood pool (long T_2) and the myocardium (short T2) [20-22]. Using the conventional design of the T_2 Prep, artifacts are accentuated at 3 T because of B1 inhomogeneity (*dashed arrows*). However, by using adiabatic RF pulses as part of the T_2 Prep (**C**), these artifacts can be significantly minimized and contrast generation between the blood pool and the myocardium increased without an exogenous contrast agent at 3 T [6]. AM—amplitude modulation; FM—frequency modulation of the radiofrequency pulse; TE—echo time of the T_2 Prep.

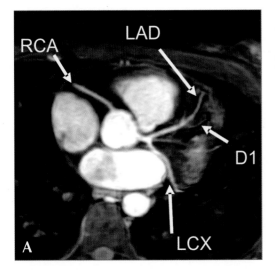

A

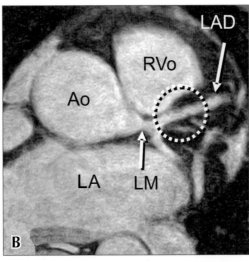

B

Figure 26-7. Whole heart and high spatial resolution coronary cardiovascular magnetic resonance (CMR) in a patient with a history of a proximal left anterior descending (LAD) dissection. **A**, Reformatted whole heart coronary CMR acquired during free breathing ~10 minutes after the administration of gadolinium [23,24]. For respiratory motion suppression realtime navigator technology was used and an adiabatic T2 Prep for contrast generation [6,20-21]. A high contrast between the coronary blood pool and the myocar-

dium is obtained and proximal to mid-coronary segments of the right coronary artery (RCA), left main (LM), LAD, and the left circumflex (LCX) together with a first order diagonal (D1). Spatial resolution is ~$1\times1\times3$ mm³ and scanning time ~8 minutes to 12 minutes depending on the heart rate and respiratory pattern of the patient. **B**, A local volume-targeted acquisition of both LM and LAD with a high spatial resolution of $0.35\times0.35\times1.5$ mm³ is displayed. Scanning duration for high-spatial resolution CMR is ~10 minutes to 12 minutes, and the higher spatial resolution is obtained at the expense of limited volumetric coverage. Minor signal variations are observed in the region of the prior dissection (*dotted circle*), but an adequate filling of the mid-LAD is observed on both the whole heart and the high spatial resolution CMR. Ao—ascending aorta; LA—left atrium; RVo—right ventricular outflow tract.

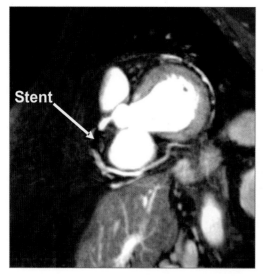

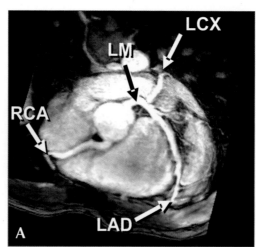

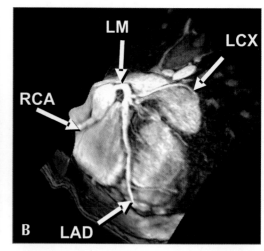

Figure 26-8. Coronary magnetic resonance angiography (MRA) in the presence of a stent. In a patient with a right coronary artery (RCA) stent, volume-targeted coronary cardiovascular magnetic resonance of the RCA was obtained after the administration of gadolinium [24]. For respiratory motion suppression, realtime navigator technology was used, as well as an adiabatic T2 Prep for contrast generation [6,20-21]. The spatial resolution was 0.7×1.0×3.0 mm³ and the scanning time ~5 minutes during free breathing. While the stent led to a local signal void in the image (*arrow*), the extent of the artifact was constrained despite the high magnetic field strength. Filling of the RCA distal to the stent can be appreciated.

Figure 26-9. Reformatted whole heart coronary cardiovascular magnetic resonance (CMR) angiography. In a healthy adult subject, whole heart coronary CMR was obtained without the use of contrast agents. For respiratory motion suppression realtime navigator technology was used, and an adiabatic T2 Prep for contrast generation [6,20-21]. The spatial resolution was 1.0×1.0×2.0 mm³ and the scanning time was ~10 minutes during free breathing. The images were reconstructed using the 'Soapbubble' tool and different orientations are shown in **A** and **B**, respectively [25]. Using whole heart coronary CMR, long and contiguous segments of the coronary arterial system can be obtained. LAD—left anterior descending; LCX—left circumflex artery; LM—left main; RCA—right coronary artery.

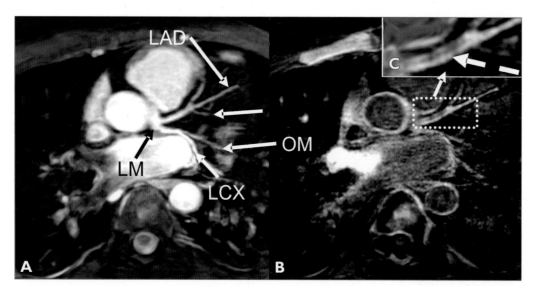

Figure 26-10. Reformatted whole heart coronary cardiovascular magnetic resonance (CMR) angiography and delayed gadolinium enhancement (LGE) of the coronary vessel wall. **A**, Reformatted whole heart coronary CMR acquired in a patient with a coronary artery bypass graft during free-breathing ~10 minutes after the administration of gadolinium [24]. For respiratory motion, suppression realtime navigator technology was used and an adiabatic T2 Prep for contrast generation [6]. A high contrast between the coronary blood pool and the myocardium is obtained, in addition to proximal to mid-coronary segments of the left main (LM), left anterior descending (LAD), left cir-cumflex (LCX), a first order diagonal (D1), and obtuse marginal (OM). The spatial resolution is ~1×1×3 mm³ and scanning time ~8 minutes to 12 minutes depending on the heart rate and respiratory pattern of the patient. **B**, The same scan was repeated ~45 minutes after the administration of the contrast agent and the adiabatic T2 Prep was replaced by an inversion-recovery prepulse with an inversion delay of ~300 ms that allows for the simultaneous signal suppression of the blood pool and the myocardium. A magnified version of the LAD is displayed in **C**. In patients, LGE of the coronary and carotid vessel wall was attributed to atherosclerosis [26-29].

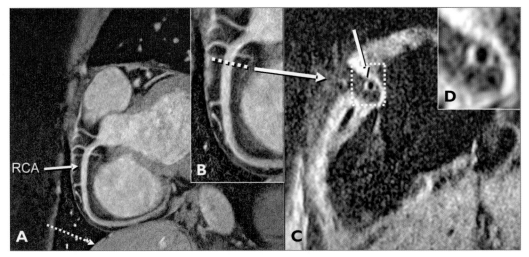

Figure 26-11. High spatial resolution coronary cardiovascular magnetic resonance (CMR) and coronary vessel wall imaging. **A**, A local volume-targeted acquisition of the right coronary artery (RCA) with a high spatial resolution of 0.35×0.35×1.5 mm³ is displayed. For respiratory motion suppression, realtime navigator technology was used and an adiabatic T2 Prep for contrast generation [6,20-21]. To support imaging at such a high spatial resolution, the period of minimal myocardial motion was automatically identified using a custom-built software ("FREEZE") and imaging was performed at the software-prescribed delay after the R-wave of the electrocardiogram [30-31]. Scanning duration for high-spatial resolution CMR is ~10 minutes to 12 minutes, and the high spatial resolution is obtained at the expense of limited volumetric coverage. Note the sharp delineation of the RCA and the visibility of smaller diameter branching vessels (*see* zoomed version [**B**]). Simultaneously, a high definition of the lung-liver interface was obtained (*dotted arrow*) suggesting effective suppression of respiratory motion during the ~10 minutes to 12 minutes scan. Perpendicular to the RCA and using a dual-inversion pulse for blood signal suppression, the coronary vessel wall can be visualized [32]. The two-dimensional acquisition in **C** and **D** (zoomed) was obtained during free breathing with a spatial resolution of 0.7 × 0.7 × 5 mm³. Scanning time per two-dimensional slice is ~2 minutes to 3 minutes. (Ustun *et al.*, [31]; with permission.)

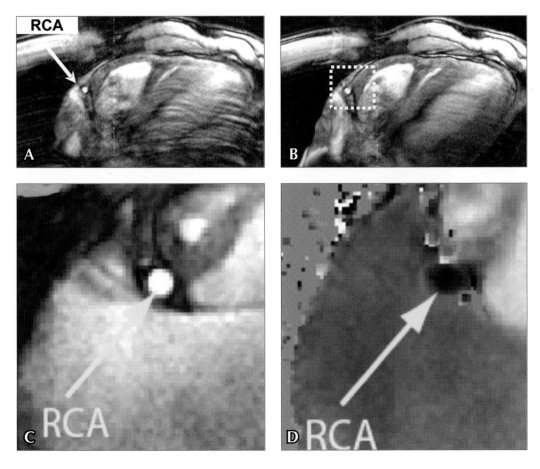

Figure 26-12. High spatial resolution coronary artery cardiovascular magnetic resonance flow measurements. Coronary flow measurements perpendicular to the proximal right coronary artery (RCA) in a healthy adult subject. In conjunction with respiratory navigator technology, respiratory motion can be effectively suppressed for coronary flow measurements (panel **A**, free breathing without navigators; **B**, free breathing with navigators) [33]. In **C**, a zoomed magnitude image showing the anatomy is displayed, and in **D**, the corresponding phase image is shown.

Continued on the next page

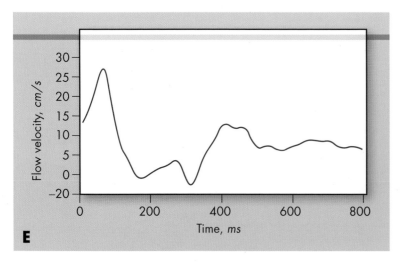

E

Figure 26-12. *(Continued)* On these phase images that are obtained with a high temporal resolution of < 20 ms and an in-plane spatial resolution of 0.7 mm, 17 pixels are available for analysis. Both spatial and temporal resolution is much higher than that previously obtained at 1.5 T. A biphasic quantitative coronary flow curve obtained in this subject is shown in **E**. (Images collected in collaboration with Dr. Christian Stehning, Philips Research Labs Hamburg, Germany, and Drs. Reza Nezafat, Ahmed Gharib, and Roderick Pettigrew, National Institutes of Health [NIBIB], Bethesda, MD.)

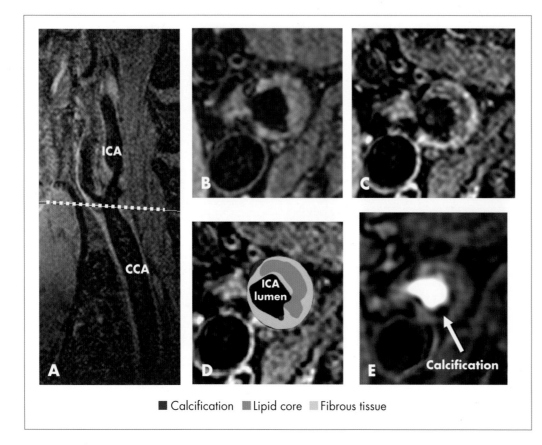

■ Calcification ■ Lipid core ■ Fibrous tissue

Figure 26-13. Pre- and postcontrast imaging of carotid atherosclerosis. Pre- and postcontrast cardiovascular magnetic resonance (CMR) through an atherosclerotic plaque involving the carotid bulb of a 68-year-old man. Black blood cardiovascular magnetic resonance (BBCMR) through the long axis of the carotid bifurcation (**A**) was used to orient a slice (*dotted line*) orthogonal to the plaque. A second oblique BBCMR was acquired with a spatial resolution of 0.35 × 0.35 × 2 mm³ both before (**B**) and then 5 minutes after (**C**) the intravenous administration of 0.1 mmol/kg gadolinium. Consistent with earlier reports, contrast enhancement is observed in areas of fibrosis including the cap overlying the lipid core (**D**) [26,27]. A reconstruction of a three-dimensional time-of-flight CMR angiogram in the same orientation confirms the presence of calcification along the luminal margin (**E**). (*Courtesy of* Dr. Bruce Wasserman, Johns Hopkins University.) CCA—common carotid artery; ICA—internal carotid artery.

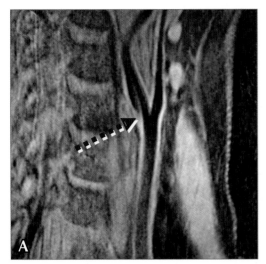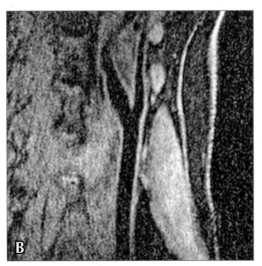

Figure 26-14. Black-blood contrast generation for carotid atherosclerosis imaging. Black-blood contrast generation perpendicular to the orientation of the carotid arteries can be obtained by the use of a dual-inversion prepulse. However, in areas of reflow (bulb), blood that is not signal-nulled reenters the area of interest thereby compromising black-blood contrast generation. Unfortunately, this area of artifactual signal enhancement occurs in regions of turbulent flow that are prone to plaque formation. As a result, this flow artifact may be misinterpreted as an eccentricity of the vessel wall. This is most commonly observed in longitudinal views of the carotid arteries. **A,** A longitudinal view of the carotid arteries obtained in a young healthy adult subject is displayed. Dual-inversion was used for black-blood contrast generation. As shown in the area of the *dotted arrow* in **A,** a focal thickening is observed, but is related to the above described flow artifact. To remove this ambiguity, stimulated echoes can be used [17]. Unfortunately, stimulated echo imaging suffers from an intrinsic 50% signal loss. Although this is unacceptable at 1.5 T, 3 T offers the opportunity to compensate for this relative loss. **B,** As a result, stimulated echo imaging is feasible at 3 T and the effective flow suppression capabilities of this technique help to remove ambiguity in the regions of flow artifacts. (Images were acquired in collaboration with Drs. Albert De Roos and Reza Dehnavi from the Leiden University, The Netherlands.)

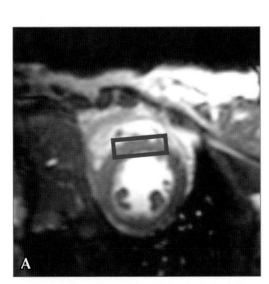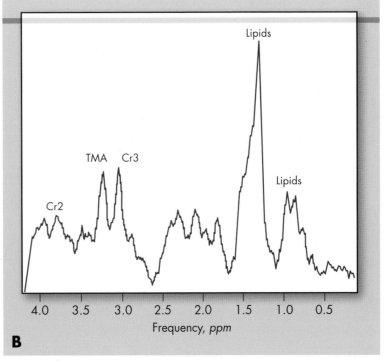

Figure 26-15. Cardiovascular magnetic resonance proton spectroscopy. This proton spectrum was obtained from the septum of a healthy adult human subject using PRESS localization [34]. The acquisition was electrocardiogram triggered at mid-diastole and realtime navigator technology was used for respiratory motion suppression (=double triggered) [35]. In **A,** a short-axis view of the heart acquired at mid-diastole during free breathing using navigator correction is shown with the spectroscopy volume placement. **B,** The spectrum obtained at that location. Peaks from methylene protons (Cr2) of creatine/phosphocreatine (Cr), trimethylammonium compounds (TMA), methyl protons (Cr3) of Cr, and lipids can be observed. (Images and spectra were acquired in collaboration with Drs. Paul A. Bottomley, Johns Hopkins University, Baltimore, MD, and Sebastian Kozerke, ETH Zurich, Switzerland.)

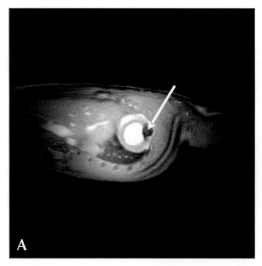

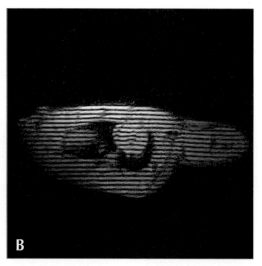

Figure 26-16. Cardiovascular magnetic resonance imaging after USPIO-labeled stem cell injection in a small animal (rat) model. With the high signal-to-noise ratio (SNR) provided by 3 T paired with the availability of integrated electrocardiogram triggering units (heart rate ~300 beats per minute in rats), imaging pulse sequences, and flexible prepulse combinations, commercial 3 T human systems are very attractive for small animal imaging. **A,** A short-axis view of a rat heart is displayed. In the region of the *arrow*, Feridex-labeled stem cells were injected that lead to a distinct signal void in the image. These cine images were obtained using spiral imaging. The temporal resolution was 12 ms and the spatial resolution 0.22×0.22×2 mm³. Both a high SNR and CNR between the ventricular blood-pool and the myocardium are obtained. Scanning time is ~2 minutes per two-dimensional slice. On the CSPAMM tagged images of **B** that were obtained in a control animal without labeled cells, the spiral imaging sequence was preceded by a tagging prepulse combination that leads to a tag line distance of 1.5 mm [36]. (Images were collected in collaboration with Drs. Roselle Abraham , Ioan Terrovitis, and Eduardo Marban, Johns Hopkins University, Baltimore, MD.)

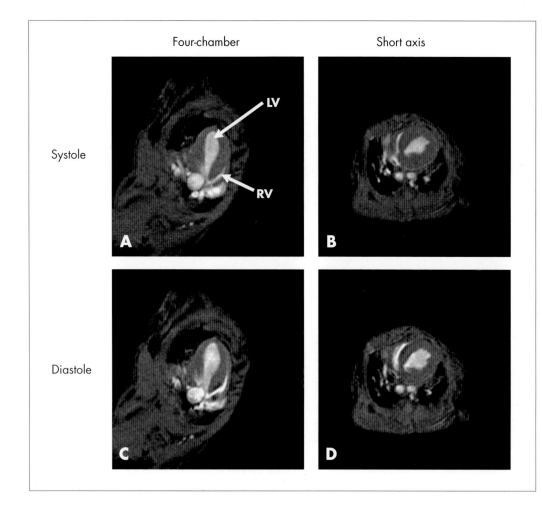

Figure 26-17. Cardiac imaging in a mouse model of transverse aorta constriction (TAC). With the high signal-to-noise ratio provided by 3 T paired with the availability of integrated electrocardiogram triggering units (heart rate ~400–600 beats per minute in mice), imaging pulse sequences, and flexible prepulse combinations, commercial 3 T human systems are very attractive for small animal imaging. End-systolic and end diastolic four-chamber views obtained in a mouse after TAC are shown in **A** and **C.** Orthogonal short-axis views are displayed in **B** and **D.** The spatial resolution was 0.2×0.2×1.0 mm³ and the temporal resolution 10 ms. Note the high blood-myocardium contrast and the thickened wall as a result of TAC. (Images collected in collaboration with Drs. V.P. Chacko and Hunter Champion, Johns Hopkins University, Baltimore, MD.) LV—left ventricle; RV—right ventricle.

REFERENCES

1. Wen H, Denison TJ, Singerman RW, Balaban RS: The intrinsic signal-to-noise ratio in human cardiac imaging at 1.5, 3, and 4 T. *J Magn Reson* 1997, 125:65–71.

2. Noeske R, Seifert F, Rhein KH, Rinneberg H: Human cardiac imaging at 3 T using phased array coils. *Magn Reson Med* 2000, 44:978–982.

3. Atalay MK, Poncelet BP, Kantor HL, *et al.*: Cardiac susceptibility artifacts arising from the heart-lung interface. *Magn Reson Med* 2001, 45:341–345.

4. Dougherty L, Connick TJ, Mizsei G: Cardiac imaging at 4 Tesla. *Magn Reson Med* 2001, 45:176–178.

5. Fischer SE, Wickline SA, Lorenz CH: Novel real-time R-wave detection algorithm based on the vectorcardiogram for accurate gated magnetic resonance acquisitions. *Magn Reson Med* 1999, 42:361–370.

6. Nezafat R, Stuber M, Ouwerkerk R, *et al.*: B1 insensitive T2 preparation for improved coronary magnetic resonance angiography at 3T. *Magn Reson Med* 2006, In Press.

7. Schar M, Kozerke S, Fischer SE, *et al.*: Cardiac SSFP imaging at 3 Tesla. *Magn Reson Med* 2004, 51:799–806.

8. Pruessmann KP, Weiger M, Scheidegger MB, Boesiger P: Coil sensitivity encoding for fast MRI. Proceedings of the International Society for Magnetic Resonance in Medicine 1998, 1:579.

9. Axel L, Dougherty L: MR imaging of motion with spatial modulation of magnetization. *Radiology* 1989, 171:841–845.

10. Zerhouni EA, Parish DM, Rogers WJ, *et al.*: Human heart: tagging with MR imaging—a method for noninvasive assessment of myocardial motion. *Radiology* 1988, 169:59–63.

11. Ryf S, Kissinger KV, Spiegel MA, *et al.*: Spiral MR myocardial tagging. *Magn Reson Med* 2004, 51:237–242.

12. Pan L, Lima JA, Osman NF: Fast tracking of cardiac motion using 3D-HARP. *Inf Process Med Imaging* 2003, 18:611–622.

13. Ryf S, Spiegel MA, Gerber M, Boesiger P: Myocardial tagging with 3D-CSPAMM. *J Magn Reson Imaging* 2002, 16:320–325.

14. Abd-Elmoniem K, Osman NF, Prince JL, Stuber M: Three-dimensional magnetic resonance myocardial motion tracking from a single image plane. *Magn Reson Med* 2007, In Press.

15. Osman NF, Kerwin WS, McVeigh ER, Prince JL: Cardiac motion tracking using CINE harmonic phase (HARP) magnetic resonance imaging. *Magn Reson Med* 1999, 42:1048–1060.

16. Osman NF, Sampath S, Atalar E, Prince JL: Imaging longitudinal cardiac strain on short-axis images using strain-encoded MRI. *Magn Reson Med* 2001, 46:324–334.

17. Frahm J, Hanicke W, Bruhn H, *et al.*: High-speed STEAM MRI of the human heart. *Magn Reson Med* 1991, 22:133–142.

18. Pan L, Stuber M, Kraitchman DL, *et al.*: Real-time imaging of regional myocardial function using fast-SENC. *Magn Reson Med* 2006, 55:386–395.

19. Stuber M, Botnar RM, Fischer SE, *et al.*: Preliminary report on in vivo coronary MRA at 3 Tesla in humans. *Magn Reson Med* 2002, 48:425–429.

20. McConnell MV, Khasgiwala VC, Savord BJ, *et al.*: Prospective adaptive navigator correction for breath-hold MR coronary angiography. *Magn Reson Med* 1997, 37:148–152.

21. Oshinski JN, Hofland L, Mukundan S, Jr., *et al.*: Two-dimensional coronary MR angiography without breath holding. *Radiology* 1996, 201:737–743.

22. Brittain JH, Hu BS, Wright GA, *et al.*: Coronary angiography with magnetization-prepared T2 contrast. *Magn Reson Med* 1995, 33:689–696.

23. Weber OM, Martin AJ, Higgins CB: Whole-heart steady-state free precession coronary artery magnetic resonance angiography. *Magn Reson Med* 2003, 50:1223–1228.

24. Zheng J, Bae KT, Woodard PK, *et al.*: Efficacy of slow infusion of gadolinium contrast agent in three-dimensional MR coronary artery imaging. *J Magn Reson Imaging* 1999, 10:800–805.

25. Etienne A, Botnar RM, Van Muiswinkel AM, *et al.*: "Soap-Bubble" visualization and quantitative analysis of 3D coronary magnetic resonance angiograms. *Magn Reson Med* 2002, 48:658–666.

26. Wasserman BA, Smith WI, Trout HH, 3rd, *et al.*: Carotid artery atherosclerosis: in vivo morphologic characterization with gadolinium-enhanced double-oblique MR imaging initial results. *Radiology* 2002, 223:566–573.

27. Yuan C, Kerwin WS, Ferguson MS, *et al.*: Contrast-enhanced high resolution MRI for atherosclerotic carotid artery tissue characterization. *J Magn Reson Imaging* 2002, 15:62–67.

28. Maintz D, Ozgun M, Hoffmeier A, *et al.*: Contrast-enhanced black-blood MRI for coronary artery plaque visualization and differentiation. Chicago. 2004; 220.

29. Maintz D, Ozgun M, Hoffmeier A, *et al.*: Selective coronary artery plaque visualization and differentiation by contrast-enhanced inversion prepared MRI. *Eur Heart J* 2006, 27:1732–1736.

30. Johnson KR, Patel SJ, Whigham A, *et al.*: Three-dimensional, time-resolved motion of the coronary arteries. *J Cardiovasc Magn Reson* 2004, 6:663–673.

31. Ustun A, Desai M, Abd-Elmoniem KZ, *et al.*: Automated identification of minimal myocardial motion for improved image quality on MR angiography at 3 T. *AJR Am J Roentgenol* 2007, 188:W283–290.

32. Botnar RM, Stuber M, Lamerichs R, *et al.*: Initial experiences with in vivo right coronary artery human MR vessel wall imaging at 3 tesla. *J Cardiovasc Magn Reson* 2003, 5:589–594.

33. Nagel E, Bornstedt A, Hug J, *et al.*: Noninvasive determination of coronary blood flow velocity with magnetic resonance imaging: comparison of breath-hold and navigator techniques with intravascular ultrasound. *Magn Reson Med* 1999, 41:544–549.

34. Bottomley PA: Spatial localization in NMR spectroscopy in vivo. *Ann N Y Acad Sci* 1987, 508:333–348.

35. Schar M, Kozerke S, Boesiger P: Navigator gating and volume tracking for double-triggered cardiac proton spectroscopy at 3 Tesla. *Magn Reson Med* 2004, 51:1091–1095.

36. Fischer SE, McKinnon GC, Maier SE, Boesiger P: Improved myocardial tagging contrast. *Magn Reson Med* 1993, 30:191–200.

27

CHAPTER

Comparison of Noninvasive Cardiac Imaging Methods

Thomas H. Hauser and Warren J. Manning

Over the past two decades, noninvasive cardiovascular imaging has exploded both in volume and with an array of new imaging options. Today, the clinician has a multitude of imaging choices, including echocardiography (*ie*, transthoracic, stress, transesophageal), nuclear, and the newest members of the noninvasive armamentarium: cardiovascular magnetic resonance and cardiac CT. Although there is considerable overlap in some of the information provided (*eg*, all provide information on left ventricular systolic function), there are considerable differences regarding the information provided in other areas (*eg*, valvular function, pericardial disease, coronary artery imaging), application of contrast agents, and exposure to ionizing radiation. In addition, there are differences in spatial and temporal resolution, as well as physician training. In this chapter, we will compare and contrast these four noninvasive cardiovascular imaging modalities.

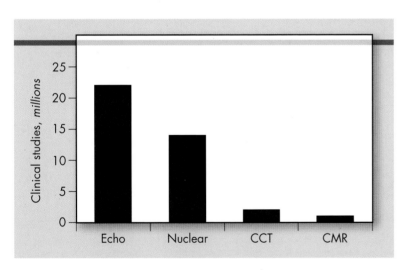

Figure 27-1. Of the four major noninvasive imaging modalities, echocardiography and nuclear cardiology are dominant with regard to the number of clinical scans performed annually. In 2006, it was estimated that over 22 million echocardiograms were performed in the United States. Stress echocardiography has shown the most growth over the last decade. In comparison, over 15 million cardiac nuclear images are performed annually, with a majority now performed outside of the hospital setting. In contrast, cardiac CT (CCT) and cardiovascular magnetic resonance (CMR) are quite small, with approximately 500,000 scans annually.

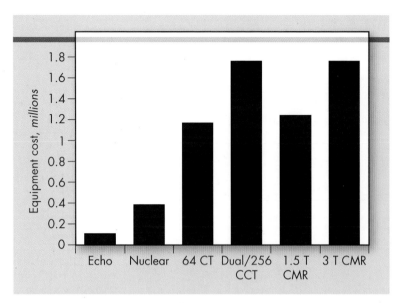

Figure 27-2. Equipment cost is a major factor when considering imaging modalities for both institutions and local practices. Because of advances in technology and migration to standardized hardware and software interfaces, the cost of medical diagnostic equipment has declined considerably. There is substantial variation among the imaging modalities. In the United States, a typical state-of-the-art echocardiograph now costs between $100 to $120,000, increasing from $150 to $200,000 for systems with three-dimensional capabilities. Dedicated laptop and portable versions of these larger units that often display impressive two-dimensional and Doppler image quality may cost more than $50,000. Nuclear cardiology cameras are somewhat more expensive ($300–$500,000), while 64-slice cardiac computed tomography and 1.5 T cardiovascular cardiovascular magnetic resonance (CMR) scanners cost over a million dollars. The most advanced models of both imaging modalities (*eg*, dual-source or 256-slice CT; high field 3 T CMR) may approach $1.8 to $2 million dollars in equipment costs. These costs do not include site placement, which is minimal for echocardiography, requires lead shielding for nuclear and CCT, and complex radio frequency electromagnetic radiation shielding for CMR.

Advantages of CMR versus CCT, Echocardiography, and Nuclear Cardiology
Excellent soft tissue contrast
Noninvasive; no ionizing radiation
Multiplane, true tomographic imaging (not reconstruction)
Dynamic/cine imaging (2D echo) with high temporal resolution; CMR tagging methods to examine local deformation
Exogenous contrast usually not needed (CMR agents are less toxic than iodinated preparations)
Blood flow/volume — quantitative
Minimal postprocessing
Potential for tissue characterization (fat, iron)
"Comprehensive" CMR examination

Figure 27-3. Advantages of cardiovascular magnetic resonance (CMR) as compared with echocardiography, nuclear cardiology, and cardiac computed tomography (CCT) are summarized in this figure. CMR offers excellent soft tissue contrast in a noninvasive environment without the need for ionizing radiation (advantage vs. nuclear and CCT). Rather than reconstructions used in CCT, multiplane, true tomographic CMR images may be acquired in any imaging plane. Dynamic and cine imaging of the beating heart with high temporal resolution and high spatial resolution may be acquired without exogenous contrast. CMR tagging methods offer the opportunity to examine local strain. When needed, CMR contrast agents (primarily gadolinium-diethylene triamine pentaacetic acid-based compounds) have a more favorable short and moderate term safety profile than the iodinated preparations used for CCT (and possibly echocardiography). CMR is also quantitative with regard to blood volume and flow, and offers the option for characterization of tissue for fat and iron (vs. echo and nuclear). Echo—echocardiography; Nuclear—nuclear cardiology.

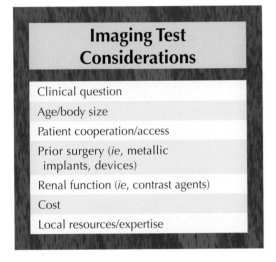

Disadvantages of CMR vs CCT, Echocardiography, and Nuclear Cardiology

Most physicians did not enjoy (or do not remember much) physics (many "fear" CMR because of its complexity)

Physicians are more comfortable (and well-trained) with CCT, echocardiography, and nuclear (CMR image interpretation is not always "intuitive")

CMR set-up is relatively complex, many options (*ie*, virtue and impediment)

CMR sequences are pathology "focused" (*ie*, fewer extracardiac findings)

Claustrophobia, exclusion (PCM, ICD)

CMR acquisition time is relatively prolonged

CMR has inferior postprocessing tools

Lack of standardization for CMR image acquisition and analysis

Not portable (Echocardiography)

Figure 27-4. Disadvantages of cardiovascular magnetic resonance (CMR) as compared with echocardiography, nuclear cardiology, and cardiac computed tomography (CCT) are summarized in this figure. Because CMR is a new modality, most clinicians did not

receive CMR training or exposure during their fellowship. The complexity of CMR image interpretation with varying appearance of similar tissue as "dark," "intermediate," or "bright" depending on the choice of sequence and prepulses is confusing to the novice CMR imager. In addition, although image orientation and plane prescription is straight forward, CMR set-up is relatively complex, including electrocardiogram and rhythm strip, receiver coil placement, etc. Because of the complexity and variability in CMR sequences, a CMR study may require 30 to 90 minutes for data acquisition, which is relatively long, as compared with CCT and echocardiography. During the CMR scan, the patient may be asked to perform multiple breath holds, a burden not acceptable to some patients. Postprocessing CMR tools are inferior to CCT, though advanced as compared with echocardiography. Cardiac specific contraindications for CMR include patients with pacemakers (PCM) and implantable cardio defibrillators (ICD), though prosthetic valves and intracoronary stents are CMR compatible. For a complete list of CMR safety issues, the reader is referred to the web site: www.mrisafety.com. While documents aiming to standardize CMR acquisition protocols and reporting have been promulgated by the Society for Cardiovascular Magnetic Resonance (*see* www.scmr.org), there remains a great deal of variability in the clinical practice of CMR acquisition protocols and reporting. Finally, like CCT, CMR is not portable, which is a benefit of echocardiography. Nuclear—nuclear cardiology.

Imaging Test Considerations

Clinical question

Age/body size

Patient cooperation/access

Prior surgery (*ie*, metallic implants, devices)

Renal function (*ie*, contrast agents)

Cost

Local resources/expertise

Figure 27-5. When considering noninvasive testing options, the clinician needs to be aware of the specific attributes of each imaging modality. Most important is the specific clinical questions that are or will be addressed. With this as the primary importance, the clinician then needs to consider the patients age and body size (echocardiography may be less successful in obese and elderly patients), patient cooperation (cardiac computed tomography [CCT] and cardiovascular magnetic resonance (CMR) both require patient cooperation with breath holding and motion restraint), implants (*eg*, acoustic shadowing for mechanical valves in echocardiography, and CMR safety issues for patients with pacemakers), renal function (iodinated contrast and gadolinium-diethylene triamine pentaacetic acid preparations), cost, and local resources or expertise. Because of training issues, local resources or expertise are likely to become more important for the newer technologies such as CCT and CMR. (*Adapted from* Tal Geva, MD.)

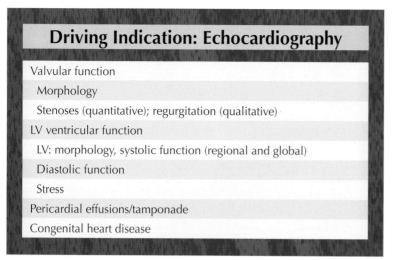

Driving Indication: Echocardiography

Valvular function

  Morphology

  Stenoses (quantitative); regurgitation (qualitative)

LV ventricular function

  LV: morphology, systolic function (regional and global)

  Diastolic function

  Stress

Pericardial effusions/tamponade

Congenital heart disease

Figure 27-6. Though echocardiography, nuclear cardiology, cardiac computed tomography (CCT), and cardiovascular magnetic resonance (CMR) can provide information regarding left ventricular (LV) systolic function, each offers advantages in other

areas or aspects of ventricular function. Because of its low cost, lack of ionizing radiation, large installed base, and ease of access, echocardiography is often at the "first line" of noninvasive cardiac imaging. The "primary" or "driving" indications for echocardiography include assessment of valvular heart disease, LV anatomy/function, pericardial disease, and congenital heart disease. Echocardiography is the most portable of the imaging modalities. While valve morphology and quantitation of stenotic valvular lesions are easily performed, quantification of valvular regurgitation is often more limited, especially in patients with eccentric jets—a situation that does not impair CMR assessment of valvular regurgitation. Regional LV systolic function is well characterized in patients with good acoustic windows, but up to 20% of adult patients will have poor visualization of ventricular segments—particularly the obese and elderly, while > 98% of cine CMR images are interpretable. Circumferential pericardial effusions and tamponade physiology are well characterized by echocardiography, but loculated effusions and pericardial thickening are better appreciated by CMR and CCT. Echocardiography does not allow for direct visualization of the coronary arteries.

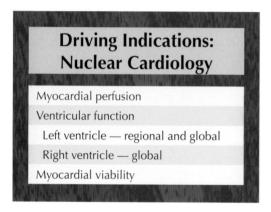

Driving Indications: Nuclear Cardiology

Myocardial perfusion

Ventricular function

  Left ventricle — regional and global

  Right ventricle — global

Myocardial viability

Figure 27-7. Driving indications for nuclear cardiology include myocardial perfusion (rest/stress), left ventricular (LV) systolic function, and myocardial viability. Single photon emission CT (SPECT) myocardial perfusion imaging provides excellent sensitivity for the detection of coronary artery disease. Reproducibility of LV ejection fraction assessment is excellent with radionuclide ventriculography (RVG). While the clinical assessment of viable myocardium using either SPECT or positron emission tomography (PET) is excellent, spatial resolution limits identification of smaller infarcts. Nuclear cardiology procedures expose the patient to considerable amounts of radiation and offers minimal information regarding the pericardium, valvular heart disease, and direct coronary artery imaging.

Driving Indication: CCT

Coronary artery lumen imaging

  anomalous coronary artery disease

  native vessel integrity

  coronary artery bypass graft patency

Epicardial calcium

Pericardial thickening/calcification

Figure 27-8. Over the last decade, cardiac computed tomography (CCT) has received considerable interest. The high spatial resolution images are aesthetically pleasing, and the data are relatively easily acquired in cooperative patients with slow heart rates (< 60/min using β blockade). The driving clinical indications for CCT include epicardial calcium assessment, coronary lumen imaging, and pericardial thickening/calcification. Regional and global LV systolic function can also be assessed with LV short- and long-axis reconstructions, but the temporal resolution is quite limited (83–200 ms) as compared with two-dimensional echocardiography and cine cardiovascular magnetic resonance. As a result, CCT estimates of LV end-diastolic volumes are often smaller, and end-systolic volume is higher (resultant lower LV ejection fraction) than these other modalities. Characterization of aortic valve stenosis was documented from planimetry of the aortic valve orifice in systole, but aortic regurgitation and mitral regurgitation flow data cannot be obtained by CCT. Left ventricular myocardial perfusion is possible with CCT, but this approach exposes the patient to considerable radiation for both rest and stress imaging.

A cardiac CT version of late gadolinium enhancement (LGE) cardiovascular magnetic resonance (CMR) using iodinated contrast was described, but requires high doses of iodinated contrast and has lower contrast-to-noise as compared with the LGE CMR approach.

LV/RV mass

LV/RV volumes, regional/global
  systolic function

Stress CMR

Myocardial viability

Valvular function (stenosis,
  quantitative regurgitation)

Pericardial disease

Congenital heart disease

Coronary artery imaging

Comprehensive cardiac examination

Figure 27-9. Though more complex, the versatility of cardiovascular magnetic resonance (CMR) incorporates nearly all of the driving indications of echocardiography, nuclear cardiology, and cardiac computed tomography (CCT) in a nonionizing environment. CMR is considered the gold standard for assessment of left ventricular (LV) and right ventricluar (RV) anatomy and function. The superiority of spatial resolution offers advantages (vs nuclear) for assessment of perfusion and viability, quantitation of valvular stenosis can be performed with both two-dimensional and phase contrast CMR, while quantitative assessment of valvular regurgitation and complex congenital heart disease is superior to echocardiography. The potential of CMR spectroscopy offers another very powerful perspective that has yet to achieve clinical role. Though coronary CCT angiography has received more attention that coronary CMR, each modality has advantages and disadvantages that need to be considered for the individual patient.

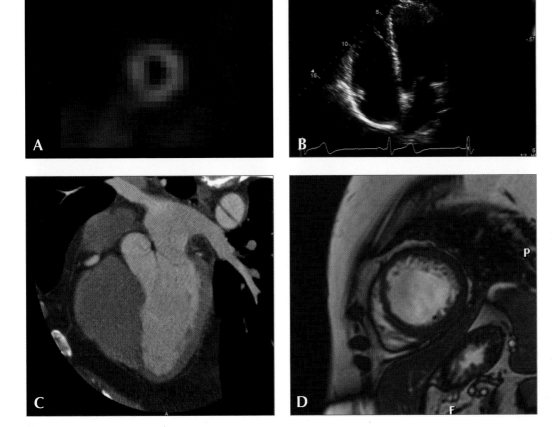

Figure 27-10. Shown are examples of short-axis and four-chamber functional images in diastole obtained by nuclear cardiology (**A**) transthoracic echocardiography (**B**) cardiac computed tomography (CCT) [**C**] and cardiovascular magnetic resonance (CMR) [**D**]. Note the low resolution images afforded by nuclear imaging with superior endocardial border definition of CMR. The CCT images are reconstructions while the echocardiographic images are often suboptimal in older and overweight subjects.

Resolution		
Modality	Temporal, *ms*	2D spatial, *mm*
Echocardiography	20–35 (2D)	1.5–2
Nuclear cardiology	16 (RVG) 125 (SPECT)	7–9
CCT	83–200	0.5
CMR	25–35	1–2

Figure 27-11. When considering function parameters, the physician needs to be aware of the temporal and spatial resolution of the imaging modalities. Cardiovascular magnetic resonance (CMR) and transthoracic echocardiography offer the greatest temporal resolution of ~25 ms to 35 ms. As a result, CMR end diastolic ventricular volumes are often larger and end systolic volumes slightly smaller. Cardiac CT (CCT) provides the greatest spatial resolution followed by CMR and two-dimensional echocardiography. Although radionuclide ventriculography (RVG) offers high temporal resolution (16 ms), there is low spatial resolution. For single photon emission CT (SPECT) imaging, both temporal and spatial resolutions are low. The coarse spatial resolution of nuclear cardiology results in its low sensitivity for identification of small myocardial infarctions.

Technical Advances	
Ultrasound	Transducers, faster processing; contrast agents (3D–hardware, software)
CCT	More detectors, faster gantry speed; postprocessing
Nuclear cardiology	Radioisotopes; postprocessing hardware; attenuation correction
CMR	Receiver coils, software (sequences); postprocessing; high field

Figure 27-12. All technologies have advanced over the last decade, though major advances differ among the noninvasive imaging modalities. Ultrasound advances are focused on minor hardware (transducer improvements), contrast agents, and postprocessing software with newer three-dimensional applications dependent on both hardware and software. In contrast, major cardiac CT (CCT) advances have been hardware modifications with more detectors and faster gantry speed. Nuclear cardiology advances have been in radioisotopes and software, while cardiovascular magnetic resonance (CMR) advances are focused on minor hardware (receiver coils) and software (sequence design, prepulses, postprocessing). Major hardware (high field 3 T) platforms are also becoming common, and responsible for over half of new systems, but 1.5 T CMR remains the dominant installed base today.

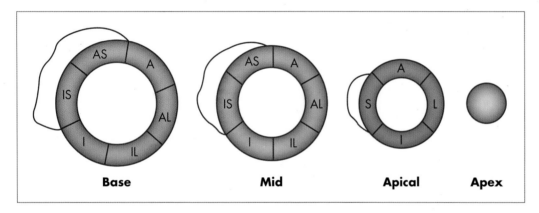

Base **Mid** **Apical** **Apex**

Figure 27-13. Though previously confusing, all of the major noninvasive imaging organizations have now agreed to use a 17-segment model for characterizing the left ventricular walls, with six basal and midventricular segments, four apical segments, and the true apex. The former posterior wall is now referred to as the inferolateral wall [1]. A—anterior wall; AL—anterolateral wall; AS—anteroseptal wall; I—inferior wall; IL—inferolateral wall; IS—inferoseptal wall; L—lateral wall; S—septal wall.

Contrast Agents: Safety Issues

Echocardiography contrast agents

  Saline

  Perflutren-albumen microsphere (Optison)

  Perflutren-lipid microsphere (Definity)

Radionuclide agents

  Thallium-201

  Technetium-99 m (MIBI)

  CCT contrantagents

  Iodinated contrast agents

CMR contrast agents

  Gadolinium-DTPA

Figure 27-14. All of the noninvasive imaging modalities use contrast, though these contrast agents vary considerably in their use and their mode of action. The use of exogenous contrast adds to the cost and complexity of most imaging studies. Echocardiographic contrast agents include agitated saline, most commonly used to assess for a patent foramen ovale/atrial septal defect, as well as agents that pass through the pulmonary bed and provide enhanced left ventricular (LV) endocardial border definition (*ie*, Optison/General Electric and Definity/Bristol Myers Squibb). Though generally very well tolerated, Definity has recently received a black box warning for acutely ill patients because of reported deaths occurring within a few hours of contrast agent administration. Unfortunately, this is a subgroup for which noncontrast echo imaging is often suboptimal. Overall, less than 5% of all transthoracic echocardiographic studies use a contrast agent. In comparison, a radiopharmaceutical is intrinsic to the performance of nuclear cardiology, with thallium-201 and technetium-99 m based agents (*eg*, Sestamibi scan) being the most commonly used agents for assessment of myocardial perfusion and viability. While not needed for assessment of epicardial calcium, both coronary cardiac computed tomography (CCT) angiography and CCT assessment of ventricular function require the use of an iodinated contrast. A volume similar to that used for diagnostic coronary angiography is often used (50–100 mL). Both allergic history and underlying renal function are important considerations. Allergic side effects manifest very early, while renal dysfunction may not manifest for a week or more. Cardiovascular magnetic resonance (CMR) contrast agents are typically gadolinium based. Minor side effects (nausea, headache, dysgusia) occur soon after administration, but a severe systemic disorder, nephrogenic systemic fibrosis (NSF) has been reported in a very small minority of patients with underlying renal dysfunction (eGFR < 30 mL/min/$1.73m^2$). This disorder, characterized by fibrosis of the skin, lungs, and other organs may not manifest for several months or up to 2 years following gadolinium administration. As a result, an assessment of renal function is performed in all patients for whom gadolinium administration is planned with a decrease in dose for those with an eGFR < 60 mLmin/$1.73m^2$. DTPA—diethylene triamine pentaacetic acid.

Safety: Radiation Exposure

Technique	mSev
Background	3/year
CXR	0.05
Dental radiograph	0.09
Diagnostic radiograph coronary	2.1–5.5 (6–12 projections)
Nuclear cardiology	6 (technetium–99 m rest and stress)
	22 (dual Thallium-201/technetium–99 m)
EBCT Epicardial calcium	0.7–1.3
Coronary CTA CCT (4, 16 slice)	1.5–6.2
CCT 16 (64)	6.7–15 (14–20)
CMR	0
Echocardiography	0

Figure 27-15. Medical sources are now the leading source of exposure to ionizing radiation in the Western World. Tremendous advances were made in radiograph technology to reduce such exposure, but for cardiac CT (CCT), nuclear cardiology, and invasive angiography, exposure can be considerable. Dual isotope (thallium-201 and technetium-99m) nuclear cardiology exposure exceeds 20 mSv while 64-slice CCT exposure is twice the exposure of a diagnostic radiograph coronary angiogram. Electrocardiogram modulation and other methods may reduce this dose, but are not always applied. Sensitivity to radiation is related to patient age and gender, with younger patients (< 40 years) and women being particularly sensitive. Neither echocardiography nor cardiovascular magnetic resonance (CMR) exposes patients to any ionizing radiation. CXR—chest x-ray; CTA—CT angiography; EBCT—electron beam CT.

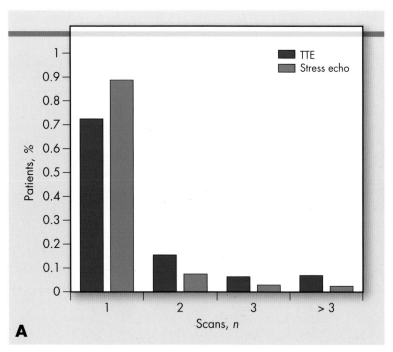

A

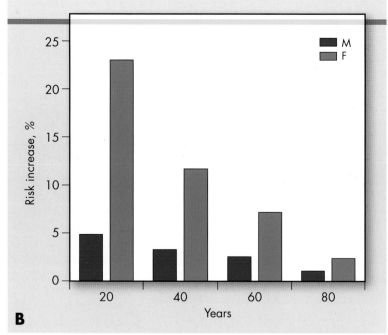

B

Figure 27-16. The issue of radiation exposure is particularly important as patients frequently have multiple tests in the evaluation and subsequent follow-up. This should be considered when choosing imaging tests. For example, a young adult with the Marfan syndrome or a young woman with atypical chest pain is likely to have numerous imaging tests during their lifetimes. Exposure to ionizing radiation is considered additive. A choice of cardiac computed tomography (CCT), cardiovascular magnetic resonance, nuclear cardiology and echocardiography would expose them to a broad range of ionizing radiation. Depicted here are data derived from BIDMC echo lab database from a 7-year period beginning in July 2000. Nearly 30% of all subjects referred for a transthoracic echocardiogram had at least one additional echocardiographic study during the subsequent period, and over 10% of patients had at least two stress echocardiograms (**A**). **B**, Shown are the estimated lifetime cancer risks for a single 64-slice coronary CCT angiogram. (*Adapted from* Einstein JAMA 2007.) Data are normalized for an 80-year-old man (risk = 1). F—women; M—men.

Fellowship Training: Imaging (Proposed)

Imaging Modality	Level	Months (Tot/Unshared)	Cases (Perform/Inter)
Echocardiography	1	3/2	75/150
	2	6/4	150/300
	3	12/6	300/750
Nuclear cardiology	1	2/1	35/100 (80 hrs)
	2	4/3	35/300
	3	10/5	35/600
CMR	1	1/0	0/50
	2	3/2	50/150
	3	10/5	100/300
CCT	1	1/0	0/50
	2	2/1	50/150
	3	6/3	100/300

Figure 27-17. Physician training in noninvasive imaging is currently "lab" specific, with fellows spending time in each laboratory to achieve Level 1 (exposure but not sufficient training to interpret), Level 2 (sufficient training to interpret studies), and Level 3 (sufficient training to interpret, direct a lab, and train others). There are numerous areas of overlap with regard to anatomy, image analysis, affording the opportunity to shorten overall training period, and create a formal noninvasive imaging track. The American College of Cardiology has recently proposed a defined noninvasive imaging track. Depicted in the figure are the proposed training months and the number of cases to achieve this goal. Note the volume of cases to achieve similar training is relatively greater for both echocardiography and nuclear cardiology. Level 1 = exposure. Level 2 = training sufficient to practice or interpret clinical studies. Level 3 = training sufficient to direct an imaging laboratory and to train others in the modality. CCT—cardiac computed tomography; CMR—cardiovascular magnetic resonance.

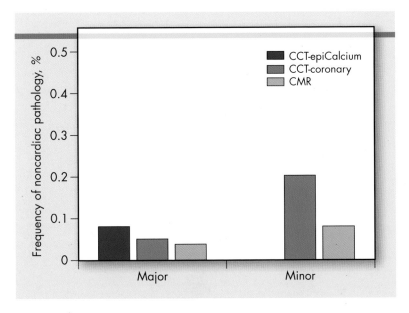

Figure 27-18. While training in cardiovascular pathology is the mainstay of all such training programs, it has become apparent that noninvasive imaging often includes visualization of noncardiac pathology. Though very unusual for nuclear and echocardiographic procedures, thoracic images acquired for both cardiac computed tomography (CCT) and cardiovascular magnetic resonance (CMR) also include neighboring structures in the mediastinum, thorax, upper abdomen, and lower neck. Most of these extracardiac findings are "minor," but major findings (eg, tumors) are sometimes seen. Limited data suggest that extracardiac findings are more common for CCT than other procedures, likely related to the use of pathology specific CMR sequences, while CCT images can be presented with bone, lung windows, etc. Cardiologists interpreting CMR and CCT need to be trained in identifying these noncardiac findings, or studies should also be interpreted by others (eg, chest radiologists) who have received such training.

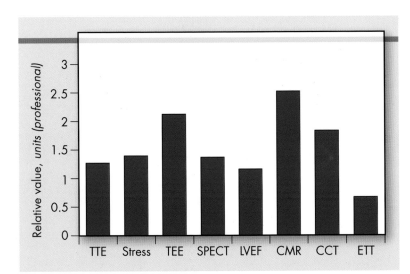

Figure 27-19. Physicians in the United States are reimbursed for their professional services based on a relative value unit (RVU) scale that incorporates training and expertise, time expenditure, and complexity of an activity. Shown are the 2008 professional RVU assigned to the common noninvasive imaging modalities. Cardiovascular magnetic resonance (CMR) and transesophageal echocardiography (TEE) are recognized as the most complex, while nuclear medicine assessment of regional and global left ventricular systolic function the least complex. For reference, data for a nonimaging exercise test (ETT) are also provided. CCT—cardiac computed tomography; LVEF—left ventricular ejection fraction; SPECT—single phone emission computed tomography; TTE—transthoracic echocardiography.

Relative Utility of Noninvasive Techniques

Cardiac anatomy	CXR	ECHO	Nuc	CCT	CMR
Chamber size	◐	◐	◐	●	●
Myocardial mass	○	◐	◐	●	●
Valvular disease	○	●	○	◐	●
Pericardial disease	○	●	◐	●	●
Coronary imaging	○	○	○	●	◐
Cardiac function					
LV systolic function	○	●	●	◐	●
RV systolic function	○	◐	○	○	●
Intracardiac shunt	○	◐	○	○	●
Myocardial stress	○	◐	●	◐	◐
Myocardial viability	○	◐	◐	◐	●

● Excellent   ◐ Very good   ◐ Limited   ○ Poor

Figure 27-20. A "Consumer Reports" style view of primary indications for cardiac imaging and the ability of cardiovascular magnetic resonance, cardiac computed tomography (CCT), echocardiography (ECHO), nuclear cardiology (Nuc), and chest radiography (CXR) for reference to provide clinically useful information. CMR provides the most comprehensive information, though with longer scan time and complexity.

REFERENCE

1. Cerqueira MD, Weissman NJ, Dilsizian V, *et al.:* Standardized myocardial segmentation and nomenclature for tomographic imaging of the heart: a statement for healthcare professionals from the Cardiac Imaging Committee of the Council on Clinical Cardiology of the American Heart Association. *Circulation* 2002, 105:539–542.

F

Familial dilated cardiomyopathy, 109
Fast Fourier transform, 6–7
Fast-spin echo, 11–12
Fat infiltration
  in arrhythmogenic RV dysplasia, 154–156, 158
Fat saturation technique, 14
Fat signal, 3, 14
Femoral artery stenosis, 243
Fibroma
  intracardiac, 101
Fibrosis
  in arrhythmogenic right ventricular dysplasia, 158
  in dilated cardiomyopathy, 106–112
Fluorine imaging, 30
Frequency encoding, 3, 5, 7
Friedreich's ataxia, 269

G

Gadofluorine, 27–28
Gadolinium-based contrast agents, 19–25
  after myocardial infarction, 70, 72–73, 76, 79
  in hypertrophic cardiomyopathy, 143–145
  in myocardial viability assessment, 89–95
Germ cell tumor
  intracardiac, 103
Ghosting artifact, 45
Gradient-recalled echo, 10, 17

H

Hand magnetic resonance angiography, 43
Heart failure, 267–268
Hemangioma
  intracardiac, 101
Hematoma
  pericardial, 176–177
High-field CMR, 281–290
Hypertensive disease
  dilated cardiomyopathy versus, 114
Hypertrophic cardiomyopathy, 133–148
  diagnosis of, 137–139
  end-stage, 146
  histology of, 134–135
  late gadolinium enhancement in, 143–145
  left ventricular obstruction in, 142–143
  myocardial viability in, 95
  overview of, 133
  pattern and distribution of, 135–136
  phenotype characterization in, 139–140
  risk of sudden death in, 141
  treatment of, 147–148
Hypoplastic left heart syndrome, 189

I

Inferior vena cava thrombosis, 214–215, 217
Intermittent claudication, 21
Interventional CMR, 273–279
  aortic, 277
  in atrial septal puncture, 277
  guidewires in, 276–277
  in passive versus active catheterization, 278
  in pre- and postprocedure evaluation, 275
  of prosthetic valves, 279
  radiography versus, 273
  in stenting, 274–275
Iron overload
  dilated cardiomyopathy versus, 115
Iron-based contrast agents, 19, 25–26
Ischemic heart disease, 264–266

K

Kawasaki disease, 252
k-space, 7–8, 12

L

Larmor frequency, 1–2
Late gadolinium enhancement, 70, 72–73, 76, 79, 89–95, 143–145
Left atrial imaging, 219–220, 222, 225
Left ventricle-pulmonary artery conduit, 21
Left ventricular aneurysm, 23, 93
Left ventricular thrombus, 93
Left ventricular imaging
  anatomic features in, 56–60
  of function, 61–65, 282–284
  in myocardial infarction, 70
LeRiche syndrome, 242

T

Tamponade, 180
Targeted contrast agents, 27–30
Tetralogy of Fallot, 186, 203–204
Thoracic aorta aneurysm, 245
Thoracic outlet syndrome, 216
Thrombus imaging, 28–29, 93, 97, 99, 214–215
Tibial artery stenosis, 243
Time-of-flight technique, 35–37, 213, 231
Time-resolved magnetic resonance angiography, 43, 234
Torsion imaging, 64
Training requirements for noninvasive imaging, 300–301
Transposition of the great arteries, 187, 205–207
Transthoracic echocardiography, 120, 124, 126, 130
Tricuspid atresia, 188, 209
Tricuspid regurgitation, 168
Truncus arteriosus, 187
Tumor thrombus, 215
Tumors
  cardiac, 97–103

V

Valvular heart disease, 163–170
  aortic stenosis and regurgitation in, 165
  bicuspid aortic valve in, 164
  mitral stenosis in, 168
  mitral valve prolapse in, 170
  overview of, 163–164
  prosthetic valve artifacts in, 170
  pulmonic stenosis and regurgitation in, 166–167
  sinus of Valsalva aneurysm in, 169
  tricuspid regurgitation in, 168
Vaso-occlusive disease, 20
Ventricular septal defect, 184, 198–199, 201, 204
Ventricular tachycardia, 129–130
Volumetric assessment
  in dilated cardiomyopathy, 106

W

Wall motion imaging
  dobutamine stress, 83–88
Whole body magnetic resonance angiography, 240
Whole heart magnetic resonance imaging, 254–255, 285–286